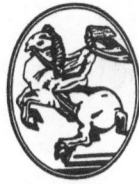

Topics in Infectious Diseases
Vol. 2

R-Factors: Their Properties and Possible Control

Symposium, Baden near Vienna, April 27-29, 1977

Edited by
J. Drews and G. Högenauer

Springer-Verlag Wien GmbH

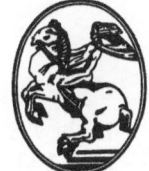

R-Factors: Their Properties and Possible Control

Sandoz-Symposium, Baden near Vienna, April 27—29, 1977

With 75 figures

Prof. Dr. Jürgen Drews
Doz. Dr. Gregor Högenauer

Sandoz Forschungsinstitut Gesellschaft m. b. H.
Vienna, Austria

© 1977 by Springer-Verlag Wien
   Originally published by Springer-Verlag/Wien in 1977
Softcover reprint of the hardcover 1st edition 1977

Library of Congress Cataloging in Publication Data

Main entry under title:

R-factors, their properties and possible control.

   (Topics in infectious diseases ; v. 2)
   Organized by Sandoz Research Institute.
   Includes index.
   1. R factors--Congresses.   I. Drews, Jürgen,
1933-   II. Högenauer, G., 1933-   III. Sandoz,
Forschungsinstitut.   IV. Series.
QR177.R2   616.01'4   77-13689

ISBN 978-3-7091-8503-2   ISBN 978-3-7091-8501-8 (eBook)
DOI 10.1007/978-3-7091-8501-8

Introduction

Ever since their discovery in 1959, bacterial R-factors have
attracted the keen interest of scientists from many fields.
R-factors have been a primary cause of concern for clinicians
and epidemiologists, but so far little has been achieved to
cope with the threat which they present to the effectiveness
of antibacterial chemotherapy. Molecular biologists and geneti-
cists have studied R-factors extensively as another class of
bacterial plasmids which, because of their small size and their
biological properties, offered certain advantages over other
more complex genetic systems. The advent of new techniques for
dissecting DNA molecules into specific segments by restriction
endonucleases and of recombining such segments artificially has
emphasized the role of R-factors as genetic models in recent
years. The discovery of transposable genetic units (transposons)
has provided a new insight into the mechanisms by which resistance properties can spread in bacterial populations and give
rise to the evolution of new phenotypes. Biochemists have un-
ravelled the enzymatic mechanisms by which the resistance genes,
carried by R-factors, inactivate antibiotics or render cells
invulnerable to the action of antibiotic substances.

A tremendous amount of data regarding each of these areas as
well as other aspects of R-factor research has accumulated over
the past 15 years. At the same time, however, the dynamic development taken by each individual line of research has somewhat
removed us from the central issue which is the containment, if
not control of R-factors in the practice of medicine.

For this reason we considered it appropriate to invite a number
of scientists widely known for their contributions to various
areas of research on R-factors and to obtain from them a full
contemporary assessment of the most important aspects of plasmid-
mediated bacterial resistance. It was then attempted to derive

recommendations regarding measures against the spread of R-factors and to consider possible pharmaceutical approaches to their control.

We strongly feel that the presentation of the proceedings of yet another symposium on bacterial R-factors could hardly be justified unless it would serve a specific purpose so far neglected in similar publications. In the present volume, this purpose is represented by the attempt to apply modern knowledge on the ecology, the phenotypic expression and the molecular biology of R-factors to the prevention of environmental hazards and to the solution of medical problems.

J. Drews   G. Högenauer

Vienna, November 1977

Contents

I. Epidemiology of R-Factors

a) The Incidence and Ecology of R-Factors in Different Environments

Evolutionary Aspects of Plasmid Mediated Resistance in a Hospital Environment

J. F. Acar, D. H. Bouanchaud*, and Y. A. Chabbert*

Epidemiologic and bacteriologic surveillance of endemic and epidemic nosocomial infections represents the usual approach to the study of the indigenous bacterial flora of the hospital. Nosocomial infections are most frequently caused by Gram-negative bacilli which are resistant to multiple antibiotics (1), although recently epidemics caused by multiple resistant Staph. aureus have been reported (2) (3) (4). Surveillance systems which are capable of detecting changes in antibiotic susceptibility or in species prevalence may alert the epidemiologist and clinician to the possibility of an outbreak of nosocomial infection caused by multiple resistant bacteria (5) (6).

Such a surveillance system may also serve to study the dissemination of R-factors mediating antibiotic resistance, whether spread from cell to cell, or spread from patient to patient by a predominant host species carrying an R-factor.

The high incidence of multiple resistant strains in hospital acquired infections has been widely documented (7) (8) (9) (10) (11) (12).

Newly admitted patients may introduce new strains of bacteria to the hospital flora, and during hospitalisation they may themselves acquire and disseminate the indigenous hospital flora. The bacterial strains which colonise hospitalised patients commonly cause infections which are serious and may be life-threatening.

---

* Bactériologie Médicale, Institut Pasteur, Paris

Multiple resistant strains isolated from nosocomial infections
may be grouped roughly into two categories: strains belonging
to species usually responsible for infections in the community
as well as in hospitalised patients, such as E. coli, Klebsiella,
Proteus mirabilis and Staph. aureus; and strains belonging to
opportunistic species regularly isolated only from in-patients
after several days of hospitalisation, such as Serratia, Entero-
bacter, Proteus rettgeri, Providencia and Pseudomonas.

E. coli, Klebsiella, Proteus mirabilis and Staph. aureus, isolated after the eighth day of hospitalisation and responsible for
nosocomial infections, are more commonly multiple resistant
than are strains isolated from outpatients or from in-patients
during the first week of hospitalisation.

Table 1 presents the results observed in 1974 at St. Joseph
Hospital (Paris).

Table 1.

Species	Total number tested	Strains resistant to more than 4 antibiotics			
		Time of isolation during day in the hospital			
		first week	percent	later than first week	percent
E. coli	2 411	134	10	282	25
Klebsiella	916	79	18	261	53
Proteus mirab.	654	17	4	69	30
Staph.aureus	1 143	64	10	227	41

Gram-negative bacteria were tested against 8 antibiotics (Ampicillin, Cephalothin, Streptomycin, Kanamycin, Gentamicin, Chloramphenicol, Tetracyclin, Sulfonamide). Staph. aureus were tested
for susceptibility to 9 antibiotics (Penicillin, Oxacillin,
Streptomycin, Kanamycin, Gentamicin, Chloramphenicol, Tetracycline,
Clindamycin, Erythromycin). The number of strains resistant to
more than 4 antibiotics is strikingly different when strains
isolated from patients during the first week of hospitalisation
are compared with those isolated from patients after the eighth
hospital day.

Opportunistic pathogens, such as <u>Serratia</u>, <u>Enterobacter</u>, <u>Proteus rettgeri</u>, <u>Providencia</u> and <u>Pseudomonas</u>, are most frequently responsible for serious nosocomial infections. Very rarely isolated from patients with community-acquired infections, these species have always been highly resistant to multiple antibiotics. <u>Pseudomonas aeruginosa</u> resistant to Carbenicillin (13) and Gentamicin (14), <u>Proteus rettgeri</u> resistant to all antibiotics commonly tested in the clinical microbiology lab (15), and <u>Serratia</u> marcescens resistant to Gentamicin (16) and even to Amikacin (17) have been reported. One of us, in a review of Gram-negative bacilli resistant to all currently available antibiotics, showed that among 364 strains found to be resistant to all drugs, <u>Serratia</u>, <u>Proteus rettgeri</u> and <u>Providencia</u> were the most frequent (18). Other studies have demonstrated that each hospital has probably a specific distribution of these resistant species (19). Thus each hospital might be considered as a reservoir of multiple resistant strains grouped in one or more ecological niches.

A high proportion of resistant strains isolated in the hospital are found to harbour R-factors. The incidence of R-factors mediating antibiotic resistance is equally high in bacteria colonising hospitalised patients and in bacteria causing nosocomial infections. From the published data (20) (21) (22) (23) (24) (25) (13) (26) (27), the incidence of R-factors in drug resistant clinical isolates, varies between 50 and 100 percent. The differences noted between hospitals are related to different methods of surveillance, to the different species studied and also to the numerous factors which influence mating experiments.
These results were usually based on mating experiments and, in some studies, on "cure" of the resistance markers. For technical reasons, no physical demonstration of R-factors in the host bacteria and the transconjugant have been carried out in epidemiological studies.

Our experience, using the same technique to detect transferable R-factors in large epidemiological studies is presented in Table 2. Successful transfers were obtained more frequently in the first study involving a single ward during an outbreak of infections caused by gentamicin-resistant bacteria, than in the second study, in which endemic infections with trimethoprim-resistant strains (MIC ⩾ 1000 mcg/ml) were followed in four different wards.

Table 2. *Frequency of transfers into E. coli K 12 from various hospital strains*

R plasmids mediating resistance to Gentamicin
1970 – 1971

Donors	Number of strains	Successful transfers
Klebsiella	17	14
Proteus mirabilis	8	8
Proteus indol +	8	7
E. coli	2	2
Citrobacter	4	3
Salmonella	1	1
Serratia	2	1
	42	36
		(84 percent)

R plasmids mediating resistance to Tp (MIC⩾1000 mcg/ml)
1974 – 1975

E. coli	12	12
Proteus mirabilis	16	14
Proteus indol +	29	6
Citrobacter	38	19
Klebsiella	24	5
Enterobacter	5	1
Serratia	7	0
	131	57
		(43,5 percent)

In nosocomial infections caused by Staph. aureus, R-factors must be studied by special mating procedures (28) (29) and physical techniques.

In a recent outbreak of infections caused by Staph. aureus resistant to aminoglycoside antibiotics, the staphylococcus was demonstrated to have a plasmid mediated resistance to one or several groups of drugs (30) (31).

Very few studies have compared hospital strains to community strains (24) (25). Hospital strains may contain more than one R-plasmid per cell. Among 16 multiply resistant strains from the hospital nine had more than one plasmid per cell (2 : 5 strains; 3 : 3 strains; 4 : 1 strain); among 6 community strains none had more than one plasmid (32).

Thus, strains isolated from hospital infections contain one or more *R-plasmids usually characterised by a large number of resistance markers*. In a two-year follow up of plasmids mediating resistance to Trimethoprim, we have isolated 35 plasmids from community acquired infections; the mean number of resistance markers was 3 (1-4); the predominant resistance patterns were Cm Tp and Su Tp. 42 plasmids were isolated from hospital infections : the mean number of resistance markers was 6 (4-8). The predominant resistance patterns were Am Sm Cm Su Tp and Sm Sm Cm Su Gk.

A comparison of the incompatibility groups of the R plasmids isolated from nosocomial infections to those isolated from outpatients demonstrated that most of the hospital R plasmids belonged to a small number of incompatibility groups.

Results of incompatibility typing in one hospital during a 4-year period are summarized in Table 3.

Table 3.

Year	Number of strains	S p e c i e s	Incompatibility groups	Number of R-plasmids
1971	2	Klebsiella		
	1	Citrobacter		
	1	Proteus rettgeri	6 - C	5
	1	Serratia marcescens		
1974	4	E. coli		
	5	Citrobacter x)	6 - C	9
	1	Proteus mirabilis	7 - M	1
	1	Proteus rettgeri	N	2
	1	Proteus morganii	F_{II}	1
1975	1	Proteus rettgeri		
	1	Proteus mirabilis	6 - C	4
	1	Salmonella typhi	F_{II}	1
	2	E. coli		
1976	1	Salmonella typhimurium		
	1	E. coli	6 - C	4
	2	Klebsiella pneumoniae		

x) one strain harboured two R plasmids.

Despite the paucity of comparative data from different hospitals,
a sort of institutional stability may be noted with interest. The
indigenous flora of hospital has R-factors belonging to its prevalent incompatibility group or groups. This finding suggests a
number of possible explanations. Many factors are probably involved, among which are: i) Constant selection pressure on the
same markers, ii) Ecological advantages of the R^+ strains,
iii) Wide host range of the R-factor, iv) High rate of direct
or indirect bacterial exchange between the patients.

Thus, the appearance in a hospital of a plasmid belonging to an
incompatibility group, rarely if ever previously noted there,
assumes a particular importance, since it might be associated
with a new outbreak of nosocomial infection.

Evolution of R plasmids

Several phenomena appear to be responsible for the evolution of
R plasmids in the hospital as well as in the community: the
appearance of resistance markers; the appearance of "epidemic"
plasmids which seem to be able to infect a large number of
strains in a short period of time, and the genetic exchange of
DNA between plasmids.

The appearance of new resistance markers has been observed many
times. During the past few years, several examples have been
reported in Staph. aureus as well as in Gram-negative bacilli.
The new marker is generally detected because of a sudden outbreak
of resistant nosocomial infections, or because of a change in
antibiotic sensitivity pattern noted during routine epidemiologic
surveillance.

In Table 4, we have summarized some of the new characters observed on R plasmids isolated from hospital infections.

As each new antibiotic becomes commercially available and before
it is extensively used, it is worthwhile to determine if a
corresponding "resistance marker" exists in already known R
plasmids, or in R plasmids from wild strains. For example, the
resistance markers "Gentamicin" and "Trimethoprim" were unknown

Table 4.

Host strain	New resistance marker	Resistance pattern of R plasmid	Year
Klebsiella	Gk (Km Tm) ANT 2"	Am Cm Su	1971 (33)
Enterobacter	Gm AAC 3 I	Sm Tc Su	1972 (34)
E. coli	Tp	Su	1972 (35)
Pseudomonas aeruginosa	Cb	Km Nm Tc	1972 (35)
Pseudomonas aeruginosa	Ak (Km Tm Si Bt) AAC 6'	x)	1974 (37)
Klebsiella	Gm (Km Tm) AAC 3 II	Am Sm Cm Tc Su	1974 (38)
Staph. aureus	Gm (Km Tm) APH 2"	x)	1975 (30)
Staph. aureus	Streptogramine A, B (Acetylation)	Km Tm Ak Lv Nm Bt	1975 (31)
Staph. aureus	Ak Km Tm Nm Lv Bt ANT 4' I	x)	1976 (39)

x) no other markers detected.

at the beginning of the clinical use of the drugs, and appeared suddenly (33) (35). On the other hand, the resistance marker "Amikacin" which governs an enzyme inactivating Kanamycin and Tobramycin, was present before the use of Amikacin and probably before the use of Tobramycin as well (17) (37).

The finding of each new resistance character leads to studies concerning the mechanism involved in the resistance. For example, the same resistance patterns to aminoglycoside antibiotics can be associated with different enzymes which represent different resistance markers (40). Resistance to Trimethoprim has been found to be associated with plasmid mediated dihydrofolate reductase resistant to Tp; two different dihydrofolate reductases can be responsible for the Tp resistance (41).

" Epidemic" plasmids have a high ability to "colonise" a large number of strains belonging to the same species or to different species. Such plasmids have been observed when they carried specific markers which are easily followed in an epidemiological survey. Table 5 illustrates some examples of such "epidemic" plasmids.

However, it is likely that some epidemic plasmids are missed because they do not encode for new resistance markers or for some other "exotic" characteristics.

The spread of an "epidemic" plasmid and subsequent epidemiologic fate of the infected strains, is probably dependent upon many factors including the selective pressure of antibiotics and the bacterial exchange between patients. A follow up of the epidemic plasmids harbouring the Gentamicin (ANT 2") resistance marker in two hospitals has shown two interesting findings. In one hospital, after two months, the strains harbouring the R plasmid (Rip 55) were isolated less frequently. New R plasmids isolated later from endemic strains in the hospital belonged to other incompatibility groups, although they had one or more resistance markers characterising the original epidemic plasmid (45). In the second hospital, the initial outbreak lasted 3 months; with limitation of antibiotic usage and isolation of infected patients, this outbreak of nosocomial infections was controlled. Resumption of the wide-spread use of Gentamicin and Ampicillin was again

Table 5.

Origin strain	Resistance pattern of the R plasmid	Incompatibility group	Species colonised by plasmid	Year
Klebsiella	Am Cm Su Gk	6	Ps.aeruginosa, E. coli, Prot. mir., Providencia, Enterobacter	1971(42)
Klebsiella	Am Cm Su Gk	6	Prot.mir., Enterobacter, E. coli, Serratia, Citrobacter, Prot.rett., Salmonella	1971(43)
Coli	Su Tp	W	Klebsiella, Prot.morganii	1972(35)
Ps. aeruginosa	Cb Km Nm Tc	P	E. coli, Prot. mir., Klebsiella	1972(44)

associated with a new outbreak of nosocomial infections. During
this second outbreak, R^+ strains belonging to four species, not
isolated during the first outbreak, were responsible for the
infections. It is therefore likely that the same plasmid remained endemic during the interval between outbreaks, and was
responsible for the second outbreak (Fig. 1) (43).

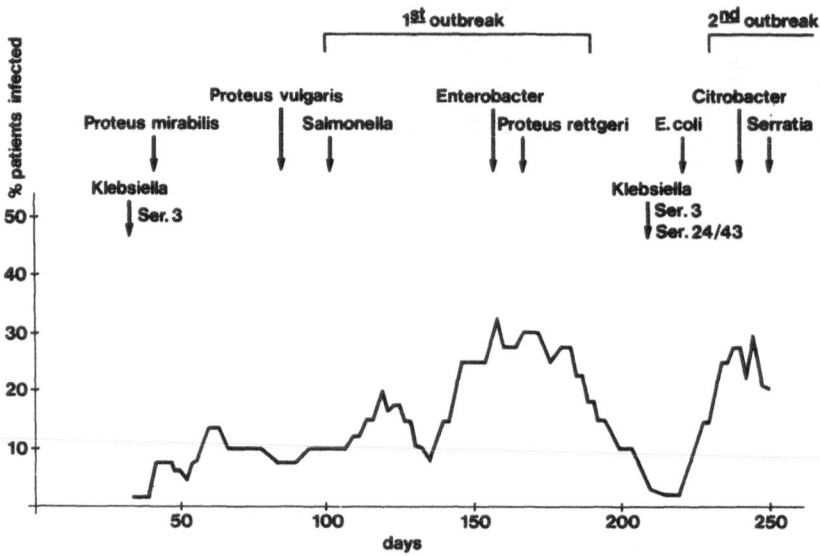

*Evolution of plasmids may be the result of changes in the structure of
DNA molecules* (acquisition or loss of properties). Proof of R-
factor recombinations <u>in vivo</u> are very rare (46). Translocation
of short pieces of DNA, referred to as transposons (47) is certainly of special interest in this regard, because this phenomenon can explain how plasmid molecules can acquire DNA fragments
without losing an equivalent length of genetic material. This
"transposon" acquisition can occur between phylogenetically unrelated molecules particularly between plasmids belonging to
different incompatibility groups.

"Transposable" characters have been recently demonstrated in some
studies. The dissemination of a Tp resistance character as a
"transposon" has been reported (48). In support of this finding,
we observed the Tp marker in 33 R plasmids belonging to six
different incompatibility groups in 1974 (49).

The epidemiological survey of R plasmids (50) (51) (52) (53) might well find a place as part of a surveillance system of nosocomial infections. Dissemination in the community of R-factors of nosocomial origin might have important implications.

For the epidemiological control of nosocomial infections, it is important to follow such factors as: the presence or absence of a resistance marker for an antibiotic to be used in the hospital; the carriage of the resistance marker by a plasmid; any other markers carried by the plasmid which could account for the selection of such a plasmid; other R plasmids harbouring the same resistance marker and their incompatibility groups; and evidence for epidemic spread of an R plasmid between strains of the same or different species.

Epidemiological surveillance and the tracing of R plasmids in a pool of bacteria would be done primarily by phenotypical observations complemented by genetic study (transferability, incompatibility grouping) and, if possible, biochemical and physical analysis.

Phenotypical observations may follow several kinds of "markers". The drug resistance markers are the most commonly used. A new drug resistance marker is of great value, but in other cases, different types of markers must be found: metal resistance (Hg, Cd, As, Ni, Ca)...(54) (55) (56) is sometimes useful in the characterisation of R plasmids. Other markers, such as colicin, hemolysin and metabolic markers are more difficult to use at present. The drug resistance marker can sometimes be defined by the enzyme which governs the resistance to the drug.

The transferability of the R plasmids is generally easy to test and can be used routinely for Enterobacteriaceae. Pseudomonas and Staph. aureus are more difficult to study (28) (57). However, the transferability depends upon many factors; thus, the epidemiological significance of an easily transferable <u>in vitro</u> R plasmid is not clear.

The incompatibility grouping (58) is of great value when the R plasmid belongs to an incompatibility group, which is uncommon in the specific institution surveyed. The groups 6-C, 7-M and

F_{II} have been most frequently found in two hospitals in Paris. This fact must be considered in interpreting the significance of the appearance of new R plasmids in these hospitals.

The physical studies are difficult to carry out in a hospital survey. New studies on molecular weight determination and restriction enzyme analysis by more simple techniques (59) may provide valuable tools for the epidemiological tracing of R plasmids in the near future.

References

1. Finland, M.: Changing Prevalence of Pathogenic Bacteria in Relation to Time and the Introduction and Use of New Anti-Microbial Agents. In "Bacterial Infections", Bayer Sympos.III., Springer-Verlag, 4-18, 1971.
2. Speller, D. C. E., Raghmath, D., Stephens, M., Viant, A. C., Reeves, D. S., Wilkinson, P. J., Broughall, J. M., Holt, H. A.: Epidemic Infection by Gentamicin Resistant Staphylococcus Aureus in Three Hospitals. Lancet i, 464-466, 1976.
3. Soussy, C. J., Dublanchet, A., Cormier, M., Bismuth, R., Mizon, F., Chardon, H., Duval, J., Fabiani, G.: Nouvelles résistances plasmidiques de Staphylococcus aureus aux aminosides N. Presse Méd., 5, 2599-2602, 1976.
4. Shanson, D. C., Kensit, J. G., Duke, R.: Outbreak of Hospital Infection With a Strain of Staphylococcus Aureus Resistant to Gentamicin and Methicillin. Lancet, ii, 1347-1348, 1976.
5. Eichkoff, T. C., Brachman, P. S., Bennett, J. V., Brown, J. F.: Surveillance of Nosocomial Infections in Community Hospitals. I: Surveillance Methods, Effectiveness and Initial Results. J. Infect. Dis., 120, 305-317, 1969.
6. O'Brien, T. F., Kent, R. L., Medeiros, A. A.: Computer Surveillance of Shifts in the Gross Patient Flora During Hospitalisation. I. Infect. Dis., 131, 88-96, 1975.
7. Lorian, V., Topf, B.: Microbiology of Nosocomial Infections. Arch. Intern. Med., 130, 104-109, 1972.
8. Isenberg, H. D., Berkman, J. I.: The Role of Drug Resistant and Drug Selected Bacteria in Nosocomial Disease. Am. N. Y. Acad. of Sc. 182, 21-39, 1971.

9. Rose, H. D., Schreier, J.: The Effect of Hospitalisation and Antibiotic Therapy on the Gram Negative Fecal Flora. Am. J. Med. Sci., 255, 228-236, 1968.

10. Pollack, M., Charache, P., Niemann, R. E., Jett, M. P., Reinhardt, J. A., Hardy, P. H.: Factors Influencing Colonisation and Antibiotic Resistance Patterns of Gram Negative Bacteria in Hospital Patients. Lancet, 2, 688-671, 1972.

11. Mc Gowan, J. E., Barnes, M. W., Finland, M.: Bacteremia at Boston City Hospital; Occurrence and Mortality During 12 Selected Years (1935 - 1972) With Special Reference to Hospital Acquired Cases. J. Infect. Dis. 132, 316-335, 1975.

12. Johanson, W. G., Pierce, A. K., Sanford, J. P., Thomas, G. D.: Nosocomial Respiratory Infections With Gram Negative Bacilli: the Significance of the Colonisation of the Respiratory Tract. Am. Int. Med., 77, 701-706, 1972.

13. Lowbury, E. J. L., Babb, J. R., Roe, E.: Clearance From a Hospital of Gram Negative Bacilli That Transfer Carbenicillin Resistance to Pseudomonas Aeruginosa. Lancet, II, 942-944, 1972.

14. Brusch, J. L., Barza, M., Bergeron, M. G., Weinstein, L.: Cross Resistance of Pseudomonas to Gentamicin and Tobramycin. Antimicrob. Ag. Chemoth., I, 280-281, 1972.

15. Kaslow, R. A., Lindsey, J. O., Bisno, A. L., Price, A.: Nosocomial Infection With Highly Resistant Proteus Rettgeri. Am. J. of Epidem., 104, 278-286, 1976.

16. Traub, W. H., Kleber, I., Pühler, A., Burkhardt, H. J.: Characterisation of a Nosocomially Significant Multiple Drug Resistant Strain of Serratia Marcescens. Chemotherapy, 22, 297-312, 1976.

17. Acar, J. F., Witchitz, J. L., Goldstein, F. W., Talbot, J. N., Le Goffic, F.: Susceptibility of Aminoglycoside Resistant Gram Negative Bacilli to Amikacin. Delineation of Individual Resistance Patterns. J. of Infect. Dis., 134 (Suppl.), 280-285, 1976.

18. Soussy, C. J., Denoyer, M. C., Duval, J., Goldstein, F. W., Guibert, J. M., Acar, J. F., Begue, P.: Les bactéries résistantes à tout existent-elles? Med. Mal. Infect., 4, 6bis, 341-348, 1974.

19. Schaeffler, S., Winter, J., Catelli, A., Greene, J., Toharski, B.: Specific Distribution of R Factors in Serratia Marcescens Strains Isolated From Hospital Infections. Applied Microb., 22, 339-343, 1971.

20. Salzman, T. C., Klenner, L.: Transferable Drug Resistance (R Factors) in Enterobacteriaceae: Relationship to Nosocomial Infections. Antimic. Ag. Chemoth., 1966 (1967 Am. Soc. for Microbiology), 212-220.

21. Kontomichalon, P.: Studies of Resistance Transfer Factors. Pathol. Microbiol., 30, 71-75, 1967.

22. Datta, N.: Drug Resistance and R Factors in the Bowel Bacteria of London Patients Before and After Admission to Hospital. Brit. Med. J. 2, 407-409, 1969.

23. Lebek, G.: Neue Aspekte der Antibiotika-Resistenz menschlicher Krankheitserreger. Schweiz. Med. Wochensch., 99, 397-400, 1969.

24. Lewis, M.J.: Transferable Drug Resistance and Other Transferable Agents in Strains of Escherichia coli From two Human Populations. Lancet, I, 1389-1393, 1968.

25. Linton, K.B., Richmond, M.H., Bevan, P., Gillespie, W.A.: Antibiotic Resistance and R Factors in Coliform Bacilli Isolated From Hospital and Domestic Sewage. J. of Med. Microb., 7, 91-103, 1974.

26. Jonnsson, M.: Resistance to Antibiotics and R Factors in Gram-negative Bacteria Isolated in a Hospital For Infectious Diseases. Scand. J. Infect. Dis., 4, 133-137, 1972.

27. Anderson, F.M., Datta, N., Shaw, E.J.: R Factors in Hospital Infection. Brit. Med. J., 2, 82-85, 1972.

28. Lacey, R.W.: Antibiotic Resistance Plasmids of Staphylococcus aureus and Their Clinical Importance. Bact. Rev., 39, 1-32, 1975.

29. Fouace, J.M.: Transfer of Resistance Plasmids in Staphylococcus aureus. Ann. Microb. (I.P.), 125 A, 517-520, 1974.

30. Soussy, J.C., Bouanchaud, D.H., Fouace, J.M., Dublanchet, A., Duval, J.: A Gentamicin Resistance Plasmid in Staphylococcus aureus. Ann. Microb. (I.P.), 126 B, 91-94, 1975.

31. Bouanchaud, D.H., Fouace, J.M., Bieth, G.: Physical Studies of a Staphylococcus aureus Plasmids Mediating Resistance to Streptogramins, Lincosamins, and Aminoglycosides. Subm. for publication.

32. Chabbert, Y.A., Witchitz, J.L., Gerbaud, G.R.: Epidemics of R Factors Mediating Gentamicin Resistance and Belonging to Different Incompatibility Groups. Progress in Chemotherapy, G. Daikos Edit., Vol. 1, 22-28, 1973.

33. Witchitz, J.L., Chabbert, Y.A.: Résistance transférable à la Gentamicine: I, Expression du caractère de résistance. Ann. Microb. (I.P.), <u>121</u>, 733-742, 1971.

34. Witchitz, J.L.: Plasmid-Mediated Gentamicin Resistance not Associated With Kanamycin Resistance in Enterobacteriaceae. J. Antibiotics, 15, 10, 622-624, 1972.

35. Datta, N., Hedges, R.W.: Trimethoprim Resistance Conferred by W Plasmids in Enterobacteriaceae. J. Gen. Microb., <u>72</u>, 349-356, 1972.

36. Sykes, R.B., Richmond, M.H.: Intergenetic Transfer of a Lactamase Between Ps. aeruginosa and E. coli. Nature, <u>226</u>, 952-954, 1970.

37. Jacoby, G.A.: Properties of an R Plasmid in Pseudomonas aeruginosa Producing Amikacin (BB-K 8), Butirosin, Kanamycin, Tobramycin and Sisomicin Resistance. A.A.C., 6, 6, 807-810, 1974.

38. Le Goffic, F., Baca, B., Soussy, C.J., Dublanchet, A., Duval, J.: ANT (4') I: une nouvelle nucleotidyltransferase d'aminoglycosides isolée de Staphylococcus aureus. Ann. Microb. (I.P.), <u>127 A</u>, 391-399, 1976.

39. Le Goffic, F., Martel, A., Witchitz, J.L.: 3-N Enzymatic Acetylation of Gentamicin, Tobramycin and Kanamycin by Escherichia coli Carrying an R Factor. Antimicrob. Ag. Chemoth., <u>6</u>, 680-684, 1974.

40. Price, K.E., Pursiano, T.A., de Furia, M.E., Wright, G.E.: Activity of BB-K 8 (Amikacin) Against Clinical Isolates Resistant to One or More Aminoglycoside Antibiotics. Antimicrob. Ag. Chemoth., <u>5</u>, 143-152, 1974.

41. Pattishall, K.H., Acar, J.F., Burchall, J.J., Harvey, R.J.: Two Distinct Types of Trimethoprim Resistant Dihydrofolate Reductase, Specified by R Plasmids of Different Compatibility Groups. J. of Biol. Chem. (to be published).

42. Witchitz, J.L., Chabbert, Y.A.: Résistance à la Gentamicine. II: Transmission et liaison du caractère de résistance. Ann. Microb. (I.P.) <u>122</u>, 367-370, 1972.

43. Acar, J.F.: unpublished results.

44. Roe, E., Jones, R.J., Lowbury, E.J.L.: Transfer of Antibiotic Resistance Between Pseudomonas aeruginosa, E. coli and other Gram-negative Bacilli in Burns. Lancet, <u>I</u>, 150-152, 1971.

45. Witchitz, J.L.: Epidemic of a Plasmid in a Hospital. (to be published).

46.Ingram, L.C., Anderson, J.D., Arraud, J.E., Richmond, M.H.:
A Probable Example of R Factor Recombination in the Human
Gastro-Intestinal Tract. J. of Med. Microb., 7, 251-257, 1974.

47.Heffron, F., Sublett, R., Hedges, R.W., Jacob, A., Falkow, St.:
Origin of the TEM Lactamase Gene Found in Plasmids. J. Bact.,
122, 250-256, 1975.

48.Barth, P.T., Datta, N., Hedges, R.W., Grinter, N.J.: Trans-
position of a Deoxyribonucleic Acid Sequence Encoding
Trimethoprim and Streptomycin Resistances From R 483 to Other
Replicons. J. Bact., 125, 800-810, 1976.

49.Acar, J.F., Goldstein, F.W., Gerbaud, G.R., Chabbert, Y.A.:
Plasmides de résistance au Trimethoprime, transférabilité
et groupes d'incompatibilité. Ann. Microb. (I.P.), 128 A,
41-47, 1977.

50.Anderson, E.S.: Ecology and Epidemiology of Transferable
Drug Resistance. Bacterial Episomes and Plasmids. J.A.
Churchill, London, 1969, 102-119.

51.Davies, J.E., Rownd, R.: Transmissible Multiple Drug Resistance in Enterobacteriaceae. Science, 176, 758-762, 1972.

52.Richmond, M.H.: R Factors in Man and His Environment.
Microbiology (Am. Soc. for Microbiology), 27-35, 1974.

53.Falkow, St.: The Transmission of R Factors In Vivo. in
"Infectious Multiple Drug Resistance", Pion Ltd., 1975,
230-252.

54.Novick, R.P., Roth, C.: Plasmid Linked Resistance to Inorganic
Salts in Staphylococcus aureus. J. Bact., 95, 1335-1342, 1968.

55.Richmond, M.H., John, M.: Cotransduction by a Staphlyococcal
Phage of the Genes Responsible for Penicillinase Synthesis
and Resistance to Mercury Salts. Nature, 202, 1360-1361, 1964.

56.Smith, D.H.: R Factors Mediate Resistance to Mercury, Nickel
and Cobalt. Science, 156, 1114-1116, 1967.

57.Jacoby, G.A.: Properties of R Plasmids in Pseudomonas
aeruginosa. Microbiology, (A.S.M.), 36-42, 1974.

58.Datta, N.: Epidemiology and Classification of Plasmids.
Microbiology (A.S.M.), 9-15, 1974.

59.Meyers, J.A., Sanchez, D., Elwell, L.P., Falkow, St.:
Simple Agarose Gel Electrophoretic Method for the Identi-
fication and Characterization of Plasmid Deoxyribonucleic
Acid. J. of Bact., 127, 3, 1529-1537, 1976.

Discussion

Falkow: As far as the strains you have studied are concerned, were they a representative collection of strains, or was there a preponderance of urinary tract strains?

Acar: The majority of the strains we studied were from hospitals, and were from urinary tract infections and from wound infections. Practically all the trimethoprim resistant strains were from urinary tract cases.

Falkow: The community strains you studied, were they also from urinary tract infections?

Acar: Yes.

Anderson: An important point to bear in mind here is that there are three classes of organisms. First, you have the non-pathogenic commensals. They accumulate R-factors. They act as a source of R plasmids for organisms that cause trouble. In themselves they cause no trouble. In the middle you have the organisms that cause a lot of trouble because they are the opportunist pathogens. They need antibiotic use in order to become epidemic. If you press with antibiotics, they come up like a flash. This has been shown time and again. pseudomas, proteus, some of the colis, citrobacters, etc., etc. Thirdly, there are the essential pathogens. They do not need antibiotic use. If they have R-factors, so much the better for them, so much the worse for the patient: the salmonellas, the typhoid bacillus. There is no need to press with antibiotics on these because they have epidemic potential, and they will spread with or without antibiotics. The critical point is the centre group. It is with this group that you must not press with the antibiotics.

Richmond: Would you agree, in Western European countries, at least, that R-factor resistance is primarily a problem of the hospitals? Would you like to comment on the level of R plasmids in the community in France? For example, what proportion of people coming into hospital carry resistant infections?

Acar: We really have no significant data on this point. Only a few isolated studies.

The second question relates specifically to ampicillin resistance. Do you have the impression, which I certainly have from talking to hospital doctors in England, that this antibiotic is becoming somewhat eroded in its effect by the high incidence of resistant strains?

Acar: Yes. We see ampicillin resistance very frequently. Even in outpatients. It is an impression based on a single study, but it is my feeling that ampicillin is now the worst drug for treating urinary tract infections. In 60 to 65% of hospital patients a superinfection with ampicillin resistant strains is observed.

Richmond: That certainly fits with data from the Bristol clinics where they reckon that about 40% of all E. coli from urinary tract infections are ampicillin resistant.

Falkow: If I can add data from the urinary tract clinic in Seattle, for those patients coming from the community we see essentially only sulphonamide resistance (about 11% currently). Once the patient is admitted to the hospital, the incidence of resistance goes up very dramatically.

Richmond: This raises the interesting question as to whether we have reached the worst point in the community, or can things get worse?

Anderson: I have strong views on this point. I think the use of antibiotics as it is now practised in the community is a calamity. It's an act of complacency to say that we have reached a steady state, and do not have to worry. We do need to worry. We need to worry about the antibiotics we have got, and the antibiotics we might get.

Acar: In a study I have done with Chabbert, which concerned isolates from the community in small towns in France, we find about 20% of strains resistant to ampicillin and 40% resistant to sulphonamide. An interesting point emerged: we found a higher incidence of tetracycline in E. coli in the community than in the hospitals. The difference was only five per cent: 30% in the community, and 25% in the hospitals.

Starlinger: What happens to the people that acquire a resistant flora in hospital and then leave?

Richmond: We have tried to answer this question, but it is ex-

tremely difficult to sample people on the day they are to
leave hospital. It is even harder to follow them into the community. Having escaped from hospital, they just do not want to
have anything to do with anything that can relate to medical
intervention.

Levy: Looking at our hospital population, I find two things:
First within a single hospital, each ward has a different pattern. And if you take an immuno-suppressed patient, their infections are not usually by "hospital" organisms. They are
usually infected with something they bring in with them.
The other point is really in the form of a question. Do you
think that continued presence of a resistant strain in a ward
is because of the continued use of an antibiotic? Or is that
particular strain part of that environment? The reason I ask is
because we know from our studies that animals kept in one place
tend to maintain the same flora, whereas, if you move them,
they tend to change their flora.

Acar: I believe the strain a patient picks up is primarily related to the strain that is prevalent in the ward, and seems
to be broadly unrelated to antibiotic use. The patients arrive
with their own E. coli, and perhaps their own R-factors. During
the first week they tend to exchange these for the strains
characteristic of the wards.

Anderson: We will probably never be able to know the various
factors precisely. The problem is too complex, and the interactions too subtle.

The Geographical Predominance of Resistance Transfer Systems of Various Compatibility Groups in Salmonellae

E. S. Anderson

Introduction

For many years we have carried out an intensive study of enterobacterial plasmids from different parts of the world, particularly in salmonellae, and specially in Salmonella typhimurium and S.typhi. The methods employed were those we have established for routine plasmid characterisation (1). Patterns of regional plasmid predominance have emerged and it is these patterns that I propose to outline in this communication.

Methods

The characters examined were as follows:

Spectra of resistance (R-types).

Level of resistance against particular drugs.

Transferability of resistance into standard hosts.

The fertility inhibition (fi) character.

Compatibility grouping (2, 3, 4, 5).

Phage restriction in standard salmonella strains.

Class of transfer systems involved: Class 1, in which the transfer factor and resistance determinant form a single covalently-bonded linkage group which is transferred intact to recipient cells and remains transferable from the new host; and Class 2, in which the transfer factor is distinct from, but mediates the transfer of, the resistance determinants, which are independent non-autotransferring plasmids (1, 6, 7, 8, 9).

Molecular characterisation: the size of the plasmid molecules, and their polynucleotide sequences as shown by reassociation studies.

The symbols used for antibiotic resistance markers are as follows:
A = ampicillin; C = chloramphenicol; K = neomycin-kanamycin;
S = streptomycin; Su = sulphonamides; T = tetracyclines.

Table 1. Compatibility group distribution of resistance plasmids in _Salmonella typhimurium_, 1968-1976

Area of origin (number of cultures examined)	Source of S.typhimurium	Total number of transfer systems	Predominant compatibility groups in order of frequency						
North West Europe Belgium (1,203) France (73) Germany (460) Finland (12)	Belgium: Human 6.2% Animal 93.8% Others: Human	1,330	I_1 $\underline{fi^-}$ Δ	41	N IKe^+ $\underline{fi^-}$	I_1 $\underline{fi^-}$ nr	I_1 $\underline{fi^-}$ Γ	I_1 $\underline{fi^+}$ nr	
			862	187	97	48	39	31	
		Per cent	64.8	14.1	7.3	3.6	2.9	2.3	
Southern Europe Greece (98) Spain (60) Italy (3) Portugal (71)	Italy: Animal Others: Human	189	I_1★ $\underline{fi^-}$ Γ	H_2★★	F_{II}	com 7	N IKe^+ $\underline{fi^-}$	F_{IV}	F_I
			56	50	30	20	17	9	4
		Per cent	29.6	26.5	15.9	10.6	9.0	4.8	2.1

★ 52 of 56 I_1 Γ type plasmids are from _S.typhimurium_ isolated in Greece. ★★ Group H_2 plasmids predominated in Spain, Portugal and Italy.

Results

For purposes of simplicity the data are tabulated under regions, within which the countries with their numerical contributions are shown, as table 1 demonstrates.

Belgian S.typhimurium cultures of animal origin were the most numerous in North West Europe. They were mainly isolated from pigs and belonged to phage type 194. The cultures were not sent to us because of their drug resistance, but because of their prevalence. The predominant resistance transfer system belonged to Class 2, the transfer factor being I_1 and fi⁻, and giving the Δ type of phage restriction in S.typhimurium (10); it did not itself code for identifiable resistances. The non-autotransferring resistance plasmid coded for tetracycline resistance. This R factor-carrying S.typhimurium remained prevalent in Belgian pigs up to the last batch of cultures received in January, 1975.

The second commonest compatibility group in North West Europe was also identified in Belgian cultures of animal origin, particularly from bovines. The cultures all belonged to a new phage type of S.typhimurium, type 207, and were clearly clonal in nature. The plasmid was originally described as belonging to compatibility group G (11), but as that designation had been used by others (12), and as we have adopted numerical compatibility group designations, we have allotted it the number 41. Its commonest R-type is ACKSSuT.

Most of the fi⁻ group N factors which rendered their host strains sensitive to the IKe phage (13) were identified in Belgian bovine S.typhimurium of a variety of phage types.

The French S.typhimurium contributions, of human origin, showed a preponderance of phage types 193 and 194, carrying an I_1 fi⁻ Δ transfer factor and a T resistance determinant transferring in a Class 2 relationship.

The German contribution, again of S.typhimurium of human origin, also shows a heavy predominance of type 194 carrying plasmids similar to those identified in Belgian porcine and French human strains: a discrete I_1 fi⁻ Δ type of transfer factor and a separate T plasmid, transferred in a Class 2 relationship.

It is clear, therefore, that much the commonest resistance transfer system in S.typhimurium in North West Europe is that in which the transfer factor is I_1, fi⁻ and gives phage restriction of the Δ type; and the non-autotransferring resistance plasmid associated with it codes for tetracycline resistance. The uniformity of the phage type, 194, establishes that this is in effect a widespread clonal outbreak and the animal source seems probably to be the pig.

Prevalence of a transfer factor of the Δ type in North West Europe is interesting in view of the earlier studies in England, which revealed the predominance of a single strain of S.typhimurium, of phage type 29, which carried a similar if not identical transfer factor (14, 15). However, the animal source of that strain was bovine.

The Southern European studies were uneven, since they involved mainly the Iberian peninsula on the one hand, and Greece on the other. The predominant plasmids reflected that distribution, since most of the I_1 fi⁻ Γ phage-restricting type of plasmids were identified in Greek cultures of phage type 205 of S.typhimurium of paediatric origin. The transfer system was of mixed Class 1 and Class 2: the Class 1 system coded for neomycin-kanamycin resistance and ColIb synthesis; this mediated the transfer of non-autotransferring A and SSu resistance determinants. The cultures concerned were of paediatric origin, like so many epidemic drug-resistant strains of S.typhimurium we have studied.

The Portuguese cultures received up to 1972 belonged mainly to phage type 193, were of paediatric origin, and carried a group H_2 plasmid of R-type CSSu, CKSSu or ACSSu, transferring its resistances in a Class 1 relationship.

The prototype H_2 plasmid was identified in 1969 from a chloramphenicol-resistant strain of S.typhi isolated from a patient infected in Spain (16). The R-type was CSSu (Class 1). Fourteen Spanish S.typhimurium cultures carried H_2 plasmids of R-type CKSSu (Class 1). These cultures were isolated from man (8), bovines (4) and birds (2) in 1973 and 1976. All but one belonged to phage type 1, which suggests that they are clonal in nature.

Group H_2 plasmids are evidently endemic to the Iberian peninsula.

Table 2 summarises the distribution of plasmids in S.typhimurium from South America. These cultures were largely isolated from severe epidemics in paediatric units, with a high morbidity rate, and a mortality rate of the order of 20 - 30%. Septicaemia and meningitis, the latter always fatal, were common complications. The striking feature of these cultures is the strong suggestion that the distribution of the various clones concerned, of which there were probably three, was limited by natural barriers. Thus the cultures of phage type 193 and related types were found in Argentina, Brazil, Uruguay and Paraguay. They carried a group N fi⁺ transfer factor which did not render its host strain

Area of origin (number of cultures examined)	Source of S.typhimurium	Total number of transfer systems	Predominant compatibility groups in order of frequency					
South America								
Argentina (93) Peru (5)	Human	413	N IKe^- $\underline{fi^+}$	$\underline{com}$ 7	F_{II}			
Brazil (372) Uruguay (73) Chile (135)* Venezuela (12)**			347	29	8			
Paraguay (6)								
		Per cent	84.0	7.0	1.9			
North America	Canada:	180	I_1☆ $\underline{fi^-}$ Γ	H_2☆	N IKe^+ $\underline{fi^-}$	I_1 $\underline{fi^-}$ nr	I_1 $\underline{fi^-}$ 145	F_{IV}
Canada (336)	Human 50.3% Animal 49.7%		61	55	15	10	9	4
Mexico (100)	Mexico: Human							
		Per cent	33.9	30.6	8.3	5.6	5.0	2.2

* 102 of 122 drug-resistant S.typhimurium (83.6%) from Chile carry non-autotransferring resistance plasmids A and SSu, mobilisable by Δ and CKT, mobilisable by X.

** The predominant serotype from Venezuela is S.saintpaul carrying I_1 Γ type plasmids.

☆ Group I_1 Γ type predominates in Mexico and group H_2 in Canada.

sensitive to the IKe phage (17). It mediated transfer of ASSu and CKT
plasmids in a Class 2 relationship. These cultures were distributed south
of the Mato Grosso and East of the Andes.

In Chile, west of the Andes, the picture changed: although the cultures
were again largely paediatric in origin, they belonged to a different
phage type of S.typhimurium, type 12. Of 119 cultures of this type, 102
carried only non-autotransferring resistance plasmids: those of R-type A
and SSu were mobilisable by the Δ (I_1) transfer factor, while a CKT
plasmid was mobilisable by X, an F_{II} transfer factor.

There is little doubt about the clonal nature of the Chilean infections,
only one strain of type 12 of S.typhimurium being involved. However, its
mode of spread from Santiago to Valdivia, 500 miles further south, where
it has caused similar outbreaks, is as yet unknown.

In Venezuela, S.typhimurium was much rarer than drug-resistant S.saintpaul,
which was again a clone that caused severe paediatric infections. It
presented as a number of R-types, of which a substantial proportion
carried the chromosomally determined nalidixic acid resistance marker.
The remainder of the resistances were plasmid in nature and were
transferred in a Class 1 relationship with an I_1 fi⁻ Γ transfer factor.

I should like to add at this point that, despite the clonal nature of
these outbreaks, a substantial degree of variation of R-type occurred in
the strains isolated. This is a general phenomenon, occurring in
resistant cultures isolated throughout the world. Stored cultures with
a wide resistance spectrum show resistance losses similar to those
encountered in nature. This is specially striking in strains carrying
Class 1 R factors. Expansion in resistance of such R factors in nature
is the result of acquisition of new R translocons; diminution of
resistance results from their deletion. Such loss or gain of translocons
may be followed by establishment of the new sublines so that they
predominate in particular areas.

The findings in North America were quite different from those in South
America. In Canada group H_2 was prevalent in S.typhimurium of both human
and animal origin. Four phage types were involved, the possible inter-
relationship of which has not so far been resolved.

One bovine S.typhimurium strain from Canada carried an $F_I$me plasmid, the
first we have identified on the American continent and also the first
found in an animal strain.

Mexico has the distinction of having presented the world in 1972-73 with
the largest typhoid outbreak on historical record. It was caused by a

Table 3. Compatibility group distribution of resistance plasmids in _Salmonella typhimurium_, 1968-1976

Area of origin (number of cultures examined)	Source of S.typhimurium	Total number of transfer systems	Predominant compatibility groups in order of frequency					
			I₁★★ fi⁻ Γ	I₁ fi⁻	F_II	N IKe⁺ fi⁻		H₂
Australia (193)	Australia:		42★	145				
	Human 54.4%							
	Animal 45.6%							
New Zealand (165)	New Zealand:	105	41	36	7	6	5	3
	Human 60.0%							
	Animal 40.0%							
	Per cent		39.0	34.3	6.7	5.7	4.8	2.9

Area of origin (number of cultures examined)	Source of S.typhimurium	Total number of transfer systems	Predominant compatibility groups in order of frequency				
			H₁	F_II	I₁ fi⁻ Γ	I₂	F_I me nt
South East Asia							
India (3) Singapore (93)	Singapore:						
	Human 46.2%						
	Animal 53.8%						
Malaysia (77)☆	Malaysia:	180	121	22	22	8	2
	Human 97.4%						
	Animal 2.6%						
Philippines (8)	Others:						
	Human						
	Per cent		67.2	12.2	12.2	4.4	1.1

★ 31 of 41 Group I₁ Γ type plasmids are from S.typhimurium isolated from processed chickens from Australia.

★★ Group I₁ Γ type plasmids predominated in New Zealand.

☆ S.typhimurium isolated in 1970 carried Group F_II and Group I₁, Γ type plasmids. Group H₁ predominated in cultures isolated in 1972-1974.

strain of the typhoid bacillus carrying an R factor belonging to group H_1 and coding for CSSuT resistances. However, no resistant Mexican S.typhimurium strains studied carried H_1 factors. The predominant S.typhimurium resistance plasmid belonged to group I_1 , was fi⁻ and gave the Γ type of phage restriction in S.typhimurium. It was a Class 1 transfer system, carrying mostly AK, but also AKSu resistances.

A new plasmid compatibility group was identified in Australia. This is shown in table 3 as group 42; it is fi⁺ and non F-like. It transfers A or AT in a Class 1 relationship. It was found in S.typhimurium, largely of phage type 170 in man, and in poultry which were the source of the human infections.

Most of the R factors in S.typhimurium cultures from New Zealand belonged to group I_1, were fi⁻ and gave the Γ type of phage restriction in S.typhimurium. They transferred T in Class 1 and an SSu non-autotransferring plasmid in Class 2. The carrier strains of S.typhimurium belonged to type 206 and were mostly of bovine and avian origin.

Singapore and Malaysia are noteworthy because of the predominance of H_1 R factors in S.typhimurium of human, porcine and avian origin. The phage type was 193 and the identity of phage type, R-type and the plasmids left no room for doubt about the clonal nature of the strain.

H_1 R factors coding for, inter alia, chloramphenicol resistance have been found in a number of phage types of S.typhi in India, Vietnam, Thailand and Indonesia, but not in Singapore or Malaysia.

As we have shown elsewhere, a detailed study of strains of S.typhimurium of Middle Eastern origin has revealed the very wide distribution of a clone of S.typhimurium carrying a main resistance plasmid which we have designated $F_I me$ (18). This plasmid occurs in autotransferring and non-autotransferring forms. The autotransferring members stimulate their carrier strains to produce F fimbriae, but the non-autotransferring members do not. Because their compatibility reactions are identical with those of the transferring members of the group, however, and because they have a very close molecular relationship to them (Willshaw, Smith and Anderson, in preparation), the non-transferring members can be confidently designated $F_I me$. Their host strains, which belong to phage type 208 or derivatives of it, also carry non-transferring small multicopy resistance plasmids of R-type A or AK and SSu.

The infections caused by these strains were predominantly paediatric, and often severe.

Table 4. Compatibility group distribution of resistance plasmids in _Salmonella typhimurium_, 1968-1976

Area of origin (number of cultures examined)	Source of S.typhimurium	Total number of transfer systems	Predominant compatibility groups in order of frequency				
Africa			$F_I$me*	I_1	H_2	I_1	I_1
	Ghana:		t	fi$^-$		fi$^-$	fi$^+$
Ghana (33) Liberia (5)	Human 18.2%			nr		r	nr
Kenya (20) Tanzania (1)	Animal 81.8%	58	20	14	12	11	1
	Others:						
	Human						
	Per cent		34.5	24.1	20.7	19.0	1.7
Middle East			$F_I$me	$F_I$me	H_2	I_1	
			nt	t		fi$^-$	
Iran (142) Iraq (2)						Δ	
Israel (163) Jordan (1)	Human	253	135	47	60	5	
Kuwait (2) Syria (1)							
Turkey (2) Other (2)	Per cent		53.4	18.6	23.7	2.0	
			72.0%				

* Autotransferring Group $F_I$me plasmids were isolated in Kenya and Liberia.

A strain of S.wien carrying an $F_I$me plasmid caused widespread and severe paediatric outbreaks in Algeria (19) and France (20). There have also been a number of incidents caused by this organism in Britain (McConnell, Leonardopoulos, Smith and Anderson, in preparation). Only one strain of S.wien is involved, which started its career in Algeria, spread from there to France, and subsequently to England.

We have had relatively few S.typhimurium strains from Africa, but 15 from Kenya were isolated from fatal infantile meningitis and five from Liberia were also involved in serious paediatric infection. These 20 strains carried $F_I$me plasmids.

The property of non-transferability predominated only in the $F_I$me plasmids of the Middle Eastern series of S.typhimurium strains, and in infections in Britain of Middle Eastern origin.

As I have indicated, other salmonellae than S.typhimurium have shown plasmid-mediated resistances, the most important, apart from S.typhi, being S.wien. However, the story of chloramphenicol-resistant S.typhi has exceptional features that warrant a brief description. The huge Mexican typhoid outbreak of 1972-73 was caused by a clone of S.typhi carrying an H_1 R factor, mostly of R type CSSuT, but since ampicillin was thrown into the fray, the A translocon appeared in a number of lines, tacked on to the CSSuT linkage group. It seems paradoxical that H_1 factors, again mostly CSSuT but also ACSSuT in R-type, have manifested themselves in the typhoid bacillus wherever chloramphenicol resistance has become a problem in this organism. It has appeared particularly in South East Asia: in India, in phage types D1-N and C5; in Vietnam in types A, D6, E7, DVS, UVS1, UVS2, UVS3, 53 and 56; in Thailand in types D1, M1 and 53; and in Indonesia in type 53 (8, 21). The H_1 factors all transferred their resistances in a Class 1 relationship.

About 80 per cent of cultures from South Vietnam, where typhoid is hyperendemic, were chloramphenicol-resistant by 1975. Because of the multiplicity of phage types involved, it is plain that the resistant organisms constitute a series of clones, as opposed to the single clone in Mexico. In South East Asia there are thus the interlocked epidemiologies to be considered of the H_1 plasmids and of the S.typhi lines they infect. There is no reason to suppose that the H_1 factors in South East Asia have a direct epidemiological relationship with that in Mexico, although a phylogenetic relationship clearly exists.

We have demonstrated the presence of H_1 factors similar to those of S.typhi in "normal" E.coli from non-typhoid patients in Vietnam and Thailand, albeit rarely. However, this was some years after the emergence of the resistant typhoid strains, so that the origin of the $\underline{E.coli}$ H$_1$ plasmids is conjectural. But it can be supposed that these plasmids were present in the normal enterobacteria before they were passed to $\underline{S.typhi}$. What is not clear is the reason for their evident special affinity for that organism.

Discussion

The international studies described above establish that particular compatibility groups of plasmids may show a regional predominance in salmonellae, especially in $\underline{S.typhimurium}$. Thus, in North West Europe the I$_1$ $\underline{fi}^-$ Δ type of factor predominates and it tends to form Class 2 resistance transfer systems. The animal origins of these systems have been clearly established. In Greece the I$_1$ $\underline{fi}^-$ Γ type predominates with Class 1 transfer and in the Iberian Peninsula H$_2$ systems, again with Class 1 transfer, are common. In South America group N IKe$^-$ $\underline{fi}^+$ plasmids predominate in $\underline{S.typhimurium}$; in Canada, group H$_2$; in Mexico, group I$_1$ $\underline{fi}^-$ Γ, both forming Class 1 transfer systems.

The natural conclusion can be drawn that in each region ecological conditions have favoured the emergence of particular strains of $\underline{S.typhimurium}$ or other salmonellae, armed with particular plasmids; that these strains have established themselves and spread; and that they may maintain their predominance for long periods. Naturally, plasmids of other compatibility groups are also scattered widely, but much more thinly.

In addition to the phenomenon of local plasmid predominance, and doubtless dependent on it, is the fact that of recent years extensive human outbreaks of severe salmonellosis in many parts of the world have been caused by strains carrying resistance plasmids. The commonest salmonella involved in these incidents has been $\underline{S.typhimurium}$, which is perhaps not surprising since it is the most ubiquitous salmonella. However, other salmonellae, such as $\underline{S.saintpaul}$ and $\underline{S.wien}$, have been involved.

Although a different phage type of $\underline{S.typhimurium}$ is involved in each region, the outbreaks have shown striking similarities: paediatric units in particular have been affected; the morbidity rate is of the order of 50% and the case mortality rate may be as high as 30%; systemic invasion and meningitis are common complications; and most of the strains concerned have five or more resistances.

Despite the similarity of the outbreaks, the organisms causing them show only a regional distribution, although large regions may be affected, as in the $\underline{S.typhimurium}$ carrying F$_I$me plasmids in the Middle East, and that carrying the group N IKe$^-$ $\underline{fi}^+$ plasmids in South America.

An unusual feature of the paediatric epidemics referred to earlier is the
fact that, although we know that human infection with S.typhimurium and
other salmonella is of animal origin, no animal source has been identified
in these paediatric outbreaks. Indeed, a limited study of S.typhimurium
currently prevalent in South American livestock, which I carried out some
years ago, showed no similarity of phage types in the animal and epidemic
human strains. Of course, there is little doubt that the ultimate source
of these strains was animal, but transmission to man may have occurred
years ago, and there is no doubt that present cycling is in the human host,
by nosocomial or other institutional spread. For this reason these
outbreaks are of long duration and are very difficult to control. It is
nowadays almost invariable that, when such outbreaks are established, the
infecting strain carries multiple plasmid-mediated resistances, probably
acquired in the human host. I have long suspected that these strains may
also be carrying plasmids augmenting communicability and virulence
(other than those of haemolysin and enterotoxin synthesis). I believe
there is a problem here awaiting solution.

Summary

Particular compatibility groups of resistance plasmids predominate in
salmonellae in different parts of the world. S.typhimurium is the most
important organism involved. In North West Europe Group I_1 $\underline{fi}^-$ plasmids,
showing the Δ type of phage restriction in S.typhimurium, predominate.
In S.typhimurium in South America Group N $\underline{fi}^+$ plasmids, which do not code
for sensitivity to the IKe phage, have caused extensive outbreaks. In
the Middle East, S.typhimurium carrying $F_I$me plasmids is widespread.

The S.typhimurium strains concerned are frequently involved in serious
outbreaks of paediatric infections, and it is clear that in such cases
the organism is cycling, and probably acquiring much of its plasmid-
borne resistance, in the human host. Other plasmids, conferring augmented
communicability or virulence, may also be involved.

References

1. Anderson, E. S. and Threlfall, E. J.: The characterisation of plasmids
    in the enterobacteria. J. Hyg. 72, 471-487 (1974).

2. Datta, N. and Hedges, R. W.: Compatibility groups among $\underline{fi}^-$ R factors.
    Nature 234, 222-223 (1971).

3. Grindley, N. D. F., Grindley, J. N. and Anderson, E. S.: R factor compatibility groups. Molec. gen. Genet. 119, 287-297 (1972).

4. Hedges, R. W. and Datta, N.: R124, an fi^+ R factor of a new compatibility class. J. gen. Microbiol. 71, 403-405 (1972).

5. Grindley, N. D. F., Humphreys, G. O. and Anderson, E. S.: Molecular studies of R factor compatibility groups. J. Bact. 115, 387-398 (1973).

6. Anderson, E. S.: The ecology of transferable drug resistance in the enterobacteria. Ann. Rev. Microbiol. 22, 131-180 (1968).

7. Anderson, E. S.: Ecology and epidemiology of transferable drug resistance. In: Ciba Foundation Symposium on Bacterial Episomes and Plasmids (eds. G. E. W. Wolstenholme and M. O'Connor) J. and A. Churchill Ltd., London, 102-119 (1969).

8. Anderson, E. S.: The ecological significance of R factor activity. Topics in Infectious Diseases 1, 59-76 (1975).

9. Anderson, E. S. and Natkin, E.: Transduction of resistance determinants and R factors of the Δ transfer systems by phage P1kc. Molec. gen. Genet. 114, 261-265 (1972).

10. Anderson, E. S.: Influence of the Δ transfer factor on the phage sensitivity of salmonellae. Nature 212, 795-799 (1966).

11. Anderson, E. S., Threlfall, E. J., Frost, J. A. and Carr, J. M.: Transferable drug resistance in animal and human infection with new phage types of Salmonella typhimurium. Proc. Soc. Gen. Microbiol. 2, 64 (1975).

12. Hedges, R. W.: R factors from Providence. J. gen. Microbiol. 81, 171-181 (1974).

13. Khatoon, H., Iyer, R. V. and Iyer, V. N.: A new filamentous bacteriophage with sex-factor specificity. Virology 48, 145-155 (1972).

14. Anderson, E. S. and Lewis, M. J.: Drug resistance and its transfer in Salmonella typhimurium. Nature 206, 579-583 (1965).

15. Anderson, E. S. and Lewis, M. J.: Characterisation of a transfer factor associated with drug resistance in Salmonella typhimurium. Nature 208, 843-849 (1965).

16. Anderson, E. S. and Smith, H. R.: Chloramphenicol resistance in the typhoid bacillus. Brit. Med. J. iii, 329-331 (1972).

17. Anderson, E. S., Threlfall, E. J., Carr, J. M. and Frost, J. A.: Transferable drug resistance in salmonellae in South and Central America. Proc. Soc. Gen. Microbiol. 1, 66 (1974).

18. Anderson, E. S., Threlfall, E. J., Carr, J. A., McConnell, M. M. and Smith, H. R.: Studies of F_I plasmids with special reference to those predominating in <u>Salmonella typhimurium</u> in the Middle East. Submitted for publication.

19. Mered, B., Benhassine, M., Papa, F., Kharti, B., Kheddari, M., Rahal, A. and Sari, L.: Epidémie à <u>S.wien</u> et <u>S.typhimurium</u> dans un service de pédiatrie. Archives d'Institut Pasteur Algérie <u>48</u>, 41-52 (1970).

20. Le Minor, S.: Apparition en France d'une épidémie à <u>Salmonella wien</u>. Médecine et Maladies Infectieuses <u>2</u>, 441-448 (1972).

21. Anderson, E. S.: The problems and implications of chloramphenicol resistance in the typhoid bacillus. J. Hyg. <u>74</u>, 289-299 (1975).

Discussion

Levy: Do you think that the outbreaks in the developing countries are because there is an unusual plasmid involved, or is
it basically a problem of sanitation, or is it because of the
uncontrolled use of antibiotics?

Anderson: I think it is a whole lot of things.

Levy: Which do you think is predominant?

Anderson: I don't think you would get these epidemics if you
did not have antibiotics lashing around. I think that is the
most important single factor. On the other hand, there are a
lot of others.

Falkow: In that regard, the outbreak of typhoid in Mexico and
the surrounding area was always somewhat of a mystery, and it
now appears that workers at CDC Atlanta have traced the source
to bottled water which was prepared by a local bottling company
and distributed throughout Mexico. It was considered to be
pasteurised, but in point of fact it was non-carbonated, and
this turned out to be the ultimate source of the epidemic.

Anderson: I'd like a signed statement about that!

Falkow: I can't give you that. But it is what I was told.

Anderson: It illustrates what I have always said. It needs only
one organism, with the right sort of plasmid, at a particular
point in time, given the opportunity for an outbreak, to unleash
something that may have gargantuan proportions.

Another point: no one has ever explained to me, and I am still
scratching my head, why it is that the H1 class of plasmids is
so much associated with typhoid all over the world? Wherever
chloramphenicol resistant typhoid is a problem, it is an H1
plasmid.

Starlinger: Has anyone tried yet to dissect H1 and to clone
pieces of it in other plasmids to see whether there are new kinds
of genes that are responsible for a plasmid to stick so closely

to a host organism? It is probably not the transfer region,
nor is it the simple replication origin, but it will be something in the "unassigned" regions.
Anderson: Please come to Colindale to find out!
Richmond: Andy, you said that H1 occurs also in Salmonella
typhimurium. Do other plasmid compatibility groups occur in
Salmonella typhi?
Anderson: Oh yes, but very rarely.
Mitsuhashi: Are there any characteristics in resistance markers
carried by types of plasmids?
Anderson: The $F1_{me}$ class of plasmids usually confers resistance
to ampicillin, but not to the cephalosporins. Some strains,
however, also carry a small, multicopy, non-autotransferring
plasmid which confers resistance both to ampicillin and to cephalosporins; and this gives you a higher overall resistance
against ampicillin. And similar things are found among the
amino-glycoside resistance patterns.
Richmond: Are the "Mexico" and the "Viet-nam" versions of H1
identical?
Anderson: Indistinguishable. One hundred percent similarity.
Starlinger: If I remember correctly, the Central American
Shigella outbreak had the same resistance pattern as the H1
plasmids, but the compatibility group was different.
Anderson: That's right, it was B.
Starlinger: Is there a similarity in the DNA specifying resistance in these two plasmids, or are they completely different?
Anderson: We have not been able to find any. The CSSu and CSSuT
marker pattern is a common one among plasmids; which is not surprising, because these are common antibiotics.
Drews: Is there any indication that these plasmids that are
widespread - like the H you have mentioned - confer any special
type of virulence or pathogenicity to the organisms they are in?
In other words, has anyone taken $H1^+$ and $H1^-$ variants and compared them in an animal situation where you could study well
defined parameters of virulence and pathogenicity and looked to
see whether there are genes which endow these organisms...
Anderson: It is difficult in typhoid because you only have a
human host. In S. typhimurium, there are worries about introducing an organism such as this into your animal house. We do
not have the necessary facilities; but this is the sort of experiment I would very much like to be done to see whether you

could demonstrate a difference in properties. As far as virulence is concerned, the evidence is there that the mortality
from the chloramphenicol resistant strains (in Mexico) was the
same, if chloramphenicol was not used, as it used to be with
chloramphenicol sensitive S. typhi: ten percent or so. Successful treatment was claimed with septrin; and others used ampicillin; but the successes with ampicillin were short-lived
since the ampicillin resistance translocon merely stuck itself
on to the end of the linkage group. There was a huge clone in
Thailand where we could predict the phage type of the strain
because it had the A translocon stuck on to the end of the H1
linkage group. Incidentally, this is another proof of the
clonal distribution. I stress that we are dealing with single
lines of organisms and single lines of plasmids. We have an
interlocked epidemiology.

Richmond: I would extend that. We are looking - as it were - at
epidemics of plasmids in bacteria as well as of bacteria in man,
but I think it is a mistake to relate this only to pathogens.

Anderson: I agree.

Falkow: I just wanted to make a comment in terms of pathogenicity. Our experience has been that, in terms of the strains
that cause meningitis, which was highly unusual and used always
to be hospital....

Richmond: Is this S. typhimurium?

Falkow:....Yes, typhimurium. These strains seemed to carry a
specific type of A-antigen that gave them adhesion. As you know
neo-natal meningitis is usually associated with E. coli carrying
K1 and other factors, and we are finding that this adhesion
factor is not dissimilar to ones we have recently found in urinary tract infections. What I feel is important from Professor
Anderson's work is that, as you increase probability of genetic
transfer, so you essentially increase the plasmid pool, and you
begin to generate all kinds of recombinations. So now you are
beginning to find increasingly Ent plasmids also carrying resistance determinants as a single unit. So you are really building
up now factors that are carrying resistance plus virulence. They
have the whole packet.

Anderson: Were your meningitides fatal?

Falkow: Yes, they appeared to be.

Anderson: Yes. Our experience is that such infections are 100%
fatal.

Effect of an Antibiotic-Supplemented Feed on the Ecology of E. coli on a Farm

Stuart B. Levy, George B. FitzGerald, and Ann B. Macone

Antibiotic resistance in microbial organisms is widespread. The emergence of these resistant organisms has resulted from the selective pressures following their use in therapy of man, animals and plants (1,2). Many of these organisms are pathogenic to man. In order to curb the increasing proportion of these resistant organisms, a re-evaluation of the use of drugs in our environment has been strongly urged and considered (2-5).

We had the opportunity to study the effect of the introduction of a tetracycline-supplemented feed on the bacterial ecology of a newly-created farm and its environs (6). The farm area was a homestead located 30 miles outside of Boston which housed the resident family consisting of husband, wife and nine children, aged four to twenty. Neighbors in five families (ten adults and fourteen children) living within a five mile radius represented a control group. Their children went to the same schools as did those in the resident family.

The purpose of the study was to monitor the bacterial environment on the farm after introduction of a tetracycline-supplemented feed (tet-feed) to livestock. For this study we chose chickens. About three hundred one-day old chickens were brought to the farm from SPAFAS (Connecticut) where they had hatched that day. The eggs came from hens raised under conditions where no antibiotic had been used for over ten years. The details of the raising of these chickens have been described (6). The absence of antibiotics in their feed was carefully monitored by testing for antibacterial activity.

At two months of age they were separated into six cages with about 50 chickens per cage. Two groups of chickens were put outside in A-frame cages of about 100 square feet and the others were housed in similar sized cages inside a 10,000 square foot barn. Two cages inside and one outside would eventually be given the tet-feed. The other cages would receive no antibiotic feed. The cages on the outside would assess the effect of an open vs. closed environment on the types of organisms and resistances which could appear after introduction of the antibiotic supplemented feed.

Changes Occurring After Introduction of Tet-feed to the Farm

Before beginning the tet-feed we performed bacteriologic studies on the feces from members of the farm family, their neighbors, and the chickens on the farm. In all groups, the numbers of tetracycline resistant coliforms excreted were low, ranging from < .1% to 10%. Regular monitoring continued throughout the course of the study. Within days, the chickens given tet-feed began to excrete large numbers of tetracycline-resistant E. coli and Proteus mirabilis. The relative amounts of E. coli and Proteus in the feces did not change, however, from that seen prior to tet-feed (6). The E. coli which emerged were initially resistant only to tetracycline or to tetracycline and sulfonamides, but over a period of three months, resistances to other antibiotics emerged: tetracycline-fed chickens inside the barn excreted large numbers of E. coli with a transferable plasmid coding for resistance to tetracycline, streptomycin, ampicillin and carbenicillin; tetracycline-fed chickens in the outside cage also began to excrete E. coli with multiple resistances as time on tet-feed lengthened, but ampicillin-carbenicillin resistance was never found among them. The origin of this latter plasmid determinant is unknown. The inside cages fed regular feed maintained low frequency (less than 10%) of resistant E. coli until four months into the study when increasing numbers of resistant E. coli were being excreted (6).

We examined the fecal flora of the people living on the farm and in the neighborhood. Similar numbers and kinds of organisms were recovered from fecal samples plated aerobically or anaerobically. During the first three months there was no detectable change in the relative amount of tetracycline resistant organisms assayed in fecal samples from farm dwellers (6). However, about four months after the introduction of tet-feed on the farm, an increasing number of farm members were excreting large numbers of tetracycline resistant organisms. Since the normal level of resistant E. coli ranged from <1-10% in this population (from studies before the introduction of the feed), we were particularly interested in those fecal samples in which greater than 80%, and in many cases 100% of the E. coli recovered were resistant to tetracycline. Five and six months after introduction of tet-feed on the farm over 31% of the fecal samples received from the farm individuals, on the average of 6-9 samples over the nine-week period, showed 80-100% E. coli resistant to tetracycline (6). In contrast, fecal samples from the neighbors and a group of Tufts University Medical School students who acted as an urban control group showed relatively low numbers of resistant bacteria (Table 1). These particular studies suggested that time was needed to attain a critical level of tetracycline in the environment before the bacterial flora of the farm dwellers was affected.

As was noted with the chickens, the numbers of antibiotic resistances in E. coli increased in the farm family as the time of tet-feed on the farm lengthened. In the farm members 36% of the fecal E. coli showed resistance to three or more antibiotics in contrast to 6% of the samples which were taken from the rural controls. Similar differences were noted in the number of individuals in which greater than 80% of the fecal bacteria were resistant to tetracycline. Seven out of the eleven farm members gave more than one sample with greater than 80% tetracycline resistant organisms while only three out of twenty-four neighbors did. Furthermore, many of the farm members excreted high numbers of resistant organisms during consecutive weeks in contrast to the more random occasions for the neighbors. The persistence of resistant

Table 1

Frequency of tetracycline resistant bacteria in fecal samples from
farm, family and control groups. Fecal samples obtained by rectal swab
(6) were streaked onto MacConkey agar and diluted by two-dimensional
spreading. Individual colonies (100-1000) of the predominant organisms
were observable and these were replica-plated onto MacConkey agar supplemented with tetracycline (25 ug/ml) in order to obtain the proportion of
tetracycline resistant organisms (expressed as % of total).

PERCENT OF FECAL SAMPLES WITH FREQUENCY OF RESISTANT BACTERIA

	Total # People	Total # Samples	Frequency of tetracycline resistant bacteria in the fecal sample				
			0-20%	21-40%	41-60%	61-80%	81-100%
Farm Family	11	83	51.8	9.6	4.8	2.4	31.3
Neighbors	24	189	82.0	6.3	2.6	2.1	6.8
Boston Students	10	65	93.9	0.0	1.5	1.5	3.1

organisms in addition to the multiplicity of resistances in the E. coli cultured
from the farm group, as compared to those found in the chickens, implied a
selection by tetracycline for these resistances, although pick-up of bacteria
from the chickens was also possible (7).

Most of these resistances were transferable together to recipient E. coli
(Table 2). Transfer from the E. coli was more frequent when the donor bacteria
expressed a number of resistances: transfer of tetracycline alone was less
than 10%, whereas transfer of multiple resistances was often 100%. In many
cases the resistances were transferred en bloc. As seen in Table 2, although

47

many resistance markers were transferred together, they could also be found
transferred separately to the recipients. This observation may indicate instability of the plasmid (and/or its resistance determinants) from the donor human
E. coli in the recipient laboratory strain of E. coli, or the presence of
multiple plasmids in the same donor E. coli. Some E. coli from chickens and
humans expressed the same resistance patterns and showed a similar transfer
frequency of the resistance markers (Table 3). However, we have no evidence
that similar plasmids were present in the E. coli of chicken and human origin.
We have reported that pick-up of plasmids and E. coli from chickens by two
handlers during this project (7), but the presence of these bacteria in these
individuals was transient.

This prospective study demonstrated a change in the bacterial flora of the
human population in contact with animals being given tetracycline-supplemented
feed. It agrees with findings from other groups which
examined farm dwellers already in contact with antibiotic-fed animals and
showed them to excrete higher levels of resistant organisms than a control
population (2,5,8-12). Our study suggests that there is a critical time
period required before selection in the non-ingesting population is seen. Selection

Table 2

Transfer of antibiotic resistances were evaluated by overnight mating
between the E. coli isolated from humans and strain DO-11 (nalidixic acid-
resistant derivative of E. coli CSH-2). Donor to recipient ratio was 1:10.
The mating mixture was plated onto different selective plates and the recombinants tested for coexistence of other transferred resistances.

Am - ampicillin; Cb - carbenicillin; Neo - neomycin; Sm - streptomycin;
SSS - sulfonamides; Te - tetracycline; Cm- chloramphenicol.

TABLE 2

TRANSFERABILITY OF ANTIBIOTIC RESISTANCES FROM E. COLI ISOLATED FROM HUMANS.

Resistances in donor bacteria	No. strains tested	No. strains showing transfer	No. strains transferring all resistances*	Resistance groups transferred*
Sm	5	3	3	Sm
Neo	2	2	2	Neo
Te	17	0	0	
Am,Cb	2	2	2	AmCb
Cm,Sm	1	1	1	CmSm
Sm,SSS	1	0	0	
Sm,Te	3	3	3	SmTe
SSS,Te	3	0	0	
Am,Cb,SSS	2	0	0	
Cm,Neo,Te	2	2	2	CmNeoTe,Te,NeoTe
Cm,Sm,SSS	1	1	1	CmSm
Sm,Neo,Te	4	1	0	Neo,NeoSm
Sm,SSS,Te	10	5	5	Te,SmTe
Am,Cb,Sm,SSS	3	2	0	AmCb
Am,Cb,SSS,Te	3	3	3	AmCbTe,AmCb
Cm,Sm,SSS,Te	7	4	2	Cm,Te,CmTe, CmSmTe,SmTe
Am,Cb,Sm,Neo,Te	1	1	0	AmCbSmNeo
Am,Cb,Sm,SSS,Te	6	6	5	AmCbSm,AmCbTe AmCbSmTe
Am,Cb,Sm,Neo,SSS,Te	9	9	9	AmCbTe,AmCbTeNeoS AmCbTeNeo,AmCbSmN AmCbTeSm

*exluding SSS which
 was not tested

TABLE 3

TRANSFER OF RESISTANCE GROUPS COMMON TO CHICKENS AND MAN

Resistances in donor E. coli	No. Transfer/No. Mated[1]	
	Chickens	Humans
Te	4/41	0/17
Sm	2/4	3/5
Te, Sm	2/14 Te 8/14 Te Sm	3/3 TeSm
Te, Sm, SSS	3/10 Te Sm	5/5 TeSm
Te, Sm, Am, Cb	15/15 Te Sm Am Cb	5/6 Te Sm Am Cb[2] 3/3 Am Cb Te[2]

[1] SSS was not tested in the recipient. Mating was performed as described in Table 2.

[2] Donor also had SSS which was not tested.

Te = Tetracycline; Sm = streptomycin; SSS = sulfonamides, Am = ampicillin; Cb = carbenicillin

for tetracycline resistance in animals and humans was associated with resistance towards many different antibiotics. The coincident transfer of the multiple resistances from the E. coli isolated from chickens suggests that these determinants reside on one plasmid. These resistances may have accumulated from their transposition (13) from other genetic elements to a more stable resident plasmid in the chicken E. coli.

Over this seven month period the neighbors who lived within a five mile radius were unaffected by the introduction of the feed to this farm. However, on the basis of the results within the farm, one cannot predict whether there would have been a wider selective effect had tetracycline feeding been continued for a longer period of time.

Changes Occurring after Removal of Tet-feed from the Farm

Following removal of the tet-feed from the chickens, the loss of resistant organisms in the chicken feces occurred at a very slow rate. In fact, two months after eliminating tet-feed from the diet the chickens continued to excrete entirely tetracycline resistant E. coli. In one cage in which the feces and litter were removed and the cage was cleaned twice including the changing of water trowels, most chickens still continued to excrete primarily resistant organisms (Figure 1). Reinfection of the chickens with the resistant organisms appeared to be the cause of the continued presence of resistant organisms in their feces. There was no apparent change in the kinds of resistances and their relative frequency (Table 4). This

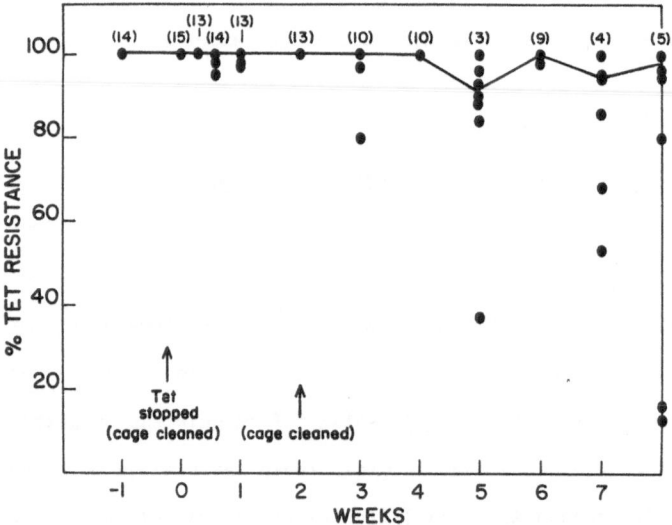

Figure 1: Effect of removal of tet-feed on the frequency of tetracycline resistant bacteria in chickens. Two months after giving tet-feed, the cage was cleaned, the tet-feed stopped and the number of resistant fecal organisms in the chickens was monitored. Numbers in parenthesis indicate the number of chickens excreting that frequency of resistant E. coli. Line designates mean frequency.

Table 4

FREQUENCY OF E. COLI IN CHICKENS WITH ANTIBIOTIC RESISTANCE PATTERN

Time (weeks) after removal of tet feed	Percent					
	Sensitive	Te	TeSSS	TeSM	TeSmSSS	AmCb Tet Sm
0	0	44.4	22.2	14.8	----	14.8
3	0	25.9	25.9	------	37.1	11.1
5	5.6	33.3	33.3	----	27.8	----
9	0	23.5	23.5	41.2	----	11.8

The sensitivity of predominant E. coli isolated from 10-15 chickens in the cage was tested over weekly intervals following removal of test-feed from the cleaned cage.

feature became evident when we placed four chickens excreting resistant bacteria with ten chickens excreting primarily sensitive organisms. There was a rapid fall in the number of resistant organisms in the four newly introduced chickens. By three weeks these same chickens were excreting less than 30% resistant E. coli.

The effect of the bacterial environment was therefore a dominant feature in the persistence of the resistant organism. The effect of drug residues was also a consideration. To eliminate this possibility we placed seven chickens in a movable cage which was cleaned and moved to areas of the barn where tet-feed had not appeared. In this case, as well, there was a rapid fall in the number of resistant organisms (Figure 2). In this instance the sensitive E. coli were presumably introduced from the ground or feed. The persistence of tetracycline-resistant E. coli in pigs in England (14) despite the elimination of tetracycline from the feed of pigs following

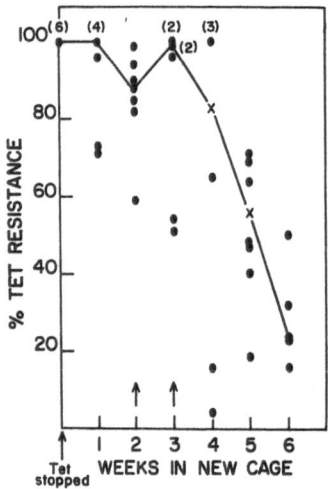

Figure 2: Effect of a change of environment on frequency of tetracycline
resistant bacteria in chickens. Seven chickens were placed
in a movable cage which was cleaned weekly and moved (arrows)
to different areas in the barn. The proportion of resistant E. coli
in each chicken was followed. Parentheses as in Figure 1. Line
designates mean frequency.

seventeen years of usage may be related to the continued presence of tetracycline residues on these farms, although continued therapeutic use of
tetracycline and/or the possible selection of a stable resistant E. coli
population are also possible explanations (14).

An assessment of loss of resistant organisms was made with the humans
living on the farm six months after the elimination of the feed. At this
time there was a marked reduction in the resistant organisms; the level
returned to that prior to the introduction of tet-feed (6).

Stability of Tetracyclines in the Environment

Weeks after excretion in the feces, oxytetracycline was still biologically active in tests against sensitive organisms. This fact reflected the

absence of a degradative mechanism for resistance to tetracycline in
Enterobacteriaceae and Group D Streptococcus which were present in great numbers
in the feces (6,15,16). This finding is very striking and indicates the long
biologic half-life of tetracycline in our environment. It is common practice
to use animal excrement as fertilizer. On this homestead the feces of the
chickens was tilled into the soil as fertilizer for the vegetable garden.
Conceivably tetracycline in the feces could be taken up by the plants and
stored in stems and leaves. These vegetables could then be potential reservoirs
for the transfer of tetracycline and/or its residues to the consumer. This
possibility is under study.

Summary

We have demonstrated that the introduction of a tetracycline-supplemented
feed to a newly established farm area will, over time, change the bacterial
flora of the residents in the area by the selection of antibiotic resistant
organisms, not only to the antibiotics given, but to other unrelated antibiotics. Loss of the resistant E. coli may be a slow process unless, 1) the
antibiotic is completely removed and 2) the environment includes a majority
of sensitive organisms. The use of a stable tetracycline in animal feed and the
absence of degradation of tetracycline by resistant organisms assure its
continued presence in our environment leading to further selection of tetracycline
resistant organisms.

Acknowledgement

These studies were supported by a grant from the Animal Health Institute,
Washington, D.C. and a Research Career Development Award to S.B.L.

REFERENCES

1. Falkow, S.: Infectious Multiple Drug Resistance. Pion. Limited, 1975.

2. Dulaney, E.L. and Laskin, A.I. (editors): The Problems of Drug-resistant
   Pathogenic Bacteria. Ann. N. Y. Acad. Sci. 182, 1971.

3. Anderson, E.S.: The ecology of transferable drug resistance in the Enterobacteria. Ann. Rev. Microbiol. 22:131-180,1968.

4. Swann, M.M., Chairman: Report of the Joint Committee on the use of anti-biotics in animal husbandry and veterinary medicine. Her Majesty's Stationery Office, London, 1969.

5. The Use of Drugs in Animal Feeds. Publication #1679, National Academy of Sciences, Washington, D.C., 1969.

6. Levy, S.B., FitzGerald, G.B. and Macone, A.B.: Changes in intestinal flora of farm personnel after introduction of a tetracycline-supplemented feed on a farm. New Eng. J. Med. 295:583-588, 1976.

7. Levy, S.B., FitzGerald, G.B. and Macone, A.B.: Spread of antibiotic-resistant plasmids from chicken to chicken and from chicken to man. Nature 260:40-42, 1976.

8. Smith, H.W.: Anti-microbial drugs in animal feeds. Nature 218:728-731, 1968.

9. Wiedemann, B. and Knothe, H.: Epidemiological investigations of R factor-bearing enterobacteria in man and animal in Germany. Ann. N.Y. Acad. Sci. 182:380-382, 1971.

10. Linton, K.B., Lee, P.A., Richmond, M.H., Gillespie, W.A., Rowland, A.J. and Baker, V.N.: Antibiotic resistance and transmissible R factors in the intestinal coliform flora of healthy adults and children in an urban and rural community. J. Hyg. Camb. 70:99-104, 1972.

11. Fein, D., Burton, G., Tsutakawa, R. and Blenden, D.: Matching of antibiotic resistance patterns of Escherichia coli of farm families and their animals. J. Infect. Dis. 130(3):274-279, 1974.

12. Siegel, D., Huber, W.G. and Dupdale, S.: Human therapeutic and agricul-tural uses of antibacterial drugs and resistance of the enterici flora of humans. Antimicrob. Agents and Chem. 8:538-543, 1975.

13. Cohen, S.N.: Transposable genetic elements and plasmid evolution. Nature 263:731-738, 1976.

14. Smith, H.W.: Persistence of tetracycline resistance in pig Escherichia coli. Nature 258:628-630, 1975.

15. Levy, S.B. and McMurry, L.: Probing the expression of plasmid-mediated tetracycline resistance in Escherichia coli. Microbiology, 1977 (in press).

16. Levy, S.B., McMurry, L., Onigman, P. and Saunders, R.M.: Plasmid-mediated tetracycline resistance in E. coli in Current Topics in Infectious Diseases II: R factors: Their properties and possible control, (Drews, J. and Högenauer, G., edit.) Wien-New York: Springer-Verlag.

Discussion

<u>Richmond</u>: One comment arising out of your talk: it seems to me
that the studies of Williams Smith that you mentioned are in-
conclusive because we just do not know how much tetracycline
continues to be used for veterinary purposes. If one talks to
Veterinary Directors of pharmaceutical companies - I know they
are never quite open about this - none have ever admitted to
me that their sales of antibiotics for veterinary purposes have
dropped since the Swann Committee recommendations were implemen-
ted. I think one must conclude that tetracycline use is continuing. It is just, I think, that the route of administration has
changed. So it is hard to interpret Williams Smith's paper.
Either - as you suggested at the end of your paper - tetracycline
resistant <u>E. coli</u> are emerging that no longer need the selective
effect of tetracycline to survive, or alternatively the selection
pressure is still, in fact, being applied.

<u>Levy</u>: I think the pressure is still there.

<u>Anderson</u>: It depends who you ask about tetracycline, because I
asked a high up chap about the possibility of a black market in
tetracycline. Not us, he said. Our tetracycline sales have fall-
en. On the other hand, I have been told by others in the pharmaceutical field that their sales of tetracycline have even
gone up since Swann. Now one does not know which of these two
stories to believe.

<u>Falkow</u>: I was interested in Williams Smith's report; although
the total incidence of R plasmids had not decreased, his feeling was that the incidence of transferability had decreased
markedly.

<u>Anderson</u>: He claimed this?

<u>Falkow</u>: Yes, and I thought it was rather interesting.
Can I just mention for the record that, as from April 15th,
1977, the Commissioner of the Food and Drug Administration in

the United States has said that he plans to publish Order to
the effect that sulphaquinoxaline, penicillins and tetracycline
will be discontinued from animal feeds in the United States.
Richmond: In Europe this has been the situation for some years
now, and on the farms we monitor, the incidence of tetracycline
resistance in any animal reared under intensive conditions,
that is veal calves, pigs and chicken, upwards of 65% of all the
E. coli you look at are tetracycline resistant.
Anderson: Because of prophylactic use, so-called.
Falkow: I just felt I should say that I thought it of some
significance that the United States had finally taken at least
some recognition of the situation.
Anderson: Might you call it the United States' swan song?
Levy: The farm we used for our study was in a very rural area,
and this farm had not been using feeds, but what was interesting
to us was that so may tetracycline resistant, I mean singly
tetracycline resistant, organisms were found. Early on only
tetracycline resistant organisms were found. Later we picked
up other resistances. We do not know whether the ampicillin and
carbenicillin were introduced, perhaps by the food carrier. It
had to come from the environment, not the feed; because the
feed was being given to both. But I am struck, and I think all
of us are, that resistance to tetracycline is so prevalent. I
am not sure that it is necessarily because we use tetracycline,
and that is the open question.
Anderson: So why do you think?
Levy: Well, I wonder that other markers may not be present
along with the tetracycline. Certainly the tetracycline plasmid
has more there than just tetracycline. And so I pose this as
a possibility.
Richmond: One of the factors undoubtedly, and I think this
varies from country to country, is that the litter that the
animals stand on is now collected up, sterilised, and may be
used itself as part of another round of feeding. And it is very
clear from some studies that Alan Linton has done in the UK
that the feed that goes to birds, although it is superficially
sterile, if you really look carefully you find you can grow up
resistant E. coli from it. So the animals are being re-fed, and
there is a recycling of resistant organisms.
Starlinger: I should like to ask something else. The first tetracycline resistant bacteria that came up in the people were rath-

er non-persistent. Do you think this was another type of plasmid or bacterium, or was this simply due to the fact that the organisms were present in smaller amounts among other bacteria at the beginning?

Levy: What I said there was that when we took random samples from the outside group, we would find that on a Monday 80% of the E. coli were resistant to tetracycline, for no apparent reason. This is obviously a tremendously high frequency of resistance in E. coli when there was no taking of the antibiotic. The next week they would go back to low level resistance. Now the question was this: in one family we had two individuals who had gone out on Saturday night for a vegetarian meal, and they had both had these enormous salads; and on the Monday after, following sampling they both had had high level resistance. Now five days later, by the time we had the results available, we examined them and the incidence of resistance had dropped down to low level. So the conclusion was either that they had picked up a large number of organisms from within the salads, organisms that had produced no pathological effects, or they had picked up tetracycline, which provided a transient selection so that, when we tested them, they showed high levels of resistance.

Anderson: Well, you have got yourself an experiment there.

Starlinger: But I mean did you keep the bacteria and compare them with those that were more persistent, and were there any differences between them?

Levy: No, we have not done that experiment.

Drews: I think that one of the disquieting features of this study is that by feeding one antibiotic, one can select for a large number of other determinants. Now does this not raise the question: if you reserve one antibiotic specifically for animal feeding, just by giving these over the years, you might well select for antibiotics that are in human use? By selecting for, I don't know what, virginiamycin resistance or bacitracin resistance, might you not select for determinants that are still of meaning to the human population?

Levy: Sure. I don't think it is clear how it is happening, nor do I know why it is, but tetracycline seems to be the one that does it most commonly. Certainly in clinical practice, which Naomi Datta and others have published on treating women with oral chemotherapy, tetracycline was an antibiotic which when

they used it they got organisms that showed more than one resistance, whereas when they treated with other drugs, they did
not seem to find it. They also, for example, treated with
chloramphenicol, and I think with ampicillin. I don't know
whether that is because tetracycline is excreted lower down in
the colon and therefore has additional selective effect. Perhaps the other drugs are present in the small intestine.

Anderson: It is just that that does not quite answer Dr. Drews'
question. What he was saying was this: and this has been suggested frequently: let us put aside certain antibiotics for
animal use, and let us keep others entirely for human use. And
it is nice and tidy, and you are not going to get a cross between
the two. But the fact is that if the "animal" organisms are at
all important in man, all you need is a mutant that is resistant
to the antibiotic you have reserved for animals, and you are
then able to select an organism that would carry a great deal
of resistance to antibiotics important to man.

Levy: No: I understand that, the question is whether all antibiotics do this - perhaps others can say.

Anderson: I am sure they can.

Davies: No, you can't say that.

Richmond: Can I just interrupt to say that there is evidence
on this. With nitrofurans, for example, the evidence is quite
clear. The use of nitrofurans very frequently produces a resistant population which also accidentally, as it were, carries
resistance plasmids. That is well documented. People have done
studies on quinoxaline di-N-oxides - be it Grofas, be it Carbadox,
be it Olaquindox - and there you do not, in general, select
gram-negative bacteria that are carrying R-factors. But whether
this situation will persist for ever, is another matter.

Falkow: The other question is that by using, for example, virginiamycin, one has a marked effect on plasmid carriage in the
streptococci. And one sees joint resistance to tetracycline and
erythromycin appearing not only in Group D but also in Group B,
so it may be that the alternatives are often these peptide kind
of things. The problem is going to shift into the gram-positives.

Richmond: The response of the pharmaceutical industry to a requirement for growth promoters, not active against gram-negatives has been to look at a number of these peptides. The first
was bacitracin, of course, but now there are many more which
are active against gram-positives. And, alright, it takes the

pressure off the gram-negatives, but we wait to see what happens.

Falkow: But there is also a new type coming up, I guess the trade name is Rumensin, which are ionophores, and these seem to shift the balance of flora in the rumen so that the animal uses its food more efficiently and you do get increased rate of growth. From their spectrum of activity, I would expect them to have very little effect on the gram-negative flora. I am not sure about the gram-positives.

Richmond: In Europe, I think I am right in saying, that there may be people here who will know, the use of sulphonamides as coccidiostats has now been limited, and people seem to be moving over to monensic acid - or some derivatives as a coccidiostat. And it will be very interesting to see whether the incidence of sulphonamide resistance falls as a result.

Anderson: If I can talk about the coccidiostat, sulphaquinoxaline, which was used extensively. The organism has a normally rather high resistance to the drug, but it was predictable that use of the drug for this purpose would produce an effect in favour of sulphonamide resistance. And it was almost like clockwork: within a year we began to have trouble with sulphonamide resistant Salmonella typhimurium. And it became transferable.

Starlinger: If it is not good to have these antibiotics in animal feeds, I should like to ask how certain the effect is. How sure is the promotion effect? In agriculture if you use improved seeds, for example, hybrid corn, half the effect is due merely to the fact that the farmers that take the trouble to buy these seeds are also taking better care of their whole operation, and the yields go up. So my question is: is the antibiotic really improving animal growth, or is it just that those farmers that take to scientific methods do better otherwise?

Levy: My information is that the difference between antibiotic fed and non-fed is about six per cent, and the claim is that that six per cent represents the profit margin for those raising the animals. And without that 6% then it does not pay to raise them. The question you raise is very apt because these studies were done 20 years ago, and I do not know of any more recent work.

Falkow: I think that there is no question that the use of antibiotics, even under filthy conditions, leads to increased feed efficiency.

Anderson: What about under clean conditions?

<u>Falkow</u>: Under clean conditions it is even better. In a new farm, for example, the difference can be as high as 12%. Even when it begins to go down, and you have more than 80% tetracycline resistance, you still see a consistent 4 1/2%. I think that is unquestionable data.

<u>Levy</u>: The other question that is raised is whether there is any other way of doing this growth promotion. That is something that perhaps we could discuss sometime.

<u>Anderson</u>: Let me ask a question. You have a spectrum of resistance there. How many plasmids have you got?

The Survival of R-Plasmids in the Absence of Antibiotic Selection Pressure

M. H. Richmond

Introduction

There is now no doubt that antibiotic use favours the emergence of resistant bacterial populations (1). This can be seen both on a worldwide scale, where the introduction of a novel antibiotic is frequently followed by the appearance of bacteria resistant to that agent, and also in individual human beings, where a therapeutic course of an antibiotic commonly results in the conversion of the bacterial population in the person's alimentary tract to a resistant state. As examples, Fig. 1 shows the emergence of hospital strains of Staphylococcus aureus resistant to benzyl penicillin in the years immediately following the introduction of that antibiotic into clinical use in 1946 (ref. 2). On the other hand, Fig. 2 shows the effect of a therapeutic course of tetracycline on the resistance of the gut coliforms in the person under treatment (3, 4). In both cases, the use of the antibiotic encourages the resistant bacteria to outgrow the sensitive, with a resulting change in the properties of the population.

Just as antibiotic use selects for resistant populations, so there is some evidence that an end to therapy leads to the reversion of the population to a predominently sensitive state. This is particularly noticeable where individual patients are involved. In general, the end of a therapeutic course of tetracycline treatment is followed by a change of the bacterial population in the patient's gut to a sensitive state, normally within a period of 10 to 14 (4) days. A similar tendency is harder to see on a worldwide scale. Nevertheless, the incidence of chloramphenicol resistance among isolates of Staphylococcus aureus in England has fallen in line with the more circumscribed use of this antibiotic for human therapy in this country (Dr. M. T. Parker - personal communication).

The emergence of resistant bacterial populations in the way that has been

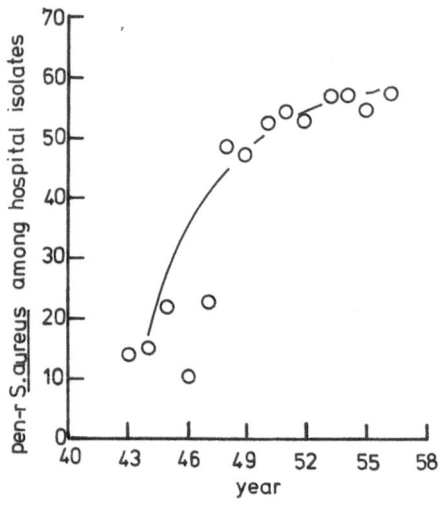

Fig. 1. The incidence of penicillinase producing S. aureus in hospital infections in the years 1943-1957. Data from the World Health Authority.

described here - and the examples used in Figs. 1 and 2 are only a few of the many that might have been chosen - has led to the view that the prevalence of resistant bacteria in the human environment is the direct result of antibiotic use (1, 5). But are there other factors that influence the survival of resistant bacteria? Surveys, in which the incidence of antibiotic resistant bacteria in people not receiving antibiotics have been followed, suggest strongly that there are; and it is the purpose of this contribution to show that this is the case and to try to define some of the factors that may be at work.

The Incidence of Antibiotic Resistant E. coli in Individuals Not Receiving Antibiotics

Examination on McConkey agar supplemented with antibiotics of samples of faeces obtained from individuals who have not been receiving antibiotics.

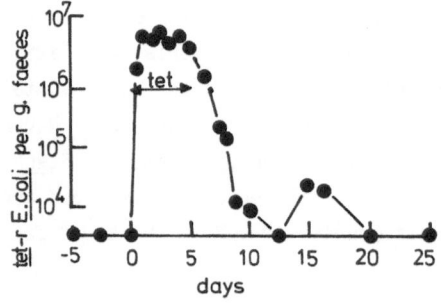

Fig. 2. Effect on the tetracycline resistant coliform flora of the gut in a single individual treated with tetracycline.

in the recent past reveals that the majority of people carry a few resistant
E. coli in their alimentary tracts at all times (6). These organisms are
almost certainly transient, in the sense that they often seem to have been
taken in with the food and be en route to elimination at the point at which
the samples are taken. The reason for believing this to be so is because
they are usually present in small numbers, and are commonly not present when
a further faecal sample is examined on the following day, or subsequently.
E. coli strains behaving in this way whether resistant or not have long been
called "transient" components of the alimentary flora (7); and it is not unreasonable that this "transience" should also be reflected among antibiotic
resistant strains.

In contrast to this pattern of events, however, it is not uncommon to find
resistant E. coli accounting for more than 10% of the faecal flora in some
samples, even though no antibiotics are being taken by the individual during
the period of the survey, and (rather less commonly) this situation may persist for long periods (8). This phenomenon first came to our notice when we
observed a student to carry an E. coli strain resistant to chloramphenicol
but to no other antibiotics for a period of over four months, even though
she had never knowingly received chloramphenicol throughout her life (8).

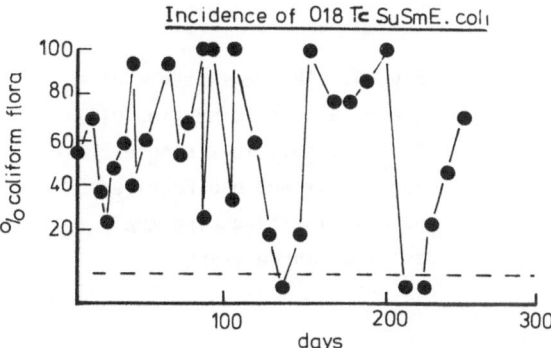

Fig. 3. The persistence of an O18 Tc Sm Su E. coli in the gut flora of a
single individual not receiving any antibiotic.

The long-term survival of individual resistant E. coli strains in the absence
of antibiotic use has now been observed by us on a number of occasions. Moreover, in some cases, the strains have persisted for upwards of nine months (9).
Fig. 3 shows a case in point: a tetracycline, streptomycin and sulphonamide
resistant (Tc Sm Su) serotype O18 E. coli formed a predominant component of
the faecal flora of a single individual for 256 days. Another example is

shown in Fig. 4. In this case, the person carried a non-lactose fermenting sulphonamide, streptomycin-resistant 018 E. coli in his faecal flora for five months, and once again no antibiotics were being taken during the period in question (V. Petrocheilou, unpublished observations).

The Effect of Antibiotic Use on the Subsequent Persistence of Resistant E. coli

These observations show clearly that resistant populations can persist for long periods in the absence of immediate antibiotic selection pressure, but can we say anything about how they arise? In the examples shown in Fig. 4, there was no known occasion of antibiotic treatment during a period of more than 2 years prior to the beginning of the survey, and in this case it seems clear that the resistant bacteria must have reached their predominant status in the flora independently of therapy. This was not so, however, for the example shown in Fig. 3. In that case, a therapeutic course of tetracycline therapy was given just before the onset of the survey (9). The 018 Tc Sm Su E. coli that became prevalent after therapy was present in small numbers before treatment began, and in this case it seems that treatment established a strain as a predominant component of the flora and once established in this way, the strain could not be displaced.

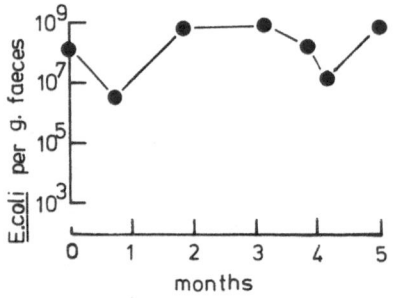

Fig. 4. The persistence of a non-lactose fermenting 018 Sm Su E. coli in a single individual who had received no antibiotics during the previous three years.

The ambiguous relationship between the persistence of resistant E. coli strains and antibiotic use is shown in a survey in which we followed the incidence of tetracycline resistant E. coli in a single individual following the end of a prolonged period of therapy with tetracycline. In this case, tetracycline had been prescribed for the treatment of acne vulgaris and had been administered to the individual under examination for a period of over a year before the phase of the study illustrated in Fig. 5 (ref. 10). Antibiotic use led to the establishment of an 075 Tc E. coli as a majority component of the faecal flora, a strain that commonly accounted for more than 95% of

all the coliforms in the alimentary tract while tetracycline therapy continued. At a point 385 days after the beginning of the survey tetracycline
therapy was stopped, never to be resumed. Despite this change, however, the
075 Tc E. coli strain persisted as a majority component of the flora for several months after tetracycline use had been discontinued. On day 425, however, a therapeutic course of ampicillin was prescribed for circumstances
unconnected with the acne, and as a result the gut flora changed dramatically.

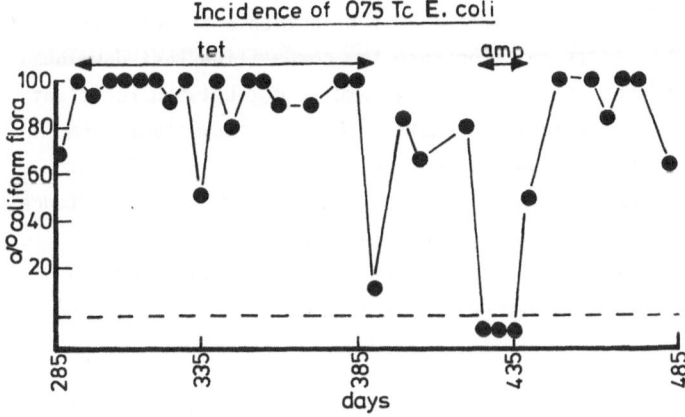

Fig. 5. The effect of an end to tetracycline therapy on the persistence of
an 075 Tc E. coli in a single individual. Note the effect of a course of
ampicillin.

The 075 Tc E. coli became undetectable on McConkey agar, except when supplemented with tetracycline, but ampicillin resistant E. coli became abundant
(see Fig. 5). The course of ampicillin therapy lasted for 10 days, and thereafter the patient received no antibiotics. Immediately the ampicillin treatment ended, the Ap resistant E. coli disappeared, but the displacing strain
was the 075 Tc E. coli that had been predominant before ampicillin was used.
In this example, therefore, the ampicillin resistant E. coli responded as
might have been anticipated to ampicillin use, but the pattern of behaviour
seen with the tetracycline resistant line was certainly unexpected and appeared unrelated to the use of tetracycline.

The Survival of Resistant E. coli in the Absence of Antibiotic Selection
Pressure

It follows from the surveys described above that the incidence of antibiotic
resistant bacteria in human beings is by no means a faithful reflection of
antibiotic use. When antibiotics are present, the possession of the approp-

riate resistance determinants is clearly helpful in allowing the bacteria to survive, but when no antibiotic selection pressure is being applied, the colonising properties of the E. coli strains seem to have a predominant influence.

There are a number of publications which show that the carriage of R-plasmids may be a disadvantage to E. coli strains that carry them, and such resistant strains are commonly outgrown by their sensitive derivatives in the absence of antibiotic pressure (11, 12). These experiments can be misleading, however, if they are used to argue that an end to antibiotic use in an individual patient must inevitably lead to a reduction in the incidence of resistant bacteria. Primarily, this seems to be because the competition that develops once the antibiotic selection pressure is withdrawn is not between resistant bacteria and their sensitive variants in another (8). In many cases, the sensitive bacteria win in such a competition, but sometimes the resistant bacterial lines, having achieved majority status by means of their resistance to selection pressure, are subsequently hard to displace. In this case, therefore, it seems that survival is independent of the resistance of the strains, and whether the bacteria are resistant or not is, under those conditions, immaterial.

On balance, at the present time, withdrawal of antibiotics tends to result in the displacement of resistant E. coli by sensitive, and this seems to be due to the fact that R-plasmids are not in general carried by those E. coli that are effective at becoming majority components of the faecal flora (8, 13). Certain E. coli O-antigen types are known to be good colonisers of the human gastrointestinal tract - antigen types O1, O2, O8, O18, O25 and O75 are notable in this respect (14), yet a survey of resistant coliforms in man has suggested that these E. coli O-antigen types are less commonly carriers of R-plasmids than are those E. coli types that survive less well (13). Nevertheless, when R-plasmids do appear in O-types of good survival potential, the resistance traits survive too: witness the surveys shown in Figs. 3, 4 and 5.

Implications for Antibiotic Therapy

The fact that the survival of antibiotic resistant E. coli in man may be the outcome of two influences - the ability of the bacteria to survive when antibiotics are present, and their ability to colonise and to compete well with other E. coli strains when antibiotics are absent - has considerable implications for our use of antibacterial agents. First, the use of an antibiotic on an individual is likely to result in the selection of resistant bacteria which will become predominant in that person's gastro-intestinal tract. At the end of treatment, these bacteria will tend to disappear (this is the experience at the moment of writing at least) but in a few cases the resistant strains will persist for long periods after the antibiotics have ceased to have selective effect. As far as the person who has been treated is concerned this may not be of great importance. Several examples are known where resistant bacteria have persisted for long periods in the gastro-intestinal tract of individuals without producing any pathological effects. Yet it seems certain that infections of the urinary tract commonly arise from patients' own gut flora (15), and the persistence of resistant bacteria in large numbers in the gut must make the probability of such infections with a resistant organism proportionally higher. In particular, those people particularly prone to such infections may well have the successful treatment of the urinary infections in the future imperilled by a resident E. coli flora in their gastro-intestinal tracts which is resistant.

Perhaps the most interesting conclusions to be drawn from these surveys, however, are in relation to the effect to be expected if the worldwide use of antibiotics is curtailed. Would this inevitably lead to a reduction in the incidence of resistance? Under those circumstances in which the R-plasmids are not commonly found in bacterial lines that are good colonisers, reduction in the use of antibiotics is likely to have a beneficial effect in terms of the incidence of resistant bacteria; but this advantage would have to be balanced against the effectiveness of treatment under the new circumstances. In a situation where the R-plasmids are commonly carried in strains that are also good colonisers, however, the effect of withdrawing antibiotics is likely to be a good deal less immediate and dramatic. This is particularly the case with certain farm animals and with poultry, where R-plasmids are commonly carried by E. coli strains that are also good colonisers of the species concerned. Experimental observations of the effect of withdrawal of antibiotics in poultry and sheep proves this to be so. These results suggest that the limitation of use of antibiotics for animal husbandry purposes would be likely to take some time to show their full effects. Indeed, this may even be the reason why high levels of resistant coliforms are still to be encountered among farm animals and poultry (16) despite the implementation - in the United Kingdom, at least - of the majority of the Swann Committee's recommendations (17).

The Colonisation Properties of E. coli

The ability of some E. coli strains to colonise man to the point at which they become majority components of the human faecal flora raises interesting questions about the means whereby the strains concerned become so predominant. We still are very ignorant in this area of work. Certain surface capsular

antigens are known to influence the ability of E. coli to adhere to the gut
epithelium in pigs (18) and calves (19) even though similar factors have not
yet been identified conclusively for man. Other E. coli - notably those with
certain types of surface appendages are known to adhere tightly to human red
cells (20). Does adhesion play an important part in colonisation? Probably
it does when the persistence of small numbers of toxinogenic bacteria are
concerned, as is the case with some enteropathogenic E. coli strains and with
the cholera vibrio. But it seems less likely that adhesion plays an important
part in the ability of an E. coli strain to become more than 10% of the faecal
coliform flora. To reach this level in the gut, the bacteria must be present
in large numbers in the lumen; and even though adhesion may play a part in
initiating such a colonisation, it is less certain that it is fully responsible for the maintenance of such large numbers of E. coli.

Another factor that may be relevant is the ability of the strains to multiply
in the gut itself. Little is known of this process and the part it plays
in gut colonisation. Certainly in certain disease states the muliplication
of bacteria is an important part of the disease process. Furthermore, some
multiplication of E. coli must occur in man under normal circumstances, since
we certainly do not ingest as many E. coli as we excrete on any given day.

In summary then, there is much to learn about the factors that allow E. coli
to reach large numbers in the human gastro-intestinal tract. And until we
know more about these it will be very hard to assess the influences, other
than antibiotic selection pressure, that lead to the survival of resistant
bacteria in the human gut. One thing seems certain however: this is one
occasion where the absolute numbers of resistant bacteria are an important
consideration since numbers will directly influence the probability with which
the E. coli may cause pathological problems to the person that carries them,
or to others that come in contact with him.

Acknowledgements

I would like to acknowledge with appreciation, the work of Drs. Hartley,
Petrocheilou, Grinsted and Bennett which has substantially contributed to
the conclusions contained in this contribution. I would also like to thank
the Medical Research Council for support.

Literature

1. Anderson, E. S.: The ecology of transferable drug resistance in the
    Enterobacteria. Annu. Rev. Microbiol. 22, 131-180 (1968).

2. Munch-Petersen, E., Boundy, C.: Yearly incidence of penicillin-resistant Staphylococci in man since 1942. Ball. Wld. Hlth. Org. 26, 241-253 (1962).

3. Smith, H. W.: The effect of the use of antibacterial drugs on the emergence of drug resistant bacteria in animals. Adv. Vet. Sci. 15, 67-100 (1971).

4. Richmond, M. H.: R-factors in Man. In: Microbiology - 1974, pp. 27-35. Washington, D.C.: American Society for Microbiology: 1975.

5. Richmond, M. H.: Some environmental consequences of the use of anti-biotics. J. Appl. Bact. 35, 155-176 (1973).

6. Datta, N.: Drug resistance and R-factors in bowel bacteria of London patients before and after admission to hospital. Br. med. J. ii, 407-411 (1969).

7. Cooke, E. M.: Escherichia coli and Man. Edinburgh and London: J. & A. Churchill (1974).

8. Hartley, C. L., Richmond, M. H.: Antibiotic resistance and the survival of E. coli in the alimentary tract. Br. med. J. iv, 71-74 (1975).

9. Petrocheilou, V., Grinsted, J., Richmond, M. H.: R-plasmid transfer in vivo in the absence of antibiotic selection pressure. Antimicrob. Agents Chemother. 10, 753-761 (1976).

10. Petrocheilou, V., Richmond, M. H., Grinsted, J.: Spread of a single plasmid clone to an untreated person receiving prolonged tetracycline therapy. Antimicrob. Agents Chemother., (submitted for publication).

11. Anderson, J. D.: The effect of R-factor carriage on the survival of E. coli in the human intestine. J. med. Microbiol. 7, 85-90 (1974).

12. Lacey, R. W.: A critical appraisal of the importance of the R-factors in the enterobacteriaceae in vivo. J. antimicrob. Chemother. 1, 25-37 (1975).

13. Hartley, C. L., Howe, K., Linton, A. H., Linton, K. B., Richmond, M. H.: The distribution of R-plasmids among O-antigen types of Escherichia coli isolated from human and animal sources. Antimicrob. Agents Chemother. 8, 122-131 (1975).

14. Wiedemann, B., Knothe, H.: Untersuchungen über die Stabilität der Koli-flora des gesunden Menschen. I. Über das Vorkommen permanenter und passanter Typen. Arch. Hyg. 4, 342-348 (1969).

15. Brumfitt, W., Faiers, M. C., Reeves, D. S., Datta, N.: Antibiotic resistant Escherichia coli causing urinary tract infection in general practice: relation to faecal flora. Lancet i, 315-317 (1971).

16. Smith H. W.: Persistence of tetracycline resistance in pig E. coli. Nature 258, 628-630 (1975).

17. Swann, M.: Report of the Joint Committee on the use of antibiotics in animal husbandry and veterinary medicine. London: Her Majesty's Stationery Office: 1969.
18. Jones, G. W., Rutter, J. M.: Role of the K88 antigen in the pathogenesis of neonatal diarrhea caused by Escherichia coli in piglets. Infection and Immunity, 6, 918-927.
19. Ørskov, I., Ørskov, F., Smith, H. W., Sojka, W. J.: The establishment of K99, a thermolabile Escherichia coli K antigen, previously called "K_{co}", possessed by calf and lamb enteropathogenic strains. Acta Microbiol. Pathol. Scand. ser. B, 83, 31-36 (1975).
20. Duguid, J. P., Anderson, E. S., Campbell, I.: Fimbriae and adhesive properties in Salmonellae. J. Pathol. Bacteriol. 92, 107-138 (1968).

Discussion

Levy: Mark, did you have evidence that a bacterium from one of the samples did colonise the gastro-intestinal tract of the humans?

Richmond: We have examined commercially bought chickens in this sort of experiment. We bought the chickens and monitored them for the types of E. coli they carried and the resistance patterns of the bacterial strains. We also monitored the gut contents of a number of people who subsequently volunteered to eat the chickens. So far Alan Linton, in our Department, has looked at about 20 chicken carcasses and followed the consequences of feeding them to the volunteers. In all but one of the cases, there was no evidence that the E. coli from the chickens ever appeared in the humans. But in the final case, the same serotypes of E. coli carrying the same plasmids that we know to be in the chicken carcasses appeared in the gut flora of the persons who ate the chickens. This is a completely clear-cut experiment. The restriction endonuclease patterns of the plasmids, and the electron microscopy of the plasmid DNA have been done, and there is no question of the fact that the plasmids that were in the chicken appeared in substantial numbers in the gut of the person who ate it. But an interesting point emerged: it was apparently the handling of the carcass in the kitchen prior to the cooking that provided the opportunity for contamination to occur. It did not appear to be the eating of the cooked bird.

Levy: But was it the coli carrier that was present, or the plasmid?

Richmond: Both.

Levy: And did it persist?

Richmond: No, it did not persist. Not beyond 14 to 18 days. By persist, I mean months rather than days. Peter Bennett, can you recall the statistics? Something like 140,000,000 chickens are eaten in Britain every year. This is about 3 per head of the population. Put that way it does not seem so unreasonable! And if you find evidence of transfer from the first 20 you look at, I can only assume that there is a significant flow from the animal reservoir, at least to the human gut. All the evidence in the literature suggests that urinary tract infections arise from the gut, and therefore I do not think that one can argue with any force now that there is no flow of resistant E. coli from the poultry reservoir to man. Whether it is major in terms of the incidence of disease in man, is more arguable.

Levy: But the question is are there two different groups, indeed many groups of E. coli? Are there, for example, E. coli that are specific for calves, E. coli that are specific for chickens?

Richmond: All we have done is to use the Kauffmann method of serotyping E. coli. I think this is the wrong way to type E. coli for this purpose. What we are trying to do now is to find a way of looking at E. coli to determine its colonisation prop- erties, and it is already absolutely clear that whether an E. coli survives in man is only partially related to its O-type. I would like to re-classify E. coli in terms of their human colo- nisation properties. When we know that we can ask whether they also colonise chickens well. Certainly some E. coli we have looked at will bind very well to many types of cell, human or not.

Falkow: This is absolutely the point. It is a question of ad- hesion. In the case of strains that cause urinary tract in- fections, it is very clear, the one common property that we have found on examination of over 500 strains from human urinary tract infections is that they possess a specific adhesion property, and certainly those that cause urinary tract infections, and those that cause pyelonephritis, for sure, are not the run-of- the-mill faecal E. coli.

Levy: And those with cystitis?

Falkow: Even those with cystitis are absolutely easily distin- guishable from the common E. coli.

Richmond: And in many of these, serotype O6 was identified as being important?

Falkow: Absolutely.

Levy: There is this recent study from the US looking at urinary tract infections. The person concerned has claimed - he is a urologist - that it is never the same E. coli that comes up in recurrent urinary tract infections, so it is always a new faecal bacterium. So if you are right and these properties are common, so also are the bacteria that carry them common.

Falkow: Serotypes don't mean anything, in this connexion.

Drews: The adherance factor: what is it? Is it pili? Is it common?

Falkow: Well, it's quite common.

Richmond: It's not pili, at least not sex-pili.

Falkow: No, that's right. It is a mannose resistance adhesion, which we assume therefore reflects a proteinaceous appendage, and whether it is even plasmid mediated is questionable. But among strains that cause urinary tract infection, well over 50% are haemolytic and they have a high proportion of certain sugar fermentation properties. They universally will kill chick embryos, they will adhere to human erythrocytes.

Richmond: And the fact is that you can notice when you look at these strains that they are often fimbriated; but that is not the whole story.

Drews: So there is really no structure that can be correlated unequivocally with adhesion yet.

Richmond: Not yet.

Goebel: What method did you use to select your replacement strains?

Richmond: Alan Linton and his colleagues have done a lot of longitudinal monitoring for the survival of E. coli strains in chickens, and he just took six strains that persisted for more than a month or so in the guts of the animals. They are certainly not tailored strains, or anything of that sort.

Mitsuhashi: Did you demonstrate a Tc Su plasmid from the wife?

Richmond: Yes.

Mitsuhashi: I have never demonstrated such a plasmid from human beings. In my hands it is very rare.

Richmond: What about you, Andy? Tc Su is quite common, isn't it?

Anderson: Yes. But I don't know how it is in Japan.

Mitsuhashi: In Japan - very few.

Richmond: But you must realise that what we find in London is totally different from what you find in Paris.

Anderson: We have been carrying out what I call horizontal studies, not longitudinal, on faeces from normal individuals in the laboratory, their contacts outside the laboratory, and their families. This survey lasted about a year and produced some very

interesting results. First of all, it was totally impossible
to predict whether you were going to find resistant organisms.
Sometimes they were there in large numbers - sometimes at less
than 0.1%. But of course with a faecal content of about 10^9/
gram., 0.1% is an awful lot of organisms. The patterns of
carried resistance were not stable, except in a few people.
Richmond: You mean they did not persist.
Anderson: They did not persist. The short-term use of antibiotics - and here I have to be careful since in none of these
patients was tetracycline used - did not make a scrap of difference.
Levy: Short-term is how long?
Anderson: A standard course - 5 days. People who were on long-
term treatment, for example chronic bronchitis, showed exactly
what you would expect. They showed the pattern of the total
spectrum of antibiotics that they had had, and more. But the
interesting thing came when we decided to look at the sensitive
organisms in a number of these people; and there we found to
our astonishment that they were very commonly carrying transfer
factors. The organisms were not resistant, but they were carrying
transfer factors that would pick up almost anything. And this
is a point we have to bear in mind because we tend to concentrate
on resistant strains. We forget the motive force is the transfer
factor - or conjugative plasmid.
Falkow: How high was it, Andy? In our studies we found that
among random faecal samples, some thirty per cent....
Anderson: That sort of percentage....
Falkow: With no sort of markers - nothing you can identify...
Anderson: Yes.
Richmond: Stanley, I guess you would agree that there must be
some correlation - genetic linkage - between R determinants
and some properties that influence colonisation.
Falkow: Some plasmids, when transferred into E. coli, have a
profound effect on the outer envelope of the organism, there is
no question about that; and that type of work has really not
been pursued at all.
Anderson: Well, we have got to the point where that is the work
that has to be done.
Falkow: Yes, that is true. The subtle changes are important. In
vivo transmission of plasmid experiments usually end up as we
have seen. The strains that receive the plasmids do not usually

persist for long periods of time. It only occurs with special ones. You have clones. You finally select a clone that can go.

Davies: Mark, in experiments in which antibiotics are fed, one is almost always looking at E. coli. What happens to the anaerobes?

Richmond: We have tried to find resistance plasmids in bacteroides species and haven't found them.

Falkow: There are plasmids aplenty, but they do not confer resistance.

Davies: But these can form a reservoir.

Richmond: And they constitute the predominant part of the gut flora.

Davies: Has anyone looked at anaerobes in the course of treatment?

Anderson: Oh yes.

Davies: And nothing has come out?

Falkow: You find lots of bacteroides, and you find lots of plasmids, and some resistance.

Davies: But do you find tetracycline resistance?

Falkow: You can do, but there is no correlation with the carriage of plasmids, and certainly no correlation with the enterics. If you look, for example, for ampicillin resistance, and ask do they have TnA? They certainly do not have a TnA; and that is in a study of well over 200 bacteroides isolates. Much to my dismay!

Richmond: Andy, did you want to make a point?

Anderson: No, the point has been made. I wanted to stress the importance of the transmissible plasmid.

Richmond: You are attaching a lot of importance to antibiotic resistance and I quite see, in relation to man and his hospitals, that that is important, but I suspect that these elements play a central and crucial role in microbial evolution in general.

Anderson: I wrote a paper about that, my dear chap, eleven years ago. Don't get me wrong: resistance is a practical problem with which we have been preoccupied, but I am perfectly satisfied that plasmids have played a very important role, and will continue to do so in bacterial evolution.

Richmond: But if they are as important and central as that, why does antibiotic use significantly increase their incidence? Take an example: let us say that adhesion is an important part of the ecology of E. coli. This will exert a continuous pressure

and should lead to a prevalence of transfer factors - on your
theory.

Falkow: I think it is that we have a change in the steady state.
In calves, for example, more than 80% of all E. coli carry
transmissible plasmids. This implies a massive shift in the
steady state.

Richmond: Can we just look at one other point? Jacques Acar was
asking last night: what studies can one conveniently do in hospitals to cover the eventualities of the type we have been dis-
cussing here?

Davies: I thought there was a very interesting parallel between
hospital experiments and Stewart Levy's experiments. If you
don't clean the cages out afterwards, it is clear that there
is a tremendous force selecting for resistance.

Richmond: I think you can put the same point another way. The
conditions under which man comes closest to animals under intensive rearing, are in hospital.

Davies: Yes: if in hospital you stop using an antibiotic, should
you also destroy everything in the ward?

Levy: As far as our hospital is concerned, the only time a room
is extensively cleaned is when we put an immuno-suppressed patient in there, unless (of course) there has been a serious
infectious disease in the room. When we do sterilise the room
chemically, it is then that we find the endogenous flora of the
patient a greater problem.

Another point: it is estimated that a great deal of antibiotic
is injected into the environment by doctors and nurses emptying
the last small bubble of air out of a syringe before injecting
the patient.

Richmond: But if that were a major factor, then the nurses
would carry more resistant E. coli in their gut flora than the
general public, and several studies show they do not.

Falkow: That is right. In nosocomial infections, where good
studies have been done, it is possible to find a focus. Antibiotic treatment may be one, possibly a respirator, things like
that.

Levy: But they are only around 8 hours of the day, whereas the
patient is around 24 hours a day.

Falkow: Yes, but it is very clear that in nosocomial infections,
and Acar showed it this morning, if you close down a ward, or
stop using antibiotics, or raise the level of consciousness of

the personnel, or reduce patient to patient contact, that noso-
comial infection generally disappears almost immediately.
Richmond: I think the key is the colonisation properties of
the organism. Of course, the antibiotics may play a part, but
I think we are shining the light too brightly on antibiotic use.
Anderson: That depends on the organism.
Levy: I don't know if we are shining the light too brightly on
antibiotics, or whether we should turn the other light on a
little more brightly.
Anderson: No: it depends on the organism.
Richmond: Okay, it depends on the organism. But for example
among E. coli there are some that are highly communicable, and
some that are not.
Falkow: Yes.
Anderson: The trouble is we talk about E. coli.

b) Molecular Factors Responsible For the Spread of R-Factors (Transposons)

Limitations on the Transposition of TnA

P. M. Bennett, M. K. Robinson, and M. H. Richmond

Introduction

In the relatively short space of time since the process of transposition has been defined with some precision (4, 13, 14, 15,
19, 22, 23), the number of transposons known to occur in Gram-
negative bacteria has increased dramatically. The initial experiments were all concerned with the ampicillin transposon
(TnA, now redesignated Tn1, Tn2, Tn3 - see ref.7), but subsequently units which specify the transposition of trimethoprim and
streptomycin resistance (Tn7)(2, 7), tetracycline resistance
(Tn10)(7, 11, 18), neomycin and kanamycin resistance (Tn5)(5, 7),
chloramphenicol resistance (Tn9)(7, 12), and mercury ion resistance (Tn501)(24) have all been characterised with a varying
degree of completeness. In all cases in which the phenomenon of
transposition has been investigated in sufficient detail, it is
known that the process occurs independently of the host's classical recombination systems (that is, the process will occur in
recA bacteria (2, 4, 11, 12, 14, 18, 19, 22, 24) and results in
the acquisition of a discrete piece of DNA by the recipient
replicon (2, 4, 5, 12, 14, 18, 19, 22, 23, 24). Thus transposition of TnA normally results in an increase in size of the recipient plasmid of a piece of DNA of molecular weight about 3.2 Mdal.

Information currently available about the mechanism of transposition of the ampicillin resistance determinant, TnA, presents
something of a paradox. On the one hand, several small, nonconjugative plasmids, of molecular size 4 to 6 Mdal have been

shown to have many sites at which TnA can insert (14, 19, 23).
This implies that transposition, at least of TnA, has little,
if any, site specificity. In contrast, TnA cannot transpose to
all plasmids with equal efficiency (4). This is an unexpected
observation if site specificity is indeed low as far as insertion
is concerned.

We have been examining this apparent contradiction and have discovered that in certain circumstances the transposition of TnA
is blocked (21). Specifically, we have studied the effect that
the acquisition of one transposon has on the insertion of a
second, whether identical or different, into the same plasmid.

Transposition Immunity

R388 is a conjugative plasmid of molecular weight about 21.5 x
10^6 dal which belongs to the W-incompatibility group and which
confers resistance to trimethoprim and to sulphonamides (10).
E. coli strains UB1731 and UB1700 carry TnA inserted in the
bacterial chromosome and are isogenic except that UB1731 is rec^+
while UB1780 carries the $recA_{56}$ mutation (4). When introduced
into these strains, R388 can acquire TnA by transposition from
the chromosome at equal frequency (4). One of these R388::TnA
recombinant plasmids (pUB310) was treated with NTG and mutant
plasmids which were unable to express their amp gene were isolated. One of these mutant plasmids, pUB501, was chosen for
further study.

The plasmid pUB501 cannot be distinguished physically from its
parent pUB310, in that the two plasmids are the same size (24.5
x 10^6) and digestion of plasmid DNA with various restriction
endonucleases failed to differentiate them. The mutation carried
by pUB501 reverts at a frequency of 5.7 x 10^{-8} and revertants
produce the same level of ß-lactamase activity as the parent
plasmid. We conclude, therefore, that pUB501 still carried a
copy of TnA but is unable to express its amp gene.

R388 und pUB501 were introduced into E. coli strains UB1731 and
UB1780 by conjugation and plasmid containing progeny were outcrossed with the recA strain JC6310 (4). Exconjugants were

selected on minimal agar supplemented with trimethoprim (25 µg/ml), to determine the frequency of plasmid transfer, or with carbenicillin (500 µg/ml). When R388 was the carried plasmid, transfer of the amp resistance determinant from both the rec$^+$ strain UB1731 and the recA strain UB1780 was accomplished at a frequency of 10^{-2} in both cases, relative to the transfer frequency of R388 itself (Table 1).

Table 1.

Frequency of Transposition of TnA From Its Chromosomal Site in E. coli UB1731 and UB1780 to R388 and pUB501

Acceptor plasmid	Transposition frequency^x	
	UB1731(rec$^+$)	UB1780(recA)
R388	1.1×10^{-2}	2.4×10^{-2}
pUB501	6.1×10^{-3}	2.8×10^{-7}

^{x}Transposition frequency = $\dfrac{\text{Transfer frequency amp}^r}{\text{Transfer frequency plasmid}}$

These data confirm our previous findings that transposition of TnA is recA independent (4). In contrast, when pUB501 was the carried plasmid transfer of the amp resistance determinant was quite clearly dependent on a functional recA gene. Thus pUB501 mediated transfer of ampicillin resistance from UB1731 (rec$^+$) to JC6310 at a frequency of approximately 10^{-2} (relative to the transfer frequency of pUB501) but at the barely detectable frequency of 10^{-7} from UB1780 (recA). These results suggested that either transposition of TnA could, on occasion, display a marked recA dependence, or alternatively, that pUB501 cannot acquire a second copy of TnA by transposition. If so, the high frequency of transfer of the amp resistance determinant mediated by pUB501 from UB1731 must be the result of reciprocal recombination events.

It is now well established that, in general, transposition involves the acquisition by the recipient replicon of additional nucleotide sequences (2, 4, 5, 11, 12, 13, 14, 18, 22, 24) and that the increase in size is normally constant (2, 4, 5, 12, 13, 14, 18, 24). In addition, the extra DNA may be inserted into one of several different sites on the replicon (4, 14, 18, 22, 23, 24). Reciprocal recombination, on the other hand, tends to be site specific and, in general, does not result in the acquisition of additional DNA. We can use these criteria to examine the recombinant plasmids which arose from the interaction of pUB501 with the chromosomal TnA elements carried by UB1731 and UB1780.

Several of these pUB501.amp recombinant plasmids, including the single example generated in UB1780, were isolated and examined. All were the same size as the parent plasmid pUB501. When these plasmids were hydrolysed with the restriction endonuclease Bam-H1, the fragmentation patterns obtained were identical. Hydrolysis of pUB501 with Bam-H1 generates four fragments with sizes 1.1×10^6, 1.3×10^6, 3×10^6 and 19×10^6 Mdal. Hydrolysis of several pUB501 amp recombinant plasmids also generated these four sizes of fragments. On the other hand, R388, the prototype plasmid, is restricted by Bam-H1 at only 3 sites and gives three fragments with sizes 1.1×10^6, 1.3×10^6 and 19×10^6 Mdal, respectively.

The presence of an additional Bam-H1 site on the puB501 and pUB501.amp recombinant plasmids when compared with R388 is consistent with the presence on these replicons of a single copy of TnA, because TnA is known to have a single site sensitive to Bam-H1 (22).

In addition, the TnA unit carried by each of these plasmids was located at the same site because hydrolysis of pUB501 and pUB501.amp recombinant plasmids with Bam-H1 always generated the same four fragments. Thus, because all pUB501.amp recombinant plasmids were the same, and were physically indistinguishable from pUB501, we concluded that they were derived by reciprocal recombination between pUB501 and one of the chromosomally integrated TnA elements, rather than by transposition. The corollary to this conclusion, is of course, that TnA does not transpose to pUB501. But pUB501 is a R388::TnA recombinant plasmid and, as we have shown, TnA transposes readily to R388. So what prevents TnA transposing to pUB501? The only difference between R388 and pUB501 is that the latter plasmid carries a copy of TnA. We conclude, therefore, that insertion of TnA into the R388 genome makes it immune to further transposition of TnA.

Is Transposition Immunity a General Phenomenon?

To determine whether transposition immunity is a general phenomenon or is limited to R388 and TnA, we looked for other examples of the inhibition of TnA transposition.

The plasmid pUB306 (formerly RP1 amp1irp1: 8, 9) is a derivative of RP1, isolated following NTG mutagenesis, which no longer expresses its amp gene nor confers intrinsic resistance to penicillins. It is the same size as RP1. The plasmid pUB307 is also derived from RP1. It lacks a nucleotide sequence of approximately 4×10^6 which includes the amp gene. Therefore, pUB306 carries TnA in mutated form while most, if not all, of this sequence is missing from pUB307. Both plasmids, nevertheless, confer resistance to kanamycin and to tetracycline.

These two plasmids were introduced separately into UB1731 and UB1780 by conjugation. Plasmid-carrying exconjugants were outcrossed with E. coli JC6310 R$^-$ and exconjugants of this cross in turn selected on minimal agar with either carbenicillin or with kanamycin, to measure the plasmid transfer frequency. Transfer of amp^r from rec$^+$ strain UB1731 mediated by pUB306 was readily detected at a frequency of 10^{-2}, in contrast to the frequency of 10^{-5} obtained with the recA strain UB1780 carrying pUB306 (Table 2).

Since the transfer of the amp resistance determinant mediated by pUB306 is recA dependent, it is likely to be the result of reciprocal recombination. On the other hand, pUB307 mobilised the chromosomally integrated TnA units at equal frequency from both UB1731 and from UB1780. From this, we conclude that TnA interaction with pUB307 is a true transposition. The fact that pUB306.amp recombinant plasmids are the same size as pUB306 itself, but that pUB307.amp recombinant plasmids are larger than pUB307 by an amount equivalent to approximately 3×10^6 Mdal is consistent with these conclusions.

Table 2.

Frequency of Transposition of TnA From Its Chromosomal Site in E. coli UB1731 and UB1780 to Derivatives of RP1 and R1

Acceptor plasmid	Transposition frequency[x]	
	UB1731(rec$^+$)	UB1780(recA)
pUB306	1.3×10^{-2}	$<1.4 \times 10^{-5}$
pUB307	2.5×10^{-2}	2.7×10^{-2}
R1drd19ampC45	4.6×10^{-6}	5.8×10^{-7}
R1drd19K1	2.4×10^{-3}	1.4×10^{-3}

^{x}Transposition frequency = $\dfrac{\text{Transfer frequency amp}^r}{\text{Transfer frequency plasmid}}$

Similar experiments, in which the frequency of TnA transposition to R1drd19K1 and to R1drd19.ampC45 from UB1731 and from UB1780 was determined, gave analogous results (Table 2). Transposition of TnA to R1drd-19K1 occurred at a frequency of approximately 2×10^{-3} regardless of the state of the recA gene in the host cell. This pattern of results correlates well with the fact that R1drd-19K1 carries an extensive deletion which has removed from R1, among other functions, the ability to confer resistance to penicillins (3). In contrast R1drd19ampC45 carries a point mutation, and expresses its amp gene so poorly that it is possible to select against it using carbenicillin (I. Crowlesmith, personal communication). Transposition of TnA to R1drd-19ampC45 in UB1780 was not detected, at a limit of detection of 6×10^{-7} (Table 2), a result completely consistent with those described previously for derivations of R388 and RP1. Thus, the relative immunity to a further transposition of TnA brought about by carriage of a single copy of TnA seems to be a general phenomenon and not one limited to a particular replicon.

How is this desensitisation to transposition achieved? Several
possibilities can be formulated, some of them already known to
be unlikely.

(1) Certain plasmids carry only one site at which TnA can insert.
(2) Transposition is, in some manner, self-inhibitory due to an
    over-abundance of TnA copies in a bacterial cell.
(3) Acquisition of two copies of TnA by a single replicon creates
    an inherently unstable situation which leads to the elimina-
    tion of one, or both, copies of TnA perhaps by recombination.
(4) Transposition of a second copy of TnA to a replicon which
    already carries one is specifically prevented.

Does R388 Have Several Sites at Which TnA Can Insert?

From previous experiments, we concluded that TnA inserts into
R388 in at least two sites (4). We have now extended those findings. Several R388::TnA recombinant plasmids, formed in either
UB1731 or UB1780, were hydrolysed using the restriction endonuclease Bam-H1. The DNA fragments so produced were separated
electrophoretically in agarose gels (Fig.1). Since TnA has a
single site sensitive to Bam-H1 (22) hydrolytic cleavage with
Bam-H1 should generate the same DNA fragments if TnA always
inserts into R388 at the same site. On the other hand, a range
of different restriction patterns would argue that TnA had inserted at different sites in R388. We found that the fragment
profiles generated from several R388::TnA recombinant plasmids
by Bam-H1 mediated hydrolysis were similar, but not identical
(Fig.1). The figure shows four different profiles and several
others have also been found. Also illustrated in this figure
is the pattern obtained when R388 itself is cleaved with Bam-H1.
Three fragments are obtained, indicating three sites on R388
sensitive to Bam-H1; that is one site less than is found on
R388::TnA recombinant plasmids. This result is in keeping with
the fact that TnA carries a single site sensitive to Bam-H1
(22). These data show that TnA can insert into R388 at several
distinct sites. Consequently, the apparent inability of TnA to
transpose to pUB501 cannot be explained by a lack of potential
insertion sites.

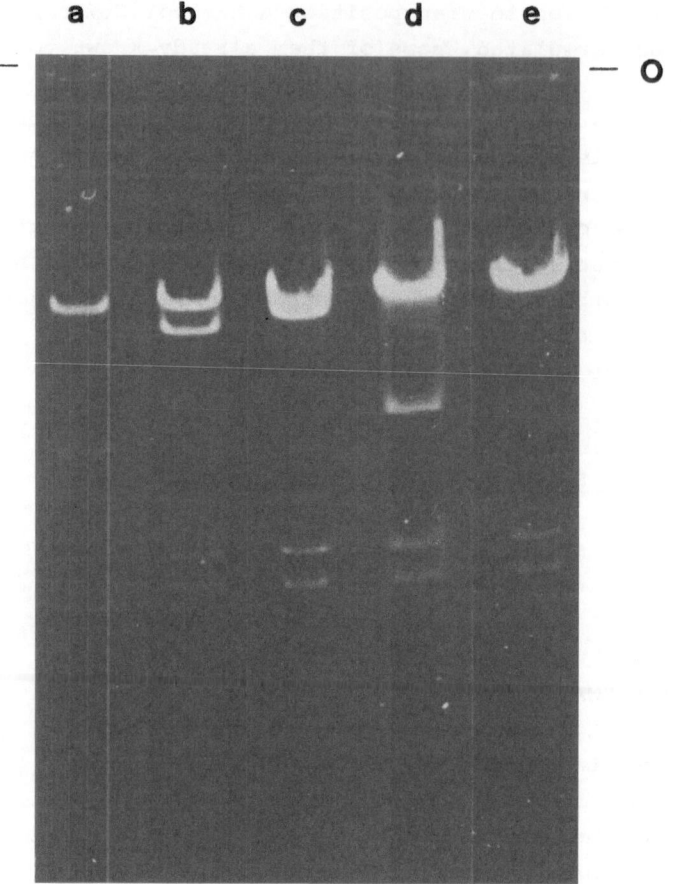

Figure 1. Bam-H1 restriction endonuclease digests of pUB310 (a),
pUB514 (b), pUB511 (c), pUB508 (d) and R388 (e) separated by electrophoresis in a 0.7% (w/v) agarose gel.
O: origin.

Is Transposition of TnA Self-Inhibitory?

If transposition of TnA to pUB501 is inhibited because of an
over-abundance of TnA units in the cell, then transposition of
TnA to plasmids other than pUB501, which are also carried by the
cell, should be inhibited; that is, the inhibition should act in
trans.

The plasmid pUB307 was introduced into sub-strains of E. coli UB1731 and UB1780 which also carried pUB501. Strains carrying both plasmids were then outcrossed to E. coli JC6310 and selection of exconjugants was made using carbenicillin. Colonies obtained in this way were then screened to determine whether they had acquired resistance to kanamycin (a character of pUB307) or to trimethoprim (a character of pUB501). In practice, all clones tested were resistant to kanamycin but sensitive to trimethoprim, and this indicates the acquisition of pUB307.

Plasmids with the properties expected of pUB307.amp were detected at a frequency of approximately 1.7×10^{-2} per pUB307 transfer event following transfer from UB1731; and from UB1780 the equivalent frequency was 2.3×10^{-3} per pUB307 transfer. These frequencies did not differ significantly and we therefore concluded that transposition of TnA to pUB307 had occurred. Furthermore, these frequencies of transposition of TnA to pUB307 in the presence of pUB501 were not markedly different from those found when pUB501 was absent (Table 2). Hence, the inhibition of transposition of TnA to pUB501 did not affect other plasmids carried by the cell and which can readily acquire TnA in the absence of pUB501. These experiments show that the inability to transpose TnA to pUB501 is not a generalised inhibition of transposition, but rather the manifestation of a specific block to additional transpositions of TnA to those replicons which already carry one copy of this transposon.

Is the Carriage of Two TnA Copies on a Single Plasmid Genetically Unstable?

The plasmid pUB501 was derived, as previously described, by transposing TnA on to R388 and then by mutating the resulting plasmid to prevent expression of its amp gene. The plasmid RSF2124 is a colE1::TnA recombinant plasmid (23). Both pUB501 and RSF2124 therefore carry a single amp gene and also have single sites which are sensitive to attack by EcoR1 restriction endonuclease. As a consequence, this property allows us to join these two plasmids together by in vitro recombination techniques and thus to test whether a plasmid carrying two TnA regions is inherently unstable.

A mixture of pUB501 and RSF2124 DNA was digested with EcoR1
endonuclease under conditions described elsewhere (21). The
enzyme was then inactivated by heating the reaction mixture to
65° for 5 min, and T4 ligase added to join the "sticky ends"
generated from the two plasmids by endonuclease action. This
DNA was then used to transform competent E. coli C600, and
transformants which carried a single plasmid derived from both
pUB501 and RSF2124 were selected on agar containing carbenicillin
and trimethoprim. One such transformant was examined in more
detail and was shown to carry a single plasmid (pUB561) molecular
weight 31.2×10^6 dal., and this size was consistent with it
being a product of the ligation of pUB501 (M.W.24.5×10^6 daltons)
and RSF2124 (M.W.7.3×10^6 daltons).

Digestion of pUB561 DNA with EcoR1 and Bam-H1 endonuclease, independently, yielded either 2 or 5 linear DNA fragments, respectively, the sizes of which were consistent with their having
arisen from a composite plasmid constructed by ligation of
RSF2124 to pUB501 via the EcoR1 sites on each plasmid. Furthermore, since pUB561 has five sites sensitive to Bam-H1, compared with 4 sites on pUB501 and a single site on RSF2124, the
composite plasmid must carry two copies of TnA, one derived
from pUB501 and the other from RSF2124.

The plasmid pUB561 confers resistance to trimethoprim, sulphonamides and to penicillins, confers immunity against colicin E1
but does not encode production of colicin E1. The plasmid is
stable in both recA and rec+ strains of E. coli and has retained
the conjugative properties of R388. Replication of pUB561 appears to be under the control of the R388 origin and not that of
ColE1, because the composite plasmid transfers readily to strains
of E. coli which carry the po1A1 mutation, a lesion which prevents replication of ColE1 (17). Furthermore, and in contrast
to ColE1 (6), replication of pUB561 is inhibited by chloramphenicol, as is the replication of R388. We conclude, therefore,
that two copies of TnA can be carried on the same replicon and
that this state is not necessarily unstable.

This conclusion was confirmed fortuitously when we isolated a
recombinant plasmid, formed in vivo, which carries two copies
of TnA. While studying transposition of TnA to pUB307, a recom-

binant plasmid with unusual physical properties, was isolated.
The particular recombinant plasmid (pUB366) is larger than other
pUB307::TnA recombinant plasmids by approximately 3×10^6. When
pUB366 DNA was digested with Bam-H1 endonuclease, two sites sensitive to this enzyme were found, in contrast to the single site
carried by the majority of pUB307::TnA recombinant plasmids. As
a result, we concluded that pUB366 might carry two copies of
TnA. Intramolecular reannealing experiments following alkali
denaturation have confirmed this conclusion. The plasmid pUB366
carries two copies of TnA, inserted in opposite orientations
and separated on the plasmid genome by a stretch of DNA of
approximately 1 Mdal. As with pUB561, pUB366 appears to be
stable. The observation that a plasmid containing two apparently
identical TnA units may be formed in vivo may seem, at first
sight, to contradict the experiments in which transposition of
TnA to a plasmid already carrying TnA was blocked. However, it must be
stressed that pUB366 may have arisen by the transposition of
two TnA units to pUB307 - a plasmid carrying no TnA - within a
short time of one another. On the other hand, the earlier experiments with pUB501 were all attempts to introduce a second
TnA into a plasmid that already carried one (21).

If this distinction is valid, it suggests that double transpositions may occur into a plasmid lacking a blocking unit, but
that this phenomenon only occurs when the two event occur within
a short time of one another. And this, in turn, suggests that
the immunity to transposition conferred by a transposon acting
cis may take some time to develop.

Does Tn10 Inhibit Transposition of TnA?

Because TnA apparently blocks its own transposition we widened
our investigations to determine if other transposons displayed
similar inhibitory tendencies. Tn10 defines the transposon
which encodes resistance to tetracycline and which originated
on the R plasmid R100-1 (11). Tn10 was transposed from a chromosomal site (11) to the R plasmid R751, which displays P type
compatibility and confers resistance to trimethoprim (4, 16).
One R751::Tn10 derivative was numbered pUB505.

R751 and pUB505 were introduced separately into E. coli strains
UB1731 and UB1780 by conjugation and plasmid carrying progeny
were outcrossed with the recA strain JC6310 (4). Exconjugants
were selected on minimal medium supplemented with trimethoprim
(25 µg/ml) to determine the frequency of plasmid transfer, or
with carbenicillin (500 µg/ml).

Table 3.

Frequency of Transposition of TnA From Its Chromosomal Site in
E. coli UB1731 and UB1780 to R751, R1-19.K1 and Derivatives
Carrying Tn10

Acceptor plasmid	Transposition frequency[x]	
	UB1731(rec$^+$)	UB1780(recA)
R751	1.1×10^{-2}	3.7×10^{-2}
pUB505 (R751::Tn10)	$<1.4 \times 10^{-6}$	$<1.5 \times 10^{-6}$
R1-19.K1	2.4×10^{-3}	1.4×10^{-3}
pUB502 (R1-19.K1::Tn10)	3.5×10^{-7}	6.3×10^{-7}
pUB505, R1-19.K1	–	6.3×10^{-4}

[x]Transposition frequency = $\dfrac{\text{Transfer frequency amp}^r}{\text{Transfer frequency plasmid}}$

TnA transposed to R751 in that the formation of recombinant
plasmid molecules was independent of a functional recA gene
product (Table 3, ref. 4). In these experiments the transposition
frequency of TnA to R751 was 1.1×10^{-2} in strain UB1731 (rec$^+$)
and 3.7×10^{-2} in strain UB1780 (recA)(Table 3). In contrast,
transposition of TnA to pUB505 was undetected in both UB1731
and UB1780 in these experiments (Table 3). But pUB505 differs
from R751 only in that it carries the extra nucleotide sequences
contained within Tn10. Hence the presence of Tn10 on pUB505
severely inhibits transposition of TnA to that replicon.

An analogous situation was observed with the R plasmids R1-19.K1
and pUB502, a derivative of R1-19.K1 which carries transposon

Tn10. Thus TnA transposed to R1-19.K1 at a frequency of approximately 2 x 10^{-3} (Table 3) but to pUB502 at the much lower frequency of approximately 10^{-6} (Table 3).

These data convincingly demonstrate that Tn10 inhibits transposition of TnA in some manner; but does the inhibition act in
a cis manner, similar to the self-inhibition displayed by TnA?
R plasmids pUB505 and R1-19.K1 were introduced into E. coli
strain UB1780 by conjugation. One isolate which carried both
plasmids was outcrossed with the recA strain JC6310. Exconjugants
were selected on minimal medium supplemented with carbenicillin
(500 µg/ml) and were then screened to determine if they were
also resistant to kanamycyin or to trimethoprim. Transfer of
pUB505 or R1-19.K1 was determined by selection with trimethoprim
(25 µg/ml) or with Kanamycin (30 µg/ml) respectively.

All exconjugants selected with carbenicillin were also resistant
to kanamycin but sensitive to trimethoprim, indicating that
TnA had transposed to R1-19.K1. The frequency at which TnA transposed to R1-19.K1 in the presence of pUB505 (6.3 x 10^{-4}) was
not much different from the value observed in the absence of this
plasmid (1.4 x 10^{-3}) (Table 3). Hence inhibition of TnA transposition by Tn10 is cis acting, a situation analogous to the
self-inhibition exhibited by TnA.

Does TnA Inhibit Transposition of Tn10?

Because Tn10 inhibits transposition of TnA it is of interest to
determine if the inhibition is mutual i.e. does TnA block transposition of Tn10?

E. coli strain UB1676 carries a copy of Tn10 inserted into the
bacterial chromosome and is also recA. E. coli strain UB5206 is
a recombination proficient (rec^{+}) revertant of UB1676. The R
plasmids R1-19.K1 and two independently isolated derivatives
which carry transposed copies of TnA were introduced separately
into strains UB5206 and UB1676. Plasmid-carrying progeny were
outcrossed with the E. coli recA strain UB5201 (UB281recA56, ref.
4). Exconjugants were selected on minimal medium supplemented
with kanamycin (30 µg/ml) to determine the frequency of plasmid
transfer, or with tetracycline (20 µg/ml).

Table 4.

Frequency of Transposition of Tn10 From Its Chromosomal Site
in E. coli UB1676 and UB5206 to R1-19.K1 and R1-19.K1::TnA
Derivatives

Acceptor plasmid	Transposition frequency[x]	
	UB5206(rec[+])	UB1676(recA)
R1-19.K1	1.2×10^{-7}	7.3×10^{-8}
R1-19.K1::TnA$_1$	7.1×10^{-8}	1.1×10^{-7}
R1-19.K1::TnA$_2$	2.6×10^{-7}	1.9×10^{-7}

[x]Transposition frequency = $\dfrac{\text{Transfer frequency Tc}^{\text{r}}}{\text{Transfer frequency plasmid}}$

Tn10 transposed to R1-19.K1 at a frequency of 10^{-7} (Table 4) and
the presence on the replicon of a copy of TnA did not inhibit
this process because Tn10 transposed to R1-19.K1::TnA$_1$ and to
R1-19.K1::TnA$_2$ at approximately the same frequency i.e. at about
10^{-7} (Table 4).

In the light of this result it is obviously pertinent to determine if Tn10 inhibits its own transposition.

Is Transposition of Tn10 Self-Inhibitory?

The plasmids pDU3 and pDU202 are derivatives of the R plasmid
R100-1 (which were kindly supplied by Dr. T. Foster, Trinity
College, Dublin). R100-1 confers resistance to chloramphenicol,
streptomycin, sulphonamides and to tetracycline. This last
resistance is encoded by Tn10, as mentioned previously (11).
pDU3 and pDU202 do not confer resistance to tetracycline, but
whereas pDU3 carries a point mutation within Tn10, pDU202 carries
a deletion which encompasses the Tn10 region of R100-1.

pDU3 and pDU202 were introduced separately into E. coli strains
UB5206 and UB1676 and plasmid-carrying progeny were outcrossed
with strain UB5201. Exconjugants were selected on minimal medium

containing chloramphenicol (50 µg/ml) to select for plasmid transfer, or with tetracycline (20 µg/ml).

Table 5.

Frequency of Transposition of Tn10 From Its Chromosomal Site
in E. coli UB1676 and UB5206 to Derivatives of R100

Acceptor plasmid	Transposition frequency^x UB5206(rec$^+$) UB1676(recA)
pDU3	7.0×10^{-5} 4.6×10^{-8}
pDU202	1.1×10^{-7} 5.0×10^{-8}

^{x}Transposition frequency $= \dfrac{\text{Transfer frequency } \underline{Tc}^r}{\text{Transfer frequency plasmid}}$

Tn10 transposed to pDU3 and to pDU202 at similar frequencies
(approximately 5×10^{-8}) as illustrated by the results obtained
using the recA donor strain UB1676 (Table 5) indicating that,
unlike transposition of TnA, transposition of Tn10 is not self-
inhibitory.

It is obvious from the data presented (Table 5) that transfer
of the tetracycline resistance determinant to pDU3 appears to
be partly recA dependent, in contrast to which transfer of the
determinant to pDU202 is recA independent. These results can be
explained by the fact that pDU3 carries Tn10 but in mutated form
and so would be expected to recombine with the chromosomal Tn10
element present in UB5206. On the other hand, Tn10 is not carried
on pDU202 and so no recombination between this plasmid and the
chromosomal Tn10 would be expected, and none is observed (Table 5).

Thus, although transposition of TnA is self-inhibitory and is
also inhibited by Tn10, inhibition is not a mutual, nor indeed
a universal, phenomenon, because TnA does not inhibit transposition of Tn10 and neither is transposition of Tn10 self-inhibitory.
The mechanism of the block remains obscure, but it is attractive

to postulate that when a replicon acquires a copy of TnA or Tn10 it may be modified in such a manner that the enzyme system responsible for mediating transposition of TnA no longer functions efficiently with that replicon. Acquisition of one of these transposons may not of itself be sufficient to exhibit the inhibitory effect because preliminary evidence suggests that the block is not expressed immediately the transposon is acquired.

Evolutionary Consequences of Transposition

The development of many outbreaks of antibiotic resistance among clinically important strains can be seen to be likely examples of gene transposition in action. Thus, for example, the celebrated outbreak of Type 29 Salmonella typhimurium infection documented by Anderson (1) showed the sequential uptake on the plasmids concerned first of SmSu resistance genes, then of Tc, then Ap, and then NeKn. All these marker patterns are now known to be carried on transposons, and it seems highly probable that the epidemic followed by Anderson showed sequential gene transposition in action.

One of the difficulties of accommodating gene transposition in an evolutionary context is the fact that the process shows such lack of specificity and, consequently, one might expect gene transposition to occur frequently and to lead to the insertion of "foreign" DNA into many replicons, including particularly the chromosome. In practice the frequency of transposition to the chromosome appears to be low. Admittedly, E. coli strains carrying TnA, specifically Tn802, (4, 20), Tn7 (2), and Tn10 (11, 18) in the chromosome have all been constructed in the laboratory. But in the case of Tn802, for example, transposition from a carried plasmid to the chromosome occurs very infrequently (4, 20). With bacteria carrying RP-1, for example, up to a dozen cycles of growth and single colony isolation from selective agar were necessary to obtain one clone in which Tn802 had now become integrated into the chromosome (20).

Although certainly not the whole story, it seems that the phenomenon of transposition immunity may have an important part to play in restricting the transposition of genes to new replicons. Moreover, the effect might be widespread if there proved

to be cross-immunity between transposons carrying a range of
markers.

If one now looks at the matter from the other side, as it were,
one can even postulate that some phenomenon analogous to transposition immunity must occur. Evolutionary progress occurs most
effectively where the population under challenge is shaped by
a balance of positive and negative effects. In this way, changes
may occur without upsetting the balance of advantage too drastically. Thus among bacterial populations one sees mutation and
repair, and restriction and modification, as two such balanced
pairs of effects. Against this background, one would certainly
expect a balancing process to gene transposition; and transposition immunity may be just such an effect.

Whatever the precise mechanisms of transposition, however, the
phenomenon must clearly have enormous evolutionary potential.
Not only does the process allow blocks of pre-refined genetic
information to pass from one replicon to another, it allows the
process to occur in the absence of normal recombination. Thus
one has a number of levels of gene exchange: conjugation and
other methods of gene transfer allow entire plasmids to pass
between bacteria; but, at a lower level of complexity, transposition allows transposons to pass between plasmids. Clearly,
"great fleas have little fleas upon their backs to bite 'em!"

Acknowledgements

The work described in this contribution was supported by a
Programme Grant from the Medical Research Council to M. H.
Richmond. M. Robinson was supported by a Scholarship for Training in Research Methods from the Medical Research Council. We
are indebted to Drs. Stanley Falkow and Fred Heffron for the
gift of the plasmid RSF 2124. Evelyn Lewis provided expert
technical help.

Literature

1. Anderson, E. S.: The Ecology of Transferable Drug Resistance in the Enterobacteria. Ann. Rev. Microbiol. <u>22</u>, 131-180 (1968).
2. Barth, P. J., N. Datta, R. W. Hedges, and J. J. Grinter: Transposition of the Deoxyribonucleic Acid Sequence Encoding Trimethoprim and Streptomycin Resistances From R583 to Other Replicons. J. Bacteriol. <u>125</u>, 800-810 (1976).
3. Beard, J. P., and J. C. Connolly: Detection of a Protein, Similar to the Sex Pilus Subunit, in the Outer Membrane of <u>Escherichia coli</u> Carrying a Derepressed F-like R Factor. J. Bacteriol. <u>122</u>, 59-65 (1975).
4. Bennett, P. M., and M. H. Richmond: Translocation of a Discrete Piece of Deoxyribonucleic Acid Carrying an <u>amp</u> Gene Between Replicons in <u>Escherichia coli</u>. J. Bacteriol. <u>126</u>, 1-6 (1976).
5. Berg, D. E., J. Davies, B. Allet, and J. Rochaize: Transposition of R Factor Genes to Bacteriophage. Proc. Natl. Acad. Sci. U.S.A. <u>72</u>, 3628-3632 (1975).
6. Clewell, D. B.: Nature of ColE1 Plasmid Replication in <u>Escherichia coli</u> in the Presence of Chloramphenicol. J. Bacteriol. <u>110</u>, 667-676 (1972).
7. Cohen, S. N.: Transposable Genetic Elements and Plasmid Evolution. Nature (Lond.) <u>263</u>, 731-738 (1976).
8. Curtis, N. A. C., M. H. Richmond: Effect of R-Factor-Mediated Genes on Some Surface Properties of <u>Escherichia coli</u>. Antimicrob. Agents Chemother. <u>6</u>, 666-671 (1974).
9. Curtis, N.A.C., and M. H. Richmond, and V. Stanisich: R-Factor-Mediated Resistance Which Does Not Involve a ß-Lactamase. J. Gen. Microbiol. <u>79</u>, 163-166 (1973).
10. Datta, N., and R. W. Hedges: Trimethoprim Resistance Conferred by Plasmids in Enterobacteriaceae. J. Gen. Microbiol. <u>72</u>, 349-356 (1972).
11. Foster, T. J., T. G. B. Howe, and M. H. Richmond: Translocation of the Tetracycline Resistance Determinant From R100-1 to the <u>Escherichia coli</u> K-12 Chromosome. J. Bacteriol. <u>124</u>, 1153-1158 (1975).
12. Gottesman, M. M., and J. L. Rosner: Acquisition of a Determinant for Chloramphenicol Resistance by Coliphage Lambda. Proc. Natl. Acad. Sci. U.S.A. <u>72</u>, 5041-5045 (1975).

13. Hedges, R. W., and A. E. Jacob: Transposition of Ampicillin Resistance from RP4 to Other Replicons. Molec. Gen. Genet. 132, 31-40 (1974).

14. Heffron, F., C. Rubens, and S. Falkow: Translocation of a Plasmid DNA Sequence Which Mediates Ampicillin Resistance: Molecular Nature and Specificity of Insertion. Proc. Natl. Acad. Sci. U.S.A. 72, 3623-3627 (1975).

15. Heffron, F., R. Sublett, R. W. Hedges, A. Jacob, and S. Falkow: Origin of the TEM Beta-Lactamase Gene Found on Plasmids. J. Bacteriol. 122, 250-256 (1975).

16. Jobanputra, R. S., and N. Datta: Trimethoprim Resistance Factors in Enterobacteria From Clinical Specimens. J. Med. Microbiol. 7, 169-177 (1974).

17. Kingsbury, D. T., and D. R. Helinski: DNA Polymerases as a Requirement for the Maintenance of the Bacterial Plasmid Colicinogenic Factor E1. Biochem. Biophys. Res. Comm. 41, 1538-1544 (1970).

18. Kleckner, N., R. K. Chan, B. Tye, and D. Botstein: Mutagenesis by Insertion of a Drug-Resistance Element Carrying an Inverted Repetition. J. Mol. Biol. 97, 561-575 (1975).

19. Kopecko, D. J., and S. N. Cohen: Site-Specific recA - Independent Recombination Between Bacterial Plasmids: Involvement of Palindromes at the Recombinational Loci. Proc. Natl. Acad. Sci. U.S.A. 72, 1373-1377 (1975).

20. Richmond, M. H., and R. B. Sykes: The Chromosomal Integration of a ß-Lactamase Gene Derived From the P-Type R-Factor RP1 in Escherichia coli. Genet. Res., Camb. 20, 231-237 (1972).

21. Robinson, M. K., P. M. Bennett, and M. H. Richmond: Inhibition of TnA Translocation by TnA. J. Bacteriol. 129, 407-414 (1977).

22. Rubens, C., F. Heffron, and S. Falkow: Transposition of a Plasmid Deoxyribonucleic Acid Sequence That Mediates Ampicillin Resistance: Independence from Host rec Functions and Orientation of Insertion. J. Bacteriol. 128, 425-434 (1976).

23. So, M., R. Gill, and S. Falkow: The Generation of a ColE1-Ap^r Cloning Vehicle Which Allows Detection of Inserted DNA. Molec. Gen. Genet. 142, 239-249 (1975).

24. Stanisich, V. A., P. M. Bennett, and M.H. Richmond: Characterisation of a Translocation Unit Encoding Resistance to Mercuric Ions That Occurs on a Non-Conjugative Plasmid in Pseudomonas aeruginosa. J. Bacteriol. (in press).

Discussion

Davies: Is the R1 that you are using carrying kanamycin resistance?
Bennett: Yes.
Davies: So there is another transposon which does not affect TnA?
Bennett: Yes. Is the kanamycin resistance transposable?
Davies: In a funny way, yes.
Anderson: In what funny way?
Davies: I'll tell you (in my talk).
Bennett: We have other examples in that context of some resistance determinants which are believed to be transposable and in some situations they show that kind of character. But none of them we have rigorously shown to be transposition elements. Until that stage has been reached, these are the only two that we can really say that are interacting in that way.
Starlinger: Have you considered the possibility that if there is a TnA on the plasmid and you supertranspose another one, the juxtaposed transposed sequences are more unstable than those that are more widely spaced?
Bennett: That is a possibility but difficult to test if the resulting unit is unstable. One would have to devise a system where the two juxtapositioned elements were stable and then transfer them to a normal situation. We have some evidence which concerns not TnA but some other transposition units and which indicates that what you are saying might be true. There may be an interaction between these two elements which leads to the elimination of one of them.

Transposable Neomycin Phosphotransferases

J. Davies*, D. Berg°, R. Jorgensen*, M. Fiandt[+], T.-S. R. Huang* ,
P. Courvalin*, and J. Schloff*

Transposable genetic elements are discrete DNA segments with the capacity to
move between independent DNA replicons within the cell. The recent dis-
coveries that certain plasmid-borne genes, which confer resistance to antibiotics and to heavy metals, are components of transposable elements has
improved our understanding of how plasmids might pick up genes from nonho-
mologous DNA molecules during their evolution and during the spread of antibiotic resistant infections in hospitals. Table 1 illustrates that many
determinants of resistance have already been found in transposable elements.
Considerable diversity is seen in this collection of elements: they vary
in their DNA sequence arrangement, in the frequency and specificity of
transposition, and in the stability of the transposed genes. Some contain
known insertion sequences.

Table 1. Transposable Resistance Elements[12]

Transposable element and plasmid of origin	Resistances	Reference
Tn1 (RP4)	β-lactams	1
Tn2 (RSF 1030)	β-lactams	2
Tn3 (R1)	β-lactams	3
Tn4 (R1)	β-lactams sulphonamide, streptomycin, (adenylyl-transferase)	3
Tn5 (JR67)	Neomycin-kanamycin (phosphotransferase)	4

Department of Biochemistry[*] and McArdle Laboratory for Cancer Research[+],
University of Wisconsin-Madison and Department of Microbiology°,
Washington University, St. Louis

Tn6 (JR72)	neomycin-kanamycin	
	(phosphotransferase)	4
Tn7 (R483)	Trimethoprim,	
	streptomycin	
	("permeability")	5
Tn9 (pSM14)	chloramphenicol (1S1)	6
Tn10 (R100)	tetracycline (1S3)	7
Tn402 (R751)	trimethoprim	8
Tn501 (pVS1)	mercuric ions	9
Tn601 (R6W)	neomycin-kanamycin	
	(phosphotransferase)	10
Taβ (R938)	β-lactams, streptomycin	
	(phosphotransferase)	11

The actual mechanisms of gene transposition are of considerable interest.
Transposition can be viewed as a form of "illegitimate recombination" (13).
It appears to require neither DNA sequence homology, nor the action of those
recombination genes which have been so far recognized to function in cross-
ingover between homologous chromosomes. The transposition event is unidirectional; insertion of an element into a new site, and its loss or excision
from any given site are detected at very different frequencies. In contrast,
the reciprocal products of homologous recombination, and also of the site
specific integrative recombinations of the lambdoid phages can be recovered
at equivalent frequencies. Experiments summarized below are addressed towards
an eventual understanding of transposition mechanisms.

We have detected and then studied transposable resistance determinants by
picking them up on bacteriophage lambda (4). Of the transposable elements
which contain genes for resistance to aminoglycoside antibiotics, three
encode aminoglycoside-3'-phosphotransferase [APH(3')] which phosphorylate
kanamycin, neomycin, and related antibiotics. Tn6 from plasmid JR72 and
Tn601 from plasmid R6W, or from the colE1 - R6W chimera pML2 that contains
a 4.5×10^6 dalton fragment of R6W (14, 15) encode APH(3')-I, an enzyme
able to modify lividomycin but not butirosin. Tn5 from plasmid JR67, encodes
APH(3')-II with a different chromatographic behavior and substrate range; it
modifies butirosin, but not lividomycin. Filter hybridization (Fig. 1) (16)
and electron microscope heteroduplex studies (see below) have shown that
the resistance genes of Tn6 and Tn601 are homologous to each other, and
that they are not homologous to the resistance gene of Tn5. Antiserum
against APH(3')-II does not cross react with APH(3')-I (17, 18).

Initial characterizations revealed very significant differences between
Tn5, Tn6 and Tn601. Electron microscope heteroduplex analyses showed that
the 5.3 kb Tn5 element and the 3 kb Tn601 element contain terminal inverted
repetitions 1450 and 1000 base pairs in length, respectively. The 4 kb
Tn6 element does not contain an inverted repetition. A comparison of Tn5
and Tn601 by restriction enzyme digestion is shown in Fig. 2. Based on

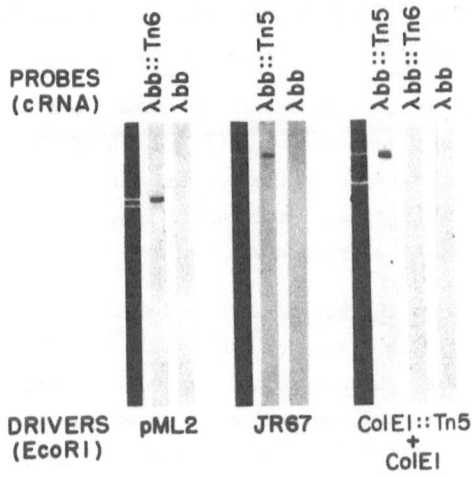

Fig. 1. Hybridization between various plasmid DNAs (on filter) and RNA
complementary to λ derivatives. (λbb ≡ $\lambda b_{515} b_{519}$)

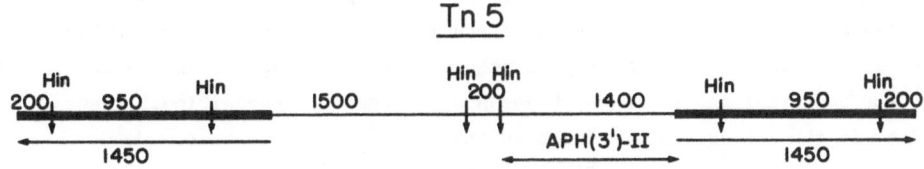

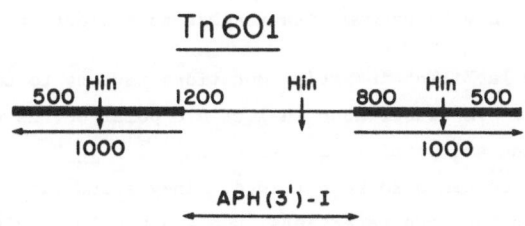

Fig. 2. HindII + III restriction endonuclease maps of Tn5 and Tn601.
Distances are in bases; the heavy lines represent the repeat sequences.

electron microscope heteroduplex studies of λ kan 3 and pML2 (Figs. 3, 4) it would appear that the loop portion of Tn601 contains almost exclusively the coding information for APH(3')-I. The size of the loop (1000bp) and the molecular weight of the enzyme ($27-54 \times 10^3$) are consistent with this, implying that the phosphotransferase gene alone is responsible for the determination of resistance to neomycin-kanamycin. (This assumes that the inverted repeat sequences of Tn601 do not code for any functions necessary for resistance.)

The Tn6 insertion in the λ phage genome is unstable. One-tenth of the progeny emerging from a single cycle of lytic growth of the phage are deleted for the kanamycin resistance trait. Tn5 and Tn601 are much more stable. Tn5 is lost from sites of insertion in phage λ or in the lac operon of E. coli at frequencies of approximately 10^{-6}.

Tn5 is transposed from λ to the bacterial chromosome, and from one chromo-somal site to another at high frequency ($10^{-2} - 10^{-3}$). Transposition of Tn6 from λ to the bacterial chromosome has not been detected to date. The behavior of Tn601 seems bizarre; instead of transposing, it apparently mediates the insertion of the λ Tn601 phage genome into the bacterial chromosome, even when the λ genes and sites necessary for phage specific integration are deleted.

The stability and rather high frequency of transposition of Tn5 have per-mitted us to undertake more detailed studies of its transposition mechanism. Tn5 is mutagenic: new auxotrophic requirements are observed in 1 - 2% of the bacterial clones in which Tn5 had undergone transposition. Inser-tions in the lac operon are found in one in 10^4 of such clones. We decided to analyze the specificity of Tn5 transposition by isolating and mapping a number of Tn5 insertions in the lac operon. As diagrammed in Fig. 5, each of 30 Tn5 insertions in the lacZ gene was found to lie at a different genetic site. From this we conclude that the choice of Tn5 insertion sites may be random with respect to nucleotide sequence.

Each of the 30 lacZ::Tn5 insertion mutations reverts to Lac$^+$ at frequencies of $10^{-6} - 10^{-7}$. Tn5 insertions in lacZ are polar on the expression of the distal lacY gene and partial revertants in which lacY$^+$, but not lacZ$^+$ function has been restored can also be obtained. They arise two to 100 fold more frequently than the true revertants, and apparently result from imprecise excision of the Tn5 element. In some, a small part of Tn5 remains as an insertion in lacZ; in others Tn5 and adjacent lacZ sequences have been lost.

Essentially all revertants are kanamycin sensitive. Thus, detectable
excision of the Tn5 element from a given site is not associated with its
transposition elsewhere in the genome. This observation reinforces the
conclusion that transposition is unidirectional.

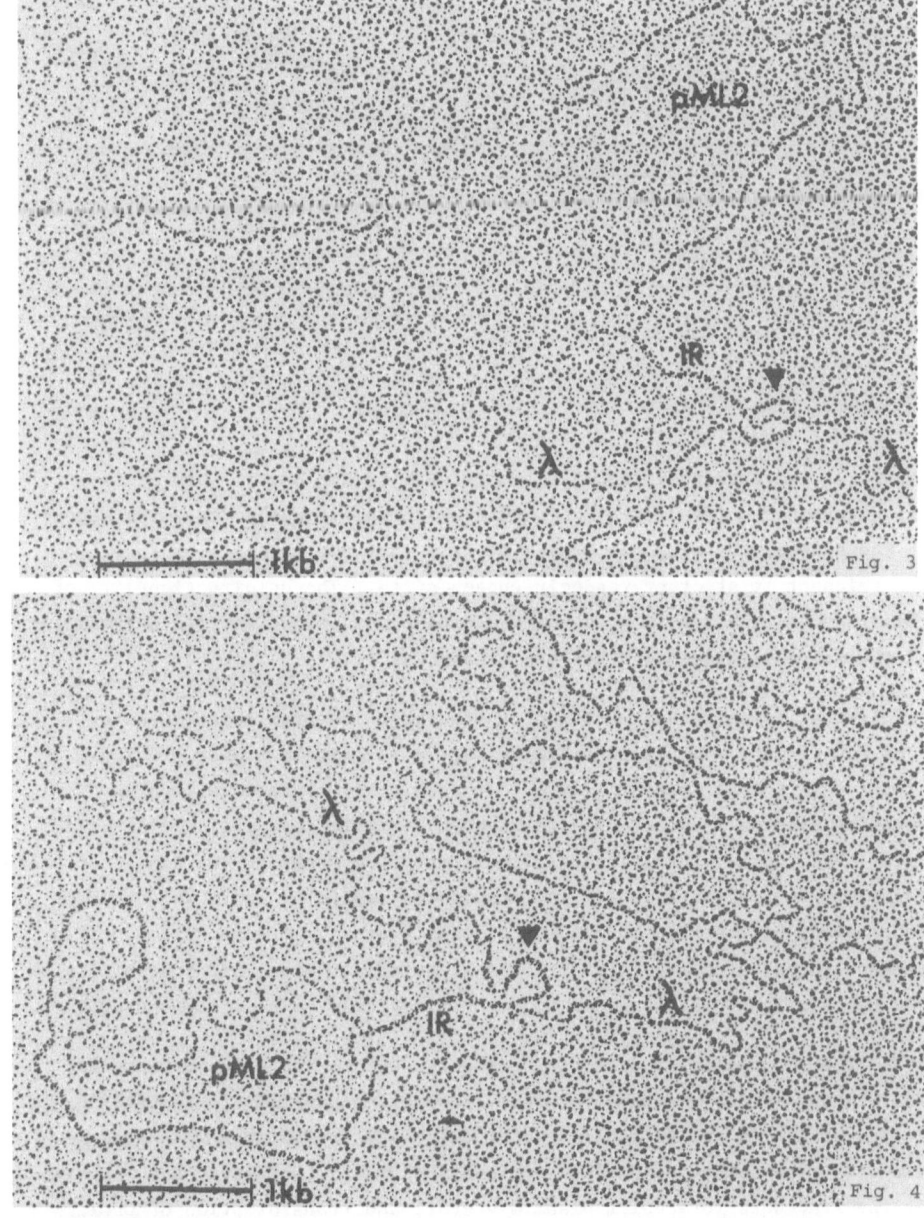

Figs. 3 and 4.
Electron microscope heteroduplexes between λkan3 and pML2 DNA. In the
upper figure pML2 is linear, in the lower figure it is circular. 1R
indicates the inverted repeat of Tn601 and the arrow indicates the
region of homology.

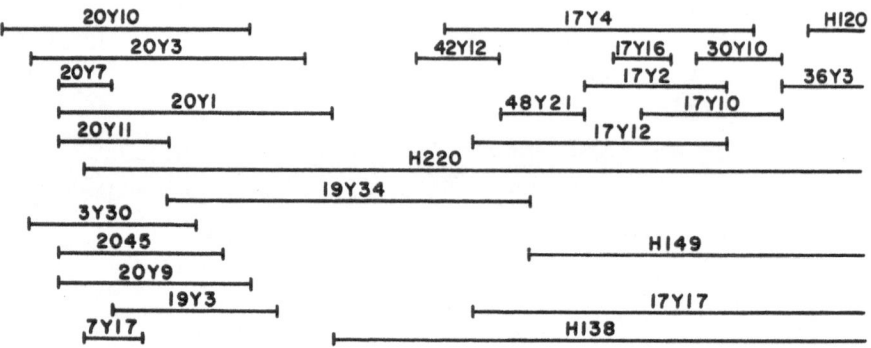

Fig. 5. Positions of insertions of Tn5 in the lacZ gene of E. coli.
The bars indicate the deletions used in mapping.

How might the transposition of elements such as Tn5 occur? One class of
explanations requires enzyme complexes which specifically recognize sequences
at the ends of the element, excise it from its original site of insertion,
and reinsert it at other randomly chosen sites. The unidirectionality of
the transposition reaction could be explained by exonucleolytic degradation
of the molecule from which Tn5 had transposed (19).

An alternative suggestion depends on the large inverted repetitions at
each end of Tn5, and the possibility that a relatively stable cruciform
structure might be formed in vivo. If such a structure were involved in
transposition only one DNA strand might be transferred to a new insertion
site. DNA repair synthesis could then completely restore the double stranded
configuration to the parental and transposed copies of Tn5. This type of
model predicts the kind of unidirectionality seen in transposition. At
present there is no evidence for or against this notion; the instability of
DNA containing single stranded sequences is likely to be a serious problem.

Both of these models predict that sequences within Tn5 are necessary for
Tn5 transposition. We have obtained encouraging preliminary results in
accord with this prediction. Several deletions of Tn5 were generated in
vitro by restriction endonuclease digestion of Tn5 containing DNA, ligation
of the fragments to a colE1 plasmid vector, and transformation of $CaCl_2$
treated E. coli. These deletions were found to be defective in transposition.

Both repeat sequences are required and deletion of the terminal 200 bases
of one of the repeat sequences abolishes the ability to transpose the drug
resistance (20). This is consistent with the notion that ends of the
inverted repeat sequences of Tn5 may be crucially involved in the synaptic
event in transposition. We are designing complementation tests to help
determine whether these deletions remove sites or diffusible functions
necessary for transposition; we also plan to generate deletions with other
breakpoints in Tn5 to define which parts of Tn5 are necessary for transposition. The availability of deletions cutting into the regulatory genes
for resistance determinants will also enable us to examine the promoter
site requirements for regulation of the expression of the resistance genes.
Synthesis of APH(3')-II from λTn5 can be readily detected following
infection of UV-irradiated E. coli with the transducing phage (S.R. Jaskunas,
personal communication).

Even though we do not yet understand the mechanism of transposition, it is
clear that this phenomenon must speed the dissemination of resistance genes
in bacterial populations. In the case of Tn5 the absence of requirements
for any particular sequence, or for homology between donor and recipient
molecules should permit the element to be passed freely between unrelated
chromosomes and plasmids existing in the same cell. The unidirectionality
of the transposition event effectively increases the frequency of Tn5
in the population of DNA molecules in the absence of selection.

In addition to aminoglycoside phosphotransferases, several other aminoglycoside-aminocyclitol resistance determinants (for example streptomycin
resistance) are carried on transposable elements (see Table 1); thus far
their nature and frequency of transposition have been little studied. Since
transposable elements for resistance have been strongly indicated as key
features in the evolution of resistance plasmids, one might expect to find
such structures in a variety of resistance plasmids from different bacterial
genera. We have examined a number of resistance plasmids from Staphylococcus
aureus and have obtained electron microscopic evidence for the typical stem-
loop (snap-back) structure (Fig. 6).

While the presence of structural gene(s) bounded by inverted repeat sequences
is strongly suggestive of the presence of transposable elements, this alone
does not constitute proof. Note that the plasmid reveals three stem-loop
structures after denaturation-renaturation; it is an interesting coincidence
that strains carrying this plasmid elaborate three known aminoglycoside-
modifying enzymes (21).

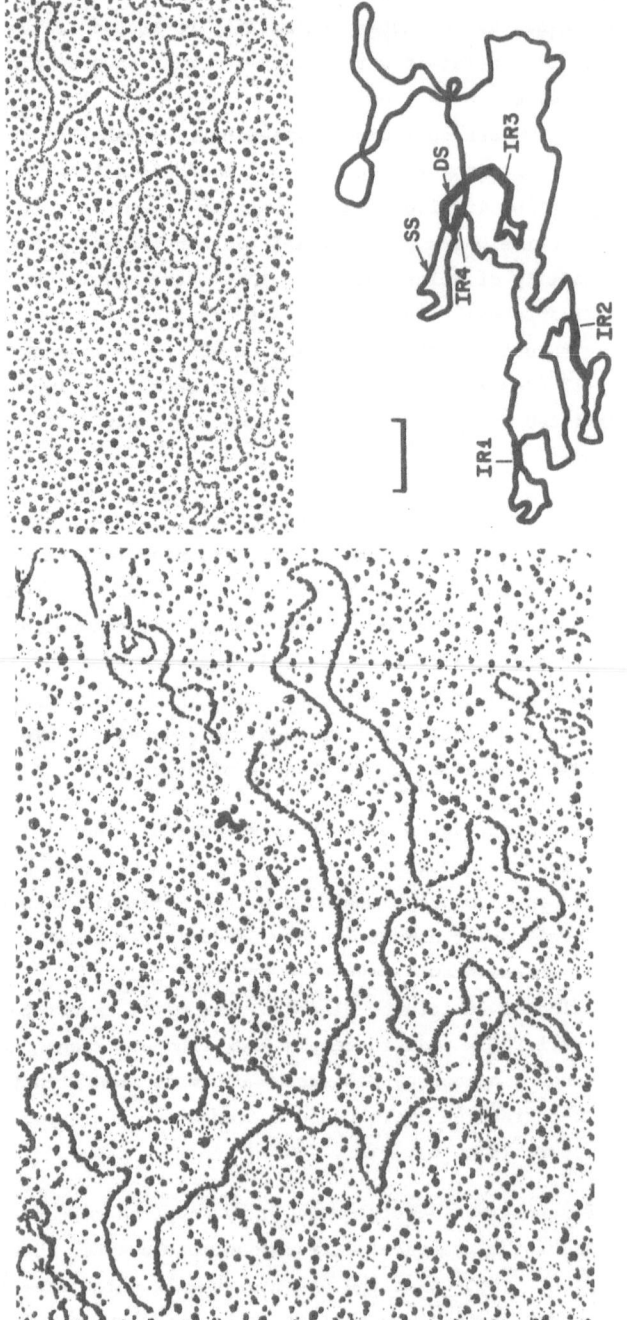

Fig. 6. Staphylococcus aureus plasmid pSJ24. On the left is native plasmid; upper right is plasmid following denaturation and renaturation; lower right is schematic drawing. The bar represents 1000 base pairs.

Acknowledgements

We are grateful for support from NIH and NSF to J. Davies, W. Reznikoff and
W. Szybalski. D. Berg was supported by a traineeship from the Viral Oncology
Training Program.

References

1. Hedges, R. W., Jacob, A. E.: Transposition of Ampicillin Resistance from
    RP4 to Other Replicons. Mol. Gen. Genet. 132, 31–40 (1974).

2. Heffron, F., Rubbens, C., Falkow, S.: Translocation of a Plasmid DNA
    Sequence which Mediates Ampicillin Resistance: Molecular Nature and
    Specificity of Insertion. Proc. Natl. Acad. Sci. U.S.A. 72, 3623–3627
    (1975).

3. Kopecko, D. J., Cohen, S. N.: Site-specific recA-independent Recombin-
    ation Between Bacterial Plasmids: Involvement of Palindromes at the
    Recombinational Loci. Proc. Natl. Acad. Sci. U.S.A. 72, 1373–1377 (1975).

4. Berg, D. E., Davies, J., Allet, B., Rochaix, J.: Transposition of
    R-factor Genes to Bacteriophage λ. Proc. Natl. Acad. Sci. U.S.A. 72,
    3628–3632 (1975).

5. Barth, P. T., Datta, N., Hedges, R. W., Grinter, N. J.: Transposition
    of a Deoxyribonucleic Acid Sequence Encoding Trimethoprim and Strepto-
    mycin Resistances from R483 to Other Replicons. J. Bacteriol. 125, 800–
    810 (1976).

6. Gottesman, M. M., Rosner, J. L.: Acquisition of a Determinant for
    Chloramphenicol Resistance by Coliphage Lambda. Proc. Natl. Acad. Sci.
    U.S.A. 72, 5041–5045 (1975).

7. Kleckner, N., Chan, R. K., Tye, B. K., Botstein, D.: Mutagenesis by
    Insertion of a Drug-resistance Element Carrying an Inverted Repetition.
    J. Mol. Biol. 97, 561 (1975).

8. Shapiro, J. A., Sporn, P.: TN402: A New Transposable Element Deter-
    mining Trimethoprim Resistance that Inserts in Bacteriophage Lambda.
    J. Bacteriol. 129, 1632–1635 (1977).

9. Stanisch, V. A., Bennett, P. M., Richmond, M. H.: Characterization of a
    Translocation Unit Encoding Resistance to Mercuric Ions that Occurs
    on a Non-conjugative Plasmid in Pseudomonas aeruginosa. J. Bacteriol.
    129, 1227–1233 (1976).

10. Berg, D. E., Davies, J., Sehloff, J.: unpublished observations.

11. Hedges, R. W., Matthew, M., Smith, D. I., Cresswell, J. M., Jacob, A. E.:
    Properties of a Transposon Conferring Resistance to Penicillins and
    Streptomycin. Gene, in press, 1977.

12. For a complete reveiw and description see "DNA Insertion Elements, Plasmids, and Episomes" (eds. Bukhari, A. I., Shapiro, J. A., Adhya, S.), Cold Spring Harbor Laboratory, 1977.

13. Franklin, N. C.: Illegitimate Recombination, in "The Bacteriophage Lambda" (ed. Hershey, A. D.), Cold Spring Harbor Laboratory, 1971, pp. 175-194.

14. Hershfield, V., Boyer, H. W., Yanofsky, C., Lovett, M. A., Helinski, D. R.: Plasmid ColEl as a Molecular Vehicle for Cloning and Amplification of DNA. Proc. Natl. Acad. Sci. U.S.A. 71, 3455-3459 (1974).

15. Cohen, S. N., Chang, A. C. Y., Boyer, H. W., Helling, D. B.: Construction of Biologically Functional Bacterial Plasmids in vitro. Proc. Nat. Acad. Sci. U.S.A. 70, 3240-3244 (1973).

16. Courvalin, P., Fiandt, M., Davies, J.: DNA Relationships Between Genes Coding for Aminoglycoside-modifying Enzymes from Antibiotic-producing Bacteria and R-plasmids, Microbiology, 1978, in preparation.

17. Matsuhashi, Y., Sawa, T., Takeuchi, T., Umezawa, H.: Immunological Studies of Aminoglycoside-3'-phosphotransferases. J. Antibiotics 29, 1127-1128 (1976).

18. Smith, D. I., Davies, J. E.: A Study of the Neomycin Phosphotransferases: Characterization and Purification, Microbiology, 1978, in preparation.

19. Berg, D. E., in reference 12.

20. Jorgensen, R., Berg, D., Allet, B., Reznikoff, W. S.: In vitro mapping of RNA Polymerase Binding Sites and Antibiotic Resistance Genes in the Transposable Elements Tn5 and Tn10, in preparation.

21. Huang, T.-S R., Crossley, K., Davies, J.: Existence of Inverted Repeated Sequences in Resistance Plasmids from Multiply Antibiotic Resistant Strains of Staphylococcus aureus, Nature, in preparation.

Discussion

Richmond: Have you analysed 601 the same way you have analysed Tn5? How much of 601 can be deleted without impairing the ability to transpose?

Davies: We have not done that yet. We should be able to do it because we have 601 on ColE1. We thought we would be able to do it starting with lambda but it does not transpose from lambda.

Falkow: In that regard what bothers me is using lambda as an acceptor. One is limited in the amount of transposons that may be inserted into lambda and it seems to me that if you are dealing with a very big transposition you may run into the problem of not getting the whole transposition packaged into lambda.

Davies: Well, with Tn10, that's a big one, this could be a problem.

Falkow: How big is the ColE1 carrying 601?

Davies: 10 million.

Falkow: You should be able to pick that up with lambda without any difficulty.

Davies: You are absolutely right.

Levy: Julian, did you want to imply that a transposon has to have inverted repeats on each side?

Davies: No, not necessarily. It depends how you define a transposon. If a transposable resistance element carries a lot of genes, they transpose much better if they have an inverted repeat rather than a direct repeat. If you take chloramphenicol resistance, for example, that transposes –

Interjection Starlinger: IS1 has an inverted repeat on itself.

Answer Davies: Well, IS1 has a little inverted repeat in itself. But I am not talking about IS-sequences which apparently even insert without having a large repeat.

Falkow: Would you consider lambda to be a transposon?

Answer Davies: No, I don't consider that to be a transposon.

Richmond: Why not?

Davies: Because lambda integrates very specifically at a single
site on the chromosome. The other thing about lambda is that it
has a set of genes required for transposition. But I am not sure
whether transposable elements have this.

Falkow: Transposable elements do not have genes required for
site-specific insertion?

Davies: Well, they have some functions that are required for
that transposition.

Falkow: What kind of proof yould you require that transposons
have genes governing their site-specific insertion?

Davies: Well, I would like to have some point mutants in some
genes in transposable elements.

Richmond: Deletions won't do?

Davies: Well, no. Because deletions can always extend to cis-
acting structural elements, like the inverted repeats at the
termini of the transposon.

Bennett: In your lambda Tn6 where you cannot observe transposition
onto the chromosome, have you hooked it to a number of lambda
derivatives so the Tn6 is in different positions? Because I have
done some studies inserting TnA into plasmids which causes the
plasmid to become nontransmissible. Therefore, I can look at re-
transposition to a transmissible plasmid present in the same
cell. The ability to transpose to this plasmid is dependent on
the position of the TnA. Some retranspose, some don't.

Davies: Well, it is just that Tn6 wasn't that interesting. Tn5
is much more interesting to study. We have looked at the plasmid
from which Tn6 was derived and there is no inverted repeat, there
is no stem-like structure.

Starlinger: Well, I want to come back to the inverted repeat.
There are some transposons that have inverted repeats on each
side and there are those that have a direct repeat on one side.
We know from sequence work that the direct repeat has a small
inverted repeat of 25 nucleotides. Thus it is possible that all
transposons have an inverted repeat. Do you think that each
transposon is transposed by a specific transposition system, or
do you consider it possible that there is a more general mechanism, which is able to recognize inverted repeats and to transpose them together with the unique DNA located between them?

Davies: Well, I don't want to exclude that necessarily. As far
as I know, if you take a lambda carrying chloramphenicol resis-

tance and you infect E. coli with it, nobody has ever demonstrated a transposition of chloramphenicol off the phage onto
anything else. It is unstable. I think that Tn9 can be lost by
recombination within or at the IS1 bordering the transposon
more easily than it can be transposed. I think that it is going
to be the same for anything that has a direct repeat. It is
more likely to loose it under the influence of the recA system
than you are able to transpose.

Richmond: It could be that the transposition events which you
detect are those that are stabilised by a secondary reaction.
I think that an inverted repeat of 25 nucleotides might be a
recognition site for an enzyme while an inverted repeat of 1400
nucleotide pairs is by far too large to be a recognition site
in its entirety.

Davies: Unless it has to code for something. This is not possible
with those transposons that carry only a small inverted repeat
at their ends, like TnA, where the inverted repeat has a length
of only about 150 nucleotide pairs. In this case, however, it is
possible that the transposon was bordered originally by a larger
inverted repeat (able to code for a transposition function), and
that part of this has been lost from one of these repeats by a
deletion.

Bennett: Are the deletions that you described in Tn5 completely
blocked in transposition, or do they retain a lower level of this
function?

Davies: We have transposition of 10^{-2} in the normal cases. We
cannot detect transposition of 10^{-7} in those cases.

Starlinger: You think that two direct repeats at the end of a
transposon, like Tn9, are unstable because of general recombination. However, the original plasmid, from which Tn9 is derived
(R100) is not very unstable.

Davies: It depends on the cell.

Starlinger: In E. coli?

Davis: In proteus.

Interjection Saedler: There are E. coli lines where R1 (the R-
plasmid R1drd19) just disintegrates. We have one of those. There
is a second point: if there are two IS1 sequences in tandem repeat, you can measure the contribution of normal recombination
to the excision versus the illegitimate one, they are in the
same order of magnitude. So I think those are two real parallel
systems.

<u>Drews</u>: What determines the site of insertion? You mentioned
that Tn5 has a multiple site of insertion. What is the molecular basis or correlate for that?

<u>Davies</u>: If there is anything which determines the site of in-
sertion, it is a site which occurs on the <u>E. coli</u> chromosome
many times.

<u>Anderson</u>: It may be one base pair.

<u>Falkow</u>: No, I think the calculation for TnA and TnT comes out to
be around 6 nucleotide base pairs.

<u>Davies</u>: I would expect that it would be less than 6.

<u>Falkow</u>: Well, it's probably between 4 and 6, much like a restric-
tion nuclease recognition site.

<u>Bennett</u>: With respect to the transposition into the lac-operon:
do you have any information whether this occurs with the same
frequency in other parts of the chromosome?

<u>Davies</u>: The only other part on the chromosome where we have
looked a little bit was the histidine operon but we did not have
all the deletions necessary to investigate this fully.

The Transposition of Ampicillin Resistance: Nature of Ampicillin Resistant
Haemophilus influenzae and Neisseria gonorrhoeae

Stanly Falkow, Lynn P. Elwell, Marilyn Roberts, Fred Heffron, and **Ron Gill**

1. Introduction

Transposable elements are discrete genetic and physical entities which can
move from one replicon to another. This event occurs in recombination-deficient (recA⁻) bacteria where homologous recombination has been eliminated
by mutation. Transposable elements include the IS insertion sequences (see
P. Starlinger, this volume; H. Seadler, this volume) and transposable antibiotic resistance genes (see P. Bennett, this volume; J. Davies, this volume).
In this paper, we shall be concerned with the transposable sequence which
includes the determinants for β-lactamase production, the so-called TnA element. The designation TnA is a general term for several independently described transposition elements that carry ampicillin resistance (Ap^r). At
least three distinct elements are known which have been designated Tn1, Tn2
and Tn3; presumably others will be described in future. Most of our discussion concerns the Tn2 transposable element, although it seems fair to assert
that all of the transposable ampicillin elements described, thus far, are
closely related and possess similar genetic and physical properties.

2. General Aspects of the Transposition of Ampicillin Resistance

Following their discovery by Hedges and Jacob /1/ discrete ampicillin elements
capable of transposition from replicon to replicon independently of the recA
functions of the cell have been described by a number of workers /2/, /3/,
/4/. These TnA elements are 4600-4800 base pairs in size and are bounded by
inverted-repeated sequences of about 140 base pairs. Insertion of TnA into
a recipient plasmid appears to depend upon recognition of a specific, but
fairly common, nucleotide sequence /3/, /5/. Moreover, TnA may be inserted
into DNA in either of two orientations and is mutagenic when inserted within
a structural gene and polar (in one orientation) when insertion occurs within
an operon /5/. The transposition of the structural gene(s) for β-lactamase

production permits us to understand why so many different plasmids of apparently diverse origin produce an identical β-lactamase protein /6/, /7/. In a broader sense the ability of drug resistance genes in general to be transposed between DNA molecules surely helps explain the evolution of R plasmids which possess varied permutations of antibiotic resistance genes. We suppose that the evolutionary "success" of R plasmids in modern society speaks most eloquently for the efficiency of transposition in nature. Nevertheless, the precise mechanisms of transposition still remains unclear, and different transposable antibiotic resistance determinants may exert similar effects by substantially different molecular mechanisms.

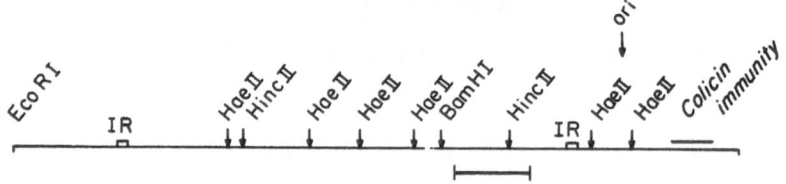

Figure 1. Restriction map of RSF1050. This plasmid is 7400 base pairs in length and specifies colicin immunity (Col) and ampicillin resistance (lower line to right of single BamHI site). IR represents the 140 base pair inverted repeated sequences which flank Tn2 and accompany its insertion. Ori designates the origin of replication. Sites cleaved by BamHI, HincII and HaeIII are represented by the appropriate arrows. The molecule is depicted as the linear sequence that would arise by cleavage with EcoRI.

3. Deletions Affecting the Transposition of TnA

If two plasmids are co-resident in the same cell it is possible to demonstrate transposition of TnA carried by one plasmid to the other /6/. A plasmid was derived in this way by transposition of the 4800 base pair (3.3×10^6 dalton) Tn2 sequence from a large conjugative R plasmid to the 1.8×10^6 dalton ColE1 derivative, pMB8 /8/. The resulting 5×10^6 dalton plasmid, RSF1050, has provided an excellent model in which to analyze deletions of Tn2 since these sequences comprise better than 50% of the total plasmid genome /8/.

Random deletions were introduced into RSF1050 by an in vitro procedure and the deleted derivatives were introduced by transformation into E. coli K-12 recA⁻ cells carrying an F Km plasmid (F Km is the classical F factor carrying resistance to kanamycin). Thus, transformant cells were expected to contain F Km as well as various deletion mutants of RSF1050. RSF1050 possesses the ColE1 replication machinery and, as such, has a strict dependence upon DNA polymerase I (polI) /9/. We exploited this property in our search for RSF1050 mutants that were transposition deficient. E. coli (F Km; RSF1050) transformants were mated with a nalidixic acid resistant [Nalʳ] polI⁻ derivative of E. coli called SF800. The mating mixtures were plated on a medium selective for Ap^r Km^r (Nal^r) colonies. Since RSF1050 could not replicate in the SF800 strain any colonies appearing on the selective medium were cells which had received F Km carrying a transposed Tn2 element. The failure to detect Ap^r Km^r [Nal^r] SF800 colonies in any given mating suggested that the RSF1050 plasmid in the donor cell was a transposition deficient mutant.

Twenty-five transposition deficient mutants were isolated in this fashion /8/ using four restriction endonucleases BamHI, EcoRI, HincII and HaeII, we have constructed a map of RSF1050 (Figure 1) by sequentially digesting RSF1050 DNA with pairs of enzymes and examining the resultant linear fragments by agarose gel electrophoresis. As anticipated, DNA from the RSF1050 transposition deficient mutants cleaved with these same enzymes showed fragment patterns that differed from the parental plasmid and so permitted the mapping of most of the deletions affecting transposition. The mapping of the deletion mutants was further facilitated by electron microscope heteroduplex analysis.

The analysis of the transposition deficient derivatives of RSF1050 permitted them to be divided into two basic classes: 1) deletions which encompassed one of the inverted-repeat (IR) sequences and 2) deletions in which only a small portion of the central region of Tn2 was lost. These findings had significant implications in the sense that they substantially reinforced the view that the terminal IR sequences were essential for transposition and that one or more essential transposition functions were encoded within the central region of Tn2. To confirm and extend these implications, complementation studies were performed. The results of the complementation studies revealed definite differences between deletions which included the terminal IR sequences and those encompassing only an internal sequence. Deletions including the terminal sequence could not be complemented. Deletions confined to the central region of Tn2 were complemented and usually transposed to F Km at a frequency 0.18-0.24 of normal. The most attractive interpretation of the data is that the IR sequences of Tn2 serve a structural role in the transposition process while the central region encodes for one or more diffusable substances which are required for transposition.

Recent studies (Gill, Heffron and Falkow, manuscript in preparation) have confirmed that the deleted Tn2 elements are indeed transposed by complementation to recipient plasmids. Moreover, it is possible to subdivide the deletions which occur in the central region of Tn2. One set of internal deletions are complemented in-trans and lead to essentially normal insertion of the deleted Tn2 into a recipient genome. The other class of internal deletions, when complemented, lead to the insertion of at least one copy of the entire RSF1050 plasmid into a recipient genome. This latter phenomenon occurs at a frequency about 5 times that seen for normal transposition of Tn2. The full importance of this latter phenomenon is not yet known. It is tempting to speculate, however, that there is a regulatory protein which controls excision and/or transposition and a second protein involved in insertion of transposed sequences. In any event, it may be of some practical significance that one or more Tn2 genes (and possibly genes of other transposable elements) have the potential to mediate recA⁻ independent recombination of an entire plasmid genome as well as the transposition of the discrete sequence on which they are carried. We have, for example, been able to generate F factors and R-plasmids of the W incompatibility group which have acquired the entire RSF1050 replicon.

4. R-plasmids of Haemophilus influenzae

During the time that we were investigating the transposition of TnA in enteric species we became aware of an increasingly serious problem of disease due to ampicillin resistant H. influenzae, type b /10/, /11/. Since it was reported /12/ that these H. influenzae isolates produced a β-lactamase very much like that produced by enteric species it seemed reasonable to examine these isolates for the presence of R plasmids. Consequently, some eighteen independently isolated ampicillin resistant H. influenzae and H. parainfluenzae strains were collected. These strains were found in normal patients and from cases of meningitis and epiglottitis; strains from Europe, Asia and the U.S.A. were examined. Sixteen of the isolates contained a 30×10^6 dalton plasmid while two contained a 4.1×10^6 dalton plasmid /13/, /14/. Typical ampicillin sensitive H. influenzae do not usually contain plasmid DNA. Of 180 Ap^S isolates examined (Elwell and Laufs, unpublished observations) only 5 contained plasmid species and these were subsequently found to be unrelated to the R plasmids by DNA-DNA hybridization. Transformation of antibiotic sensitive H. influenzae to ampicillin resistance could be accomplished with both 30×10^6 dalton and 4.1×10^6 dalton plasmid DNA showing conclusively that the structural gene for β-lactamase resided on these plasmid species /13/, /14/.

The question then before us was whether these R plasmids of H. influenzae carried the TnA sequence of enteric species. By both DNA-DNA hybridization studies (Table 1) and electron microscope heteroduplex analysis we could, in fact, show that the 30×10^6 dalton plasmid contained a complete TnA sequence while the 4.1×10^6 dalton plasmid contained but 40% of the TnA sequence /13/, /14/. In the latter instance the TnA included one of the IR sequences and including the single BamHI site of TnA (see Figure 1). Subse-

Table 1.

Source of DNA	Relative DNA Sequence Homology with TnA
E. coli (R-TnA)	100
E. coli	1
H. influenzae	1
H. influenzae (R-Ap^r; 30 x 10^6)	100
H. influenzae (R-Ap^r; 4.1 x 10^6)	40

The degree of DNA-DNA duplex formation was determined between RSF1050 and
H. influenzae plasmid. pMB8-TnA (RSF1050) is a ColE1 derivative carrying
the complete TnA sequence. pMB8-TnA ^{3}H-DNA, but not pMB8 ^{3}H-DNA, showed
about 52% actual DNA binding (taken as 100) when reacted with plasmid DNA
containing the entire TnA sequence

Table 2.

Source of DNA	% Relative DNA Sequence Homology with R-Ap From H. influenzae	% Relative DNA Sequence Homology with R-Pen^r from N. gonorrhoeae
H. influenzae	1	1
H. influenzae (R-Ap^r, 4.1 x 10^6)	100	96
N. gonorrhoeae	1	1
N. gonorrhoeae (R-Pen^r, Far East)	90	100
N. gonorrhoeae (R-Pen^r, England)	64	70

Relationship between R plasmids of H. influenzae and N. gonorrhoeae. ^{3}H-
plasmid DNA from H. influenzae and N. gonorrhoeae were reacted with DNA isolated from the indicated bacterial strains. The actual extent of binding
between ^{3}H-R-Ap^r plasmid DNA and unlabelled H. influenzae (R-Ap^r) DNA was
70% (taken as 100) and all values normalized to give % relative homology.
The actual extent of binding between ^{3}H-R-Pen^r plasmid DNA and unlabelled
N. gonorrhoeae (R-Pen^r) DNA was 80%.

quent studies revealed that both of these H. influenzae R plasmids possessed
an overall guanine + cytosine (G + C) content of 40%, very much like that of
the H. influenzae chromosome and unlike that of most known enteric R plasmids
/14/. Since R plasmids often possess G + C contents similar to their species
of origin, one might suppose that the transposition of TnA to some indigenous
H. influenzae plasmid had occurred.

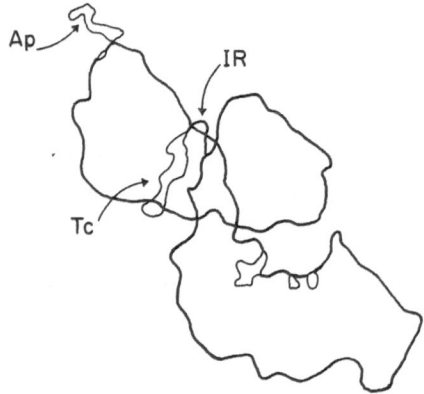

Figure 2. Diagram of heteroduplex molecule formed between H.
influenzae R-plasmids RSF007 (Ap[r]) and pUB701 (Tc[r]). The thick line
represents homologous double-stranded DNA. The thin line represents non-
homologous single-stranded DNA. Ap, ampicillin transposition sequence, TnA.
Tc, tetracycline transposition sequence and its associated inverted-repeated
sequence, IR.

More recently, R plasmids have been identified in H. influenzae which encoded
for tetracycline (Tc) /15/ as well as tetracycline and chloramphenicol (Tc +
Cm) /16/. We have, in collaboration with Jon Saunders, University of Liverpool, England and M. H. Richmond, University of Bristol, England shown that:
1) these resistances are plasmid mediated, 2) these plasmids contain very
similar or identical antibiotic resistance transposition sequences as those
found in enteric species, and 3) that the ampicillin; tetracycline and tetra-
cycline-chloramphenicol R plasmids of H. influenzae all contain a common core
of DNA sequences. Indeed, as illustrated in Figure 2, electron microscope
heteroduplex analysis reveals that Ap and Tc plasmids are virtually identical except for the inserted antibiotic resistance sequences.

While these findings are most in accord with the idea that transposition of
resistance genes have occurred to an indigenous Haemophilus plasmid, there
is no definitive data to differentiate between an alternative explanation,
namely that the R plasmids in H. influenzae represent the direct extension

of a specific incompatibility group of existing R plasmids from another bacterial group. Whatever their source, the data illustrate the ubiquity of the transposable antibiotic resistance elements.

5. R plasmids of the Gonococcus

In the spring and summer of 1976, numerous isolations of penicillin-resistant, β-lactamase-producing Neisseria gonorrhoeae were encountered in U. S. military personnel in the Far East /17/. Shortly, thereafter, a report was published from London /18/ showing the presence of a β-lactamase producing gonococcus from a woman suffering from pelvic inflammatory disease and a report was published from Liverpool /19/ documenting numerous cases of penicillin-resistant gonococcal infection. Representative strains from all of these outbreaks were sent to us by Dr. Clyde Thornesberry, Center for Disease Control, Atlanta, Georgia and we set out to examine these strains for R plasmids.

Fortunately, we had recently developed an agarose gel electrophoresis technique which permitted the rapid identification and partial chracterization of bacterial plasmids /20/. Previous studies /21/, /22/ (Elwell and Falkow, in press) have established that most gonococci harbored an indigenous 2.6×10^6 dalton plasmid while some 5% of gonococci also harbored a 24.5×10^6 dalton plasmid. Examination of the penicillin-resistant gonococci /23/ revealed novel plasmid species, however. Gonococcal isolates from U. S. Military personnel and their sexual contacts possessed a 4.4×10^6 dalton plasmid in addition to the expected indigenous plasmid(s). Examination of the gonococci from London and Liverpool revealed that they possessed a 3.2×10^6 dalton plasmid in addition to the 2.6×10^6 dalton indigenous plasmid, no 24.5×10^6 dalton plasmid has been found to date in any gonococcal isolate received from Great Britain.

It has been possible to transform E. coli (but surprisingly not (gonococci); to Ap^r with isolated plasmid DNA from penicillin resistant gonococci /24/. The transformed E. coli possess a single plasmid species of 4.4×10^6 daltons or 3.2×10^6 daltons depending on the source of transforming plasmid DNA.

Of course, our immediate course of action was to determine whether these gonococcal plasmids possessed TnA. This was found to be the case, although the entire TnA sequence was not found. Rather, very much like that observed for the small Ap^r plasmid of H. influenzae, only about 40% of the TnA sequence was present. Despite their difference in size the 3.2×10^6 dalton and 4.4×10^6 dalton plasmids were highly related when tested in DNA-DNA hybridization studies (Table 2).

When purified R plasmid DNA of gonococci were examined in more detail we discovered that they possessed a G + C content of 40%. In contrast, the indigenous plasmid species and chromosomal DNA of Neisseria have a 50% G + C content /21/. Obviously, the nearly exact coincidence in size, TnA content and G + C between the gonococcal plasmids and the small H. influenzae plasmids led us to examine their possible relationships. As shown in Table 2, the H. influenzae plasmids and the gonococcal R plasmids are highly related.

The fact that two gonococcal R plasmids are closely related to an R plasmid previously characterized in Haemophilus does not necessarily suggest that a Haemophilus species was the direct source. Indeed, it seems more likely that they represent the extension of the enteric R plasmid pool. We suggest that as the gram negative enteric bacilli R plasmid reservoir increased, a particular plasmid species emerged which had the ability to cross a previously invulnerable biological barrier protecting Neisseria and Haemophilus from R plasmid intrusion. It seems of some significance that the β-lactamase plasmids of the gonococcus and the small Haemophilus Ap^r plasmid do not appear to be related to the most common non-conjugative plasmids of enteric species which specify ampicillin resistance. Recent studies from this laboratory by Crosa et al., /25/ have shown that the prototype ampicillin plasmid described by Anderson and Lewis /26/ as well as similar plasmids found in epidemic strains of Shigella dysenteriae, many Salmonellae and E. coli strains are 5.5×10^6 daltons in mass and possess a G + C of 54%. The only common evolutionary thread shared by the plasmids of Neisseria and Haemophilus and the plasmids of the more robust enteric species is the ubiquitous TnA sequences. The gonococcal and the small Haemophilus plasmids possess only a portion of TnA and it is likely these TnA sequences themselves will not be transposable. However, it is this specific feature which may provide a clue to the possible common ancestor(s) of these new, R plasmids.

6. Transfer of Gonococcal R plasmids by Conjugation

While studying the β-lactamase-producing gonococci from the Far East, we noted that they differed in nutritional requirements and in other ways. These findings suggested to us that there had been considerable dissemination of the 4.4×10^6 dalton R plasmid rather than simply the spread of a single ancestral clone. The examination of the total plasmids of Far East strains provided us with an important clue. Whereas the incidence of the 24.5×10^6 dalton indigenous plasmid of N. gonorrhoeae was about 5% in antibiotic-sensitive strains, the incidence of this large indigenous plasmid in Far East strains was on the order of 40%. Was it possible that this large indigenous

123

plasmid might possess sex factor activity and that R plasmid transmission between gonococci might be mediated by conjugation?

By using appropriate mating methods /24/ we found that indeed it was possible to transfer the 4.4×10^6 dalton gonococcal R plasmid from N. gonorrhoeae to other N. gonorrhoeae and even from N. gonorrhoeae to E. coli /24 /. However, successful transfer of the R plasmid was observed only when the donor gonococcal strain possessed the 24.5×10^6 dalton plasmid as well as the R plasmid. Strains from Great Britain do not harbor the 24.5×10^6 dalton plasmid and cannot act as donor strains, nor do strains of Far East origin which lack the 24.5×10^6 dalton plasmid act as donors.

Even though at least one of the R plasmids of gonococci has the capability of being disseminated by conjugation, one of the most important factors in evaluating the possible spread of the gonococcal R plasmids is their intrinsic stability. Under selective conditions of daily passage on antibiotic-containing media no apparent instability was noted over an eight week period. However, if representative clinical isolates were passaged every other day on a non-selective medium for a three week period and then individual clones examined for β-lactamase production or their ability to grow on a penicillin-containing medium, plasmid loss was noted. Clinical isolates carrying the 4.4×10^6 dalton plasmid showed a plasmid loss ranging from 30% to 89%, while clinical isolates carrying 3.2×10^6 dalton plasmid showed a plasmid loss ranging from 36% to 99.9%. It is perhaps of interest that, in general, clinical isolates which contain the 24.5×10^6 dalton conjugative plasmid appear to maintain the R plasmid at a higher level than clinical isolates which do not. This higher level of stability may reflect the reinfection, by mating, of cells which have lost the plasmid. Of course, we have only studied plasmid stability in the laboratory environment and it is not clear if this accurately reflects plasmid stability in nature. Nonetheless, our studies do suggest that in the absence of antibiotic pressure there is a definite tendency for gonococci to lose their R plasmids at a higher frequency than one usually sees with R plasmid-containing enteric species.

Acknowledgement

This work was supported by grant (PCM) 75-14174 from the National Science Foundation, grant AI00191-03 from the National Institute of Allergy and Infectious Diseases and by Contract DADA-72-C-2149 from the U. S. Army Research and Development Command. L. P. Elwell is supported by Public Health Service Grant AI05328-01; Ron Gill is a predoctoral fellow of the National Science Foundation.

Literature

1. Hedges, R. W., Jacob, A.: Transposition of Ampicillin Resistance from RP4 to Other Replicons. Mol. Gen. Genet. 132, 31-40 (1974).

2. Bennett, P. M., Richmond, M. H.: The Transposition of a Discrete Piece of DNA Carrying an Amp Gene Between Replicons in Escherichia coli. J. Bacteriol. 126, 1-6 (1976).

3. Heffron, F., Rubens, C., Falkow, S.: The Translocation of a Plasmid DNA Sequence which Mediates Ampicillin Resistance: Molecular Nature and Specificity of Insertion. Proc. Natl. Acad. Sci. U.S.A. 72, 3623-3627 (1975).

4. Kopecko, D. J., Cohen, S. N.: Site-specific recA⁻ Independent Recombination Between Bacterial Plasmids: Involvement of Palindromes at the Recombinational Loci. Proc. Natl. Acad. Sci. U.S.A. 72, 1373-1377 (1975).

5. Rubens, C., Heffron, F., Falkow, S.: Transposition of a Plasmid Deoxyribonucleic Acid Sequence that Mediates Ampicillin Resistance: Independence from Host rec Functions and Orientation of Insertion. J. Bacteriol. 128, 425-434 (1976).

6. Heffron, F., Sublett, R., Hedges, R., Jacob, A., Falkow, S.: Origin of the TEM Beta-lactamase Gene Found on Plasmids. J. Bacteriol. 122, 250-256 (1975).

7. Matthew, M., Hedges, R. W.: Analytical Isoelectric Focusing of R factor Determined β-lactamases: Correlation with Plasmid Compatibility. J. Bacteriol. 125, 713-718 (1976).

8. Heffron, F., Bedinger, P., Champoux, J. J., Falkow, S.: Deletion Affecting the Transposition of an Antibiotic Resistance Gene. Proc. Natl. Acad. Sci. U.S.A. 74, 702-706 (1977).

9. Kingsbury, D. T., Helinski, D. R.: DNA Polymerase as a Requirement for the Maintenance of the Bacterial Plasmid Colicinogenic Factor E1. Biochem. Biophys. Res. Commun. 41, 1538-1542 (1970).

10. Khan, W., Ross, S., Rodriquez, W., Controri, G., Saz, A. K.: Haemophilus influenzae type b Resistant to Ampicillin. A Report of Two Cases. J. Am. Med. Assoc. 229, 298-301 (1974).

11. Tomek, M. O., Starr, S. E., McGowen, J. E., Terry, P. M., Nakmias, A. J.: Ampicillin-resistant Haemophilus influenzae type b Infection. J. Am. Med. Assoc. 229, 295-297 (1974).

12. Farrar, W. E., O'Dell, N.: β-lactamase Activity in Ampicillin-Resistant Haemophilus influenzae. Antimicrob. Agents Chemother. 6, 625-629 (1974).

13. Elwell, L. P., de Graaff, J., Seibert, D., Falkow, S.: Plasmid-linked Ampicillin Resistance in Haemophilus influenzae, type b. Infec. Immun. 12, 404-410.

14. de Graaff, J., Elwell, L. P., Falkow, S.: Molecular Nature of Two Beta-Lactamase-Specifying Plasmids Isolated from Haemophilus influenzae type b. J. Bacteriol. 126, 439-446 (1976).
15. Dang Van, A., Beith, G., Bouanchaud, D. H.: Résistant Plasmidique à la Tetracycline chez H. influenzae. C. R. Acad. Sci. 280, 1321-1323 (1975).
16. Van Klingeren, J., van Embden, J., Dessens-Kroon, M.: Plasmid-mediated Chloramphenicol Resistance in Haemophilus influenzae. Antimicrob. Agents Chemother. 11, 383-387 (1977).
17. Ashford, W. A., Golash, R. G., Hemming, V. G.: Penicillinase-producing Neisseria gonorrhoeae. Lancet 2, 657-658 (1976).
18. Phillips, I.: Beta-Lactamase-Producing Penicillin-Resistant Gonococcus. Lancet 2, 656-657 (1976).
19. Percival, A., Corkill, J., Aryo, O., Rowlands, J., Alergant, C., Ross, E.: Penicillinase-Producing Gonococci in Liverpool. Lancet 2, 1379-1382 (1976).
20. Meyers, J., Sanchez, D., Elwell, L. P., Falkow, S.: A Simple Agarose Gel Electrophoretic Method for the Identification and Characterization of Plasmid Deoxyribonucleic Acid. J. Bacteriol. 127, 1529-1537 (1976).
21. Mayer, L. W., Holmes, K. K., Falkow, S.: Characterization of Plasmid Deoxyribonucleic Acid from Neisseria gonorrhoeae. Infect. Immun. 10, 712-717 (1974).
22. Stiffler, P. W., Lerner, S. A., Bohnhoff, M., Morello, J. A.: Plasmid Deoxyribonucleic Acid in Clinical Isolates of Neisseria gonorrhoeae. J. Bacteriol. 122, 1293-1300 (1975).
23. Elwell, L. P., Roberts, M., Mayer, L. W., Falkow, S.: Plasmid Mediated Beta-Lactamase Production in Neisseria gonorrhoeae. Antimicrob. Agents Chemother. 11, 528-533 (1977).
24. Roberts, M., Falkow, S.: Conjugal Transfer of R Plasmids in Neisseria gonorrhoeae. Nature 226, 630-631 (1977).
25. Crosa, J. H., Olarte, J., Mata, L. S., Luttropp, L. K., Penaranda, M. E.: Characterization of an R Plasmid Associated with Ampicillin Resistance in Shigella dysenteriae type 1 Strains Isolated in Epidemics. Antimicrob. Agents Chemother. 11, 553-558 (1977).
26. Anderson, E. S., Lewis, M. S.: Characterization of a Transfer Factor Associated with Drug Resistance in Salmonella typhimurium. Nature 208, 843-845 (1965).

Discussion

Anderson: One obvious thing which one might want to know regarding these new plasmids is whether there is a relationship between those isolated from gonococci and haemophilus and those harboured by the enterobacteriacae. We have already an indication that this is the case. The other interesting feature is the different stability of the plasmids. In one instance (3.2×10^6 dalton R-plasmid) it seems pretty unstable unless it is made stable by pressure and the other (4.2×10^6 dalton R-plasmid) seems to achieve a steady state of about 50%. What is going to be the outcome? Are we going to end up with organisms that are stiff with resistance? I understand that vigorous epidemiological action has shown some signs of containment. I am also interested whether in the meningococci plasmids have been found.

Falkow: Meningococci have no indigenous plasmids. Because of the close relationship of these two organisms I think the meningococcus will eventually end up with a plasmid carrying ampicillin resistance.

Anderson: You have not tried to do any conjugational experiments?

Falkow: No.

Humphreys: The fact that some of the strains you have gotten from the Far East have got the transfer factor and some had not, brings up the question whether they are all the same auxotypes or not.

Falkow: No, they are not all the same auxotype. It is interesting that all the strains which we received from Great Britain required arginine while those from the Far East are of different auxotypes. Some Far East strains do have a large plasmid and some don't. The absence of the large plasmid may be one of the reasons that the strains are more easily controlled in Great Britain than the strains from the Far East and USA, aside from the fact that we handle the disease differently in the United States than in Great Britain.

Humphreys: Another question I want to ask you: is there any indication of a rescue of the penicillin resistance gene by the chromosome in the case of the instable situation which you mentioned or is it always lost completely?

Falkow: I don't think we have studied it enough in order to be able to say so. We have concentrated more on the strains from the Far East than on those from Great Britain. Our impression is that gonococcal R-plasmids isolated late in the Liverpool outbreak were more stable than those isolated earlier.

Davies: Why did it take such a long time for the resistance plasmids to get into haemophilus?

Falkow: Well, obviously one does not know. But if there is continual selection for a large reservoir for R-factors in nonpathogenic bacteria, sooner or later there will be a spill-over into pathogenic bacteria. It probably took a long time for the evolution of a plasmid that could bridge the genetic barrier. In the cases where TnA has been showing up in both haemophilus and gonococcus, one would have thought that the whole length of the TnA would be there. The question is: why isn't that so? In relation to our map of TnA (Fig. 1), part of the inverted repeat is preserved and the Bam-site seems to be always preserved in haemophilus and gonococcus R-plasmids.

Starlinger: I have a question to all three speakers: Do you know why, in the light of all these mechanisms, these resistance mechanisms are always confined to plasmids?

Falkow: Well, in one strain of haemophilus that has been described by Jon Saunders it appears the tetracycline transposon is in the chromosome. And then H. Williams Smith has described a naturally occurring phage that carries TnA. I would not be surprised if, in many instances, a strain possesses TnA on a plasmid and in the chromosome as well. I don't know whether this would or would not be the case. I don't think we have looked at enough strains.

Bennett: Could we extend this question by asking why resistance elements are not accumulating on the chromosome? Why are they actually maintained in plasmids where they can be lost?

Falkow: Well, there may be some advantage in "being" extrachromosomal.

Starlinger: Couldn't we ask the question the other way around? Why aren't there chromosomal genes found more often on plasmids?

Falkow: Well, I think one does. Plasmids that give the ability to ferment lactose, are found at an increasing rate.

Starlinger: Do you think that this is something that is occurring naturally with a high frequency?

Falkow: I don't think it has been looked at in enough detail. We have done some experiments with K 88. These are the first experiments which contradict the notion that plasmid mobilisation occurs without the formation of a covalent linkage, as in the early experiments by Dr. Anderson. We have found that the K 88 is part of the plasmid about 50 megadaltons which is nonconjugative but can be mobilised. After mobilisation to K 12 it forms, with a 40 megadalton transmissible plasmid, a new plasmid which is 90 megadalton in size. In a new host it dissociates into its components and we believe that this is some sort of transpositional or complex recombinational event.

Levy: I think one of the reasons that argue against the insertion into the chromosome is that these transposable elements cause mutations and deletions and, unless the site where they insert is fairly stable, one would have a natural selection against transposition into the chromosome.

Falkow: Don't forget the data that Dr. Anderson was presenting this morning. The plasmids of medical importance are epidemic plasmids, often clones. You see, insertions may be happening to plasmids all the time. Sometimes it's good, sometimes it's bad, but one does see the emergence of distinctive kinds of plasmids like the small nonconjugative plasmid which codes for the TEM β-lactamase. It is an extraordinarily common plasmid. If one collects a number of small Ap^r plasmids from all over the world, they are mostly all the same. Also many staphylococcal plasmids are often the same. Also in haemophilus one sees that the different R-plasmids are really a variation of the same theme. It's not just a matter of inserting a resistance determinant in any kind of transfer factor and the generation of an instant R-factor; rather there is going to be the slow evolution for rather special ones.

Levy: No, my point was: why do we so often find resistance genes on plasmids and not more often on the chromosome?

Falkow: Well, I don't think anybody can answer that question.

Richmond: You can turn things on its head and say that one may consider it an evolutionary advantage if, in the presence of selection pressure, a bacterial population becomes decimated except for just one plasmid carrying cell.

Falkow: The probability of a 'special' plasmid evolving 20 years ago was less than it is now. We are dealing with probabilities now which involves many more resistant organisms. Yet these are really low frequency events. In theory no plasmid coding for TEM ß-lactamase should ever have occurred in gonococcus because if it occurred as a single event, it should have been killed by ordinary therapeutic doses of penicillin. It was a very low probability event. But it happened. People in the Far East were taking subtherapeutic amounts of ampicillin and that selected out these strains.

Richmond: What about the ampicillin resistant gonococci from other places like Hongkong?

Falkow: They may be clones of the same plasmid. In the older literature, there are papers from the late sixties that may indicate that the strain now commonly found in Great Britain was prevalent in parts of Africa. This strain may have evolved some time ago. We are trying to get hold of these early strains - if anybody still has them.

Properties of DNA Insertion Elements of E. coli

Heinz Saedler and **Debabrota Ghosal**

The presence of IS elements in the chromosome of E.coli was
originally revealed by the transposition of these DNA elements
from their natural positions into indicator systems, resulting
in a recognizable mutant phenotype. If, for example, the gal
operon is used as an indicator system, mutations can be isolated in which not only one of the three structural genes of the
galactose operon is inactivated, but the expression of the promoter distal genes is also abolished. These mutations therefore
are strongly polar. The analysis of the nature of such mutations
is facilitated by the existence of the gal transducing phage λ
and the development of techniques for examining heteroduplex
DNA in the electron microscope. With the help of these tools
it is possible to inspect hybrid DNA molecules consisting of
one DNA strand carrying the strongly polar mutation and a complementary strand of λ dgal in the electron microscope. The strongly
polar mutation is seen as a single stranded DNA loop emerging
from a position of the double stranded heteroduplex molecule,
which corresponds to the map position of the mutation. Analysing
various independently isolated strongly polar mutations with
the above technique, revealed the existence of different categories of IS elements. The elements were numbered according to
the sequence of their detection. IS1 is about 800 nucleotide
pairs long, while IS2, IS3, IS4 and IS5 are each approximately
1400 basepairs long. For review see Starlinger and Saedler, 1976.
In the following paragraphs we will concentrate on the topics
listed below.

A) Detection of mini insertion DNA elements (D. Ghosal and H.
   Saedler, manuscript in preparation).

B) IS elements are natural components of the E.coli chromosome
   (Saedler and Heiss 1973; I. Chow 1977; Deonier and Hadley
   1976).
C) Chromosomal rearrangements mediated by IS1 (Reif and Saedler
   1975, 1977, Nevers, Reif and Saedler 1977).
D) IS elements are also found in strategical positions on certain
   plasmids (Hu et al., 1975).

A) Detection of Mini Insertion DNA Elements

The detection of IS elements using the heteroduplex technique
is limited to certain sizes of integrated DNA elements. If the
size of an IS element is an order of magnitude smaller than for
example IS1 through IS5 the heteroduplex technique is not sensitive enough to reveal the presence of such small insertions. To
analyse these mutations another technique seems to be more ade-
quate. If suitable restriction fragments are available from a
gene carrying and not carrying an integrated IS element, electrophoresis of these fragments in agarose or polyacrylamide gels
will show the difference in molecular weight due to the integrated IS element. We subjected DNA fragments of two mutants
we had genetic reason to believe that there were due to the
integration of DNA, to gel electrophoresis. Figure 1 gives the
pattern of a HindII, HindIII double digest of various plasmid
DNAs. Slot 3 shows the pattern of the parental plasmid pDG1,
which is gal positive. Slot 4 gives the pattern of pDG12, in
which an IS2 is integrated in the control region of the gal
operon, thus a cell carrying this plasmid has a gal negative
phenotype. Note the appearance of two new bands (e and f) and
the shift in molecular weight of one band (from a to b), due to
the integration of IS2. Slots 1 and 5 show the pattern of two
independent gal positive revertants obtained from plasmid pDG12.
Note the increase in molecular weight of only band e in both
mutants. This can only be interpreted if an insertion has occurred
in band e thus not affecting other bands. Using the markers
(slot 2) as references, the increase in molecular weight can
be calculated. Mutation 1 (slot 5) is due to the integration of
about a 115 basepair long piece of DNA, while the other mutation (slot 1) is about a 60 basepair insertion. The former is
given the name IS6 and the latter is termed IS7.

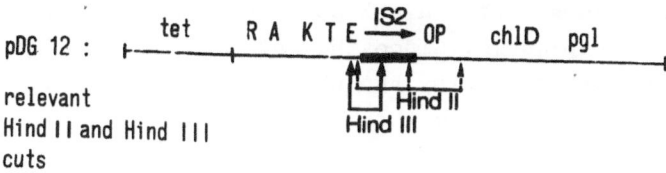

pDG 12 :

relevant
Hind II and Hind III
cuts

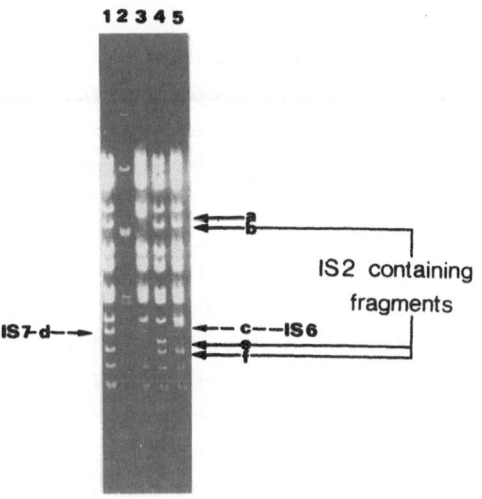

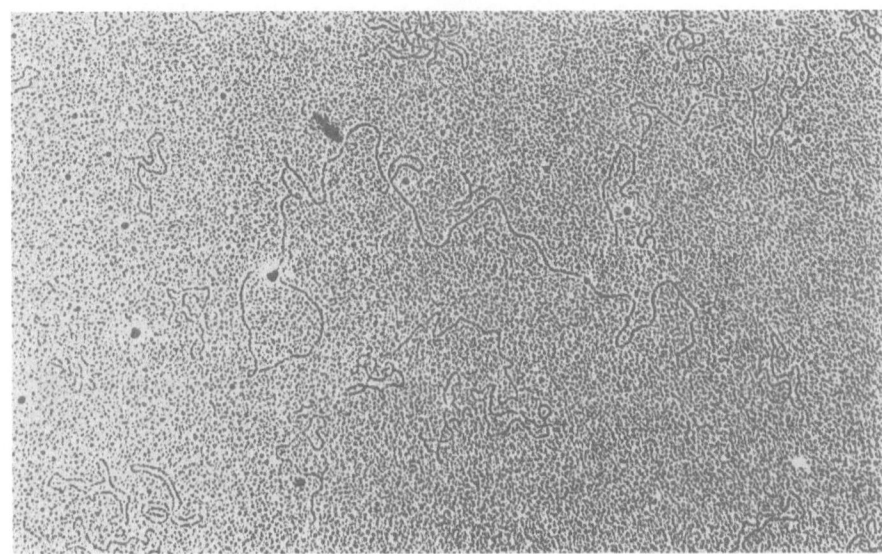

Fig. 1: Identification of the mini insertions IS6 and IS7

Both insertions confer a gal positive phenotype to the cell
carrying the plasmid. Since they seem to have integrated into
IS2, they either destroy the polar signal on IS2 or, what is
more likely, they carry their own turn on signal.

B) IS Elements Are Natural Components of the E.coli Chromsome

Some years ago we showed by DNA-DNA hybridization that at least
IS1 and IS2 are natural components of the E.coli chromosome,
where they occur in multiple copies. We found about 8 copies of
IS1 and about 5 copies of IS2 per chromosome (Saedler and Heiss
1973).

The accurate positions of the various copies in the chromosome
and their orientation are unknown, but in principle they either
can occur in direct or inverted orientations. The latter can be
seen in the electron microscope. If two copies of identical
DNA sequences occur in the chromosome in inverted orientations
they should hybridize with each other forming a double stranded
DNA stem in a single stranded DNA loop. The size of the stem is
indicative for the IS-element involved and the lengths of the
loop is a measure for the distance between the duplication genetic material. Figure 2 shows 3 different examples of this kind.
The stem in the right hand picture is of the size of IS1, and
the loop is about 22 kilobase pairs long. The stem in the middle
picture is equal to the size of IS2, IS3, IS4 or IS5. The loop
is about 120 kilobase pair long. In the left molecule multiple
interactions are seen with lengths varying from 100 to 300
basepairs. The smaller ones might correspond to IS6.

However, none of these stems has been proven to be homologous
to one of the known IS-elements. A more detailed analysis using
this technique has been done by Chow (1977), and Deonier and
Hadley (1976) showing that the stems and the loops fall into
discrete size classes. This could indicate that the multiple
copies of IS-elements are not distributed randomly in the E.coli
chromosome.

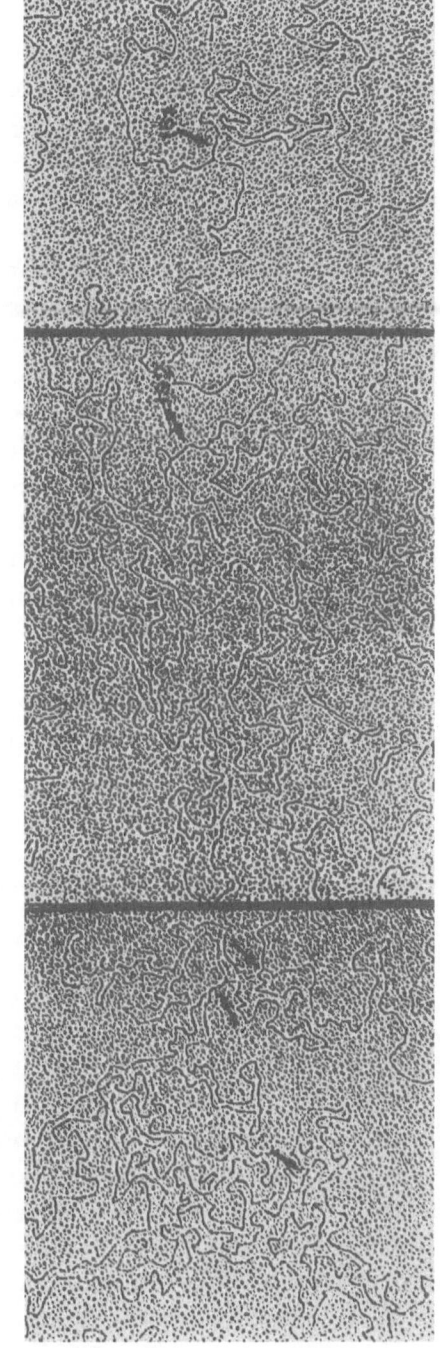

Fig. 2: Duplication of genetic material in the chromosome of E. coli K 12

C) Chromosomal Rearrangements Mediated by IS1

The formation of new chromosomal sequences can result from
translocation, duplication, inversion or deletion of genetic
material. All these events seem to play a role in the evolution
of plasmids as well as chromosomes. IS-elements seem to be
responsible for such chromosomal rearrangements.

Non-adjacent chromosomal regions can be brought together by
deletion of the intermittent genetic material, resulting in a
new chromosomal order. This reaction has been studied extensively in IS1 induced deletion formation (Reif and Saedler, 1975,
1977). The termini of the integrated IS1 elements are most important in this process. IS1 is retained in the deletion, thus
allowing further rounds of rearrangements. It is not yet clear,
however, which enzymes are involved in this rather unusual type
of recombination. Apparently the normal recombination pathways
of E.coli are not involved. However, recently a mutant was
isolated, which is deficient in IS1 induced deletion formation.
Such mutants may be helpful in the analysis of the enzymes involved in illegitimate recombinational events. IS1 can be
considered as a generator for deletions (Nevers and Saedler,
1976).

D) IS Elements Are Also Found in Structural Positions on Certain
    R-Factors

The R-factors of the fi$^+$ class are composed of two units, each
capable of replicating autonomously if dissociated from each
other. The RTF unit codes all functions necessary for cell to
cell contact, thus allowing the transfer of the plasmid. The
r-determinant carries most of the antibiotic resistance genes.
An IS1-element separates the RTF unit from the r-determinant
at each junction. Both IS1 elements are oriented in the same
direction (Hu et al., 1975, Ptashne and Cohen, 1975). This
finding suggests a model to explain the formation and dissociation of R-factors as well as the amplification of the antibiotic resistance genes. Rownd and Mickel 1971 showed that
R-factors can dissociate into the RTF and the r-determinant

in Proteus mirabilis.Dissociation may occur by recombination between the two homologous IS1 substrates of the co-integrate plasmid generating two units each containing an IS1. Fusion results from the reverse reaction. Amplification of antibiotic resistance genes might be due to recombination between the homologous IS1 elements of different r-determinant molecules leading to integrate plasmid with repeated r-determinant units.

In addition to IS1 other IS-elements are also observed on R-factors, either as mutations or as integral parts of the molecule. For example in R6 or R 100-1 IS2 is found at a position within the transfer genes, where it does not cause a transfer defective mutation but rather contributes to the transfer positive character of the plasmids (Hu et al., 1975). IS3 on the other hand is seen to border the tetracycline gene in inverted orientation (Ptashne and Cohen, 1975). Many of the antibiotic resistance genes, including tetracycline, can transpose to the various other DNA molecules (Cohen and Kopecko, 1976).

In the evolution of R-plasmids IS-elements, therefore, seem to play an important role.

Conclusions

IS elements are natural components of the E.coli chromosome. They can translocate from one position in the chromosome to another. Besides stimulating a number of illegitimate recombinational events, like deletion and transposition of other genes, which are considered to be important in evolution, they also carry signals necessary for gene expression (Saedler et al., 1974). Similar events are also known to occur in higher organisms. (Nevers and Saedler, manuscript in preparation).

References

1. Chow,L.T.: in DNA Insertion Elements, Plasmids and Episomes (edit. by Bukhari, A.I., Shapiro, J. and Adhya, S.)(Cold Spring Harbor Laboratory New York) in the press.
2. Cohen, S.N., Kopecko, D.J.: Structural Evolution of Bacterial Plasmids: Role of Translocating Genetic Elements and DNA Sequence Insertions, Federation Proceedings 35, 2031 (1976)

3. Deonier, R.C., Hadley, R.G.: Distribution of Inverted IS
   Length Sequences in the E.coli K-12 Genome. Nature 264, 191
   (1976).

4. Hu, S., Ohtsubo, E., Davidson, N., Saedler, H.: Electron
   Microscope Heteroduplex Studies of Sequence Relations Among
   Bacterial Plasmids. XII. Identification and Mapping of Insertion. Sequences IS1 and IS2 in F and R plasmids. J. Bacteriol.
   122, 764 (1975).

5. Nevers, P., Reif, H.J., Saedler, H.: A Mutant of E.coli Defective in IS1 Mediated Deletion Formation. DNA Insertion Elements
   Plasmids and Episomes (edit. by Bukhari, A.I., Shapiro, J.,
   and Adhya, S.) (Cold Spring Harbor Laboratory, New York, in
   press).

6. Ptashne, K., Cohen, S.N.: Occurrence of Insertion Sequence (IS)
   Regions on Plasmid Deoxyribonucleic Acid as Direct and Inverted Nucleotide Sequence Duplications. J. Bacteriol. 122, 776
   (1975).

7. Reif, H.J., Saedler, H.: IS1 is Involved in Deletion Formation
   in the gal Region of E.coli K-12. Molec. Gen. Genetics 137
   17 (1975)

8. Reif, H.J., Saedler, H.: Chromosomal Rearrangements in the
   gal Region of E.coli K-12 after Integration of IS1. In: DNA
   Insertion Elements, Plasmids and Episomes (edit. by Bukhari,
   A.I., Shapiro, J., and Adhya, S.) (Cold Spring Harbor Laboratory New York) (in the press).

9. Rownd, R., Mickel, S.: Dissociation of RTF and r-Determinants
   of the R-Factor NR1 in Proteus mirabilis. Nature New Biol.
   234, 40 (1971)

10. Saedler, H., Heiß, B.: Multiple Copies of the Insertion-DNA
    Sequences IS1 and IS2 in the Chromosome of E.coli K-12. Molec.
    Gen. Genetics 122, 267 (1973).

11. Saedler, H., Reif, H.J., Hu, S., Davidson, N.: IS2, a Genetic
    Element for Turn-Off and Turn-On of Gene Activity in E.coli.
    Molec. Gen. Genetics 132, 265 (1974).

12. Starlinger, P., Saedler, H.: IS-Elements in Microorganisms
    Current Topics in Microbiology and Immunology 75, 111 (1976).

Discussion

Falkow: Are the properties of the ß-galactosidase transposon identical with those of K-12? Are they constitutive?

Saedler: They are clearly inducible. There is a difference between the RP 1 lac hybrid and the original pGC1 with respect to the inducibility by a factor of approx. 4. Structurally, they are completely homologous.

Davies: Are you suggesting that a gene in Escherichia coli is producing deletions?

Saedler: I think so. However, since we have not knocked out the deletion forming activity completely in our del-mutant, there might be an additional mechanism also generating these deletions.

Bennett: When you take your derivative that has the epimerase gene embraced by two to IS-1s and you look for derivatives that have lost galE by exact excisions of this structure, do you rescue the epimerase gene in all cases? You said you end up with pro⁻ which is about 30 %. What happens to the other 70 %?

Saedler: We have not looked at at it. I should mention that we are using an artificially constructed transposon, which contains nothing else but galE flanked by the IS1 sequence in direct orientations.

Anderson: Perhaps you could speculate on the evolutionary significance of transposons.

Saedler: There are actually very few data available on the distribution of IS sequences in prokaryotes. The species which have been investigated all contain IS sequences. The species include salmonella, citrobacter, shigella and Bacillus subtilis. These bacteria all contain IS1 but, e.g. already salmonella and citrobacter do not contain IS2 sequences. It might be that these elements are natural components of the chromosome. In those bacteria that don't have them, these sequences may be introduced by plasmids and then later on they could have incorporated them into their genome.

Richmond: Sorry, did you look for them in gram-positives?

Saedler: No, we didn't.

Davies: The Yersinia-coli cross did not take place at 37°C but it would take place at 30°C.

Saedler: Yes, this pGC1 system is temperature-sensitive with respect to transfer.

Levy: The H2 is a temperature sensitive transfer plasmid.

Anderson: Sorry, which H2 plasmid are you talking about, because we have a group of plasmids called H2 which are temperature-sensitive.

Answer by both Levy and Saedler: Yes, this plasmid belongs to this group.

Saedler: I should mention that the incompatibility group of that plasmid has not been tested. Plating behaviour of T5 and T7 phages indicate it is related.

Studies on IS DNA

J. Besemer, H. Chadwell, P. Habermann, D. Kubai-Maroni, D. Pfeifer,
F. Schmidt, and P. Starlinger

IS-elements are unique, transposable DNA sequences lacking a
trans-acting phenotype. They are detectable by the effects they
exert in the cis position on adjacent genes at sites to which
they are transposed by a rare illegitimate recombination event.
These effects include mutation (of a gene, into which the IS-
element is integrated), polar effects (of genes located distal to the IS-element, but in the same transcription unit),
initiation of transcription of a silent gene (if an IS-element
carrying a promoter is integrated in front of a gene that has
lost its own promoter) and an increase in the frequency of a
variety of chromosomal aberrations occurring in the vicinity
of IS-elements. IS-elements play a role in the integration of
plasmids into chromosomes (e.g. in the formation of Hfr strains
by the integration of the F-plasmid) and some of them have
been identified as part of transposons (= transposable DNA
sequences carrying one or more genes, most of them coding for
resistance to an antibiotic, and usually bordered by a DNA
sequence, repeated at the end of the transposon directly or
in inverted form). This repeated sequence has been identified
as an IS-element in some cases. The properties of IS-elements
have been reviewed in more detail elsewhere (1,2,3,4).

IS-elements were first detected by genetic methods. Early attempts to visualize them physically included demonstration of
an increase of buoyant density of bacteriophage carrying an
IS-element in its DNA (5,6), hybridization of RNA transcribed
from DNA carrying an IS-element to DNA preparations with or
without this IS-element (7), and inspection with the electron

microscope of DNA heteroduplexes prepared from DNA molecules
with or without IS-elements (8).

A technique, originally used in the preparation of pure lac
operon DNA (9) could be applied in those cases, where two mutant phages carried the same IS-element, but in opposite orientations. In these cases, hybridization of identical rather than
complementary DNA strands of the two phages produced molecules
that were double-stranded in the region of the IS-element, and
single-stranded everywhere else.

Using these techniques, it could be shown that a limited number
of IS-elements are found in a number of unrelated genes of
E. coli and its phage λ (lo,11).

Initial studies, in which all mutations caused by the integration of IS-elements were looked at indiscriminately, gave the
impression that these elements integrated at many sites with
equal or, at least, similar probabilities (12). The picture
became more complicated when the integration properties of
single IS-elements were investigated. It now appears that
different IS-elements have different integration properties.
This can be illustrated by reference to the gal operon of
E. coli. IS1 has been found in several locations both in the
leader sequence and in the second gene of this operon, galT
(the first and third gene of the operon were not investigated
in detail for technical reasons) (lo,11). IS2 has so far only
been found in the leader sequence (lo,11), and IS4 has been
detected at a single site in galT, which also serves as an
unusual integration site for bacteriophage λ (11,13,14,15).

Several independent isolates containing IS1 and IS2 in the
leader sequence of the operon have been described, and all of
them seem to occur at the same site, as no wildtype recombinants between them can be detected in genetic crosses. Also
heteroduplex molecules prepared from the DNA of several pairs
of these mutants show substitution loops instead of two inser-
tion/deletion loops separated by a short double-stranded region. IS1 is found at this site in both possible orientations,
and IS2 is found in only one orientation (8,lo,14).

IS4 has been found repeatedly in both orientations, within galT. By the same criteria that were used in the preceding paragraph, all mutants appear to be at one single site (13).

DNA sequence analysis was employed in order to see, whether the IS-elements found in these clusters were in fact integrated at a single site, as this method gives better resolution than genetic crosses or heteroduplex analysis.

These studies made use of pure IS DNA isolated from heteroduplex molecules, in which only the IS-elements were in double-stranded form, as described above. The heteroduplex molecules were digested with single-strand specific endonuclease S1, and the IS DNA was purified from contaminating DNA fragments by sucrose gradient centrifugation or polyacrylamide gel electrophoresis (16).

The IS DNA was hybridized to purified single-stranded DNA from different λ dgal phages carrying independent IS-caused mutations in the leader sequence of the gal operon. The IS DNA served as a primer for elongation with DNA polymerase I under ribosubstitution conditions (17). The elongated material was digested by S1, and the double-stranded material containing the elongated primer was purified by gel electrophoresis, digested by pancreatic RNase, and fingerprinted (18).

This procedure, when applied to templates carrying different IS-elements in identical or closely spaced positions, should give largely identical fingerprints. Only the newly synthesized oligonucleotide immediately adjacent to the primer should be different with different mutant templates, if the IS-elements were at slightly different sites. These oligonucleotides could be released from the primer, if the latter was digested with high concentrations of S1 endonuclease. This treatment removed 3'-terminal dC from the IS1 primer which was replaced by rC during the elongation reaction.

Using this method, it could be shown that at least three different sites in the leader sequence of the gal operon are used for the integration of IS1, and that IS2 is almost certainly at a fourth site, the exact position of which has yet to be

determined, but which is closer to the promoter, than the
IS1 sites. The distance between the sites, at which IS1 is integrated, are, in one case, as small as 3 nucleotides.

We do not yet know the mechanism of integration of IS-elements.
Our experiments exclude a mechanism, in which integration occurs
via recombination within a short region of homology shared by
the IS-element and its recipient DNA. If such a homology region
were involved, every integrated IS-element would be flanked
by a direct repeat of this region. This repeated homology region would be isolated along with the IS-element in our isolation procedure.

Hybridization of a primer consisting of the IS-element and its
flanking homology regions to an integrated IS-element which is
also flanked by these regions of homology will yield the same
adjacent oligonucleotides in an elongation reaction, regardless of the site, at which the recombination event between
the IS-element and the recipient DNA has occurred in the integration process. Therefore, the presence of different sequences adjacent to independently integrated IS-elements cannot
be explained by this model.

The clustering of IS-integration sites could be explained by
assuming a common recognition site for an integration enzyme,
which would then allow the integration to occur at different
sites in its vicinity. An analogous situation has been observed in the case of restriction enzymes of class I. These enzymes are able to recognize very specifically sites on their
substrate DNA molecules. These sites, however, are not cleavage sites. Cleavage occurs at a variety of sites both to the
right and to the left of the recognition site (19). It is
conceivable that similar mechanisms are operative in the first
steps of IS-integration.

This work was supported by Deutsche Forschungsgemeinschaft
through SFB 74.

Literatur

1. Starlinger, P., Saedler, H. IS-elements in microorganisms.
   Current Topics in Microbiol. and Immunol. 75, 111 (1976)

2. Starlinger, P. Transposable elements of DNA. In: Genetic Engineering, ed. A.M. Chakrabarty, in press

3. Davidson, N., Deonier, R.C., Ohtsubo, E. The DNA sequence organization of F and F-primes and the sequences involved in Hfr formation. In: Microbiology (D. Schlessinger, ed.) 1974, American Society for Microbiol. Washington D.C. p. 56, 1975

4. Cohen, S.N. Transposable genetic elements and plasmid evolution. Nature 263, 731 (1976)

5. Jordan, E., Saedler, H., Starlinger, P. O^O- and strong polar mutations in the gal operon are insertions. Molec. Gen.Genet. 1o2, 353 (1968)

6. Shapiro, J.A. Mutations caused by the insertion of genetic material into the galactose operon of Escherichia coli. J.Mol.Biol. 4o, 93 (1969)

7. Michaelis, G., Saedler, H., Venkov, P., Starlinger, P. Two insertions in the galactose operon having different sizes but homologous DNA sequences. Molec.Gen.Genet. 1o4, 371 (1969)

8. Hirsch, H.J., Saedler, H., Starlinger, P. Insertion mutations in the control region of the galactose operon of E. coli. II. Physical characterization of the mutations. Molec.Gen.Genet. 115, 266 (1972)

9. Shapiro, J.A., MacHattie, L., Eron, L., Ippen, K., Beckwith, J. Isolation of pure lac operon DNA. Nature (Lond) 224, 768 (1969)

1o. Hirsch, H.J., Starlinger, P., Brachet, P. Two kinds of insertions in bacterial genes. Molec.Gen.Genet. 119, 191 (1972)

11. Fiandt, M., Szybalski, W., Malamy, M.H. Polar mutations in lac, gal and phage λ consist of a few DNA sequences inserted with either orientation. Molec.Gen.Genet. 119, 223 (1972)

12. Jordan, E., Saedler, H., Starlinger, P. Strong polar mutations in the transferase gene of the galactose operon in E. coli. Molec.Gen.Genet. 1oo, 296 (1976)

13. Pfeifer, D., Kubai-Maroni, D., Habermann, P. Specific
    sites for integration of IS-elements within the trans-
    ferase gene of the galactose operon of E. coli. In: DNA
    insertions, plasmids and episomes, eds. A. Bukhari,
    J. Shapiro, S. Adhya, New York, Cold Spring Harbor
    Laboratory

14. Shapiro, J.A., Adhya, S.L. The galactose operon of E. coli
    K-12. II. A deletion analysis of operon structure and
    polarity. Genetics 62, 249 (1969)

15. Shimada, K., Weissberg, R.A., Gottesman, M.E. Prophage
    lambda at unusual chromosomal locations. II. Mutations
    induced by bacteriophage lambda in Escherichia coli K12.
    J.Mol.Biol. 8o, 297 (1973)

16. Schmidt, F., Besemer, J., Starlinger, P. The isolation of
    IS1 and IS2 DNA. Molec.Gen.Genet. 145, 145 (1976)

17. Sanger, F., Donelson, J.E., Coulson, A.R., Kössel, H.,
    Fischer, D. Determination of a nucleotide sequence in
    bacteriophage f1 DNA by primed synthesis with DNA poly-
    merase. J.Mol.Biol. 9o, 315 (1974)

18. Brownlee, G.G., Sanger, F. Chromatography of ^{32}P-labelled
    oligonucleotides on thin layers of DEAE-cellulose. Eur.
    J.Biochem. 11, 395 (1969)

19. Horiuchi, K., Zinder, N.D. Cleavage of bacteriophage f1
    DNA by the restriction enzyme of Escherichia coli B.
    Proc.nat.Acad.Sci. (USA) 69, 322o (1972)

Discussion

<u>Saedler</u>: What do you think about the integration site of IS 4? Is that similar to the IS 1s in the control region? Are they spaced rather than being at an identical site?

<u>Starlinger</u>: We have isolated IS 4 and hope to do the same experiments with it as we did with IS 1 in the control region. There is no reason to believe, that all IS-elements will behave identically with regard to integration. Several laboratories have observed with TnA that integration sites are clustered in some regions on plasmid DNA molecules. The distance between the integration sites may be larger than in the case of IS 1 in the leader sequence of gal. Stan Cohen also mentioned the analogy of this behaviour to restriction enzymes of class I.

<u>Davies</u>: IS 4 has only been found in one place. Is there no experiment by which one can introduce IS 4 into a cell and ask whether you can generate mutants from that?

<u>Starlinger</u>: The question you would have to ask is whether there is an increase in the rate of insertion caused mutations over the natural rate.

<u>Davies</u>: That's right.

<u>Starlinger</u>: We could do this experiment in cells that do not contain IS 4 in another place in the chromosome. Whether there are such strains, will first have to be found out.

II. Molecular and Biochemical Aspects

a) **Phenotypic Effects of R-Factor Genes**

The Coding of Small RNA Molecules by the Resistance Factor R 1

Gregor Högenauer, Gabriella Hartmann, and Christine Ruf

The genetic and evolutionary origin of the resistance determinants of
R-factors is unknown. The genes which code for the synthesis of resistance functions are expressed in different bacterial hosts at high
levels. This could mean that the transcriptional and translational
machinery of bacterial species is a priori capable of efficiently
expressing genes which may have evolved in other organisms. Alternatively, the rate at which the foreign genes are expressed in bacteria
may depend on the complementation of the chromosomally coded protein
synthesis system of the host with components coded for by the R-factor.
One type of molecule that may have to be supplied by the R-factor in
order to promote optimal translation of its genes might be tRNA because the tRNA composition is in a given species probably related to
the overall spectrum of DNA code words.

The idea of a modified translation system was tested in a series of
experiments using the hybridization technique. If R-factors would
code for different tRNA molecules their presence should be demonstrable by specific attachment to complementary regions on plasmid
DNA while tRNA from a sensitive, isogenic strain which contains exclusively chromosomally coded tRNA would be expected to show no such
binding. For these studies the R-factor R1 was chosen because it is
one of the larger plasmids and can, therefore, accomodate a large
number of genes on its DNA. It also contains multiple resistance determinants, some of which may have originated in different organisms.
Another reason for choosing this R-factor was the fact that it is
genetically well characterized.

Hybridization Experiments

The RNA of an E. coli J5 strain containing this R-factor, was extracted in parallel with its R⁻ strain, after growing these bacteria in a nutrient containing radioactive phosphate. It was separated
from the large ribosomal RNA by chromatography on DEAE-cellulose and
subsequently purified by electrophoresis on polyacrylamide gels. Both
the 4S and 5S RNA bands were cut out. After elution from the gels the
RNA was hybridized in the presence of formamide at $37^{\circ}C$ (1) to the
DNA immobilized on the nitrocellulose filters.

The potential of these RNA fractions to hybridize was first tested
by assays using the filter discs which were loaded with chromosomal
DNA (2). The result was in accord with the values published in the
literature. If R-factor DNA was used in subsequent experiments a component of the 4S fraction, which was isolated from the R⁺ strain and
contains all the tRNAs was found to hybridize to the filters. Under
the same conditions the 4S RNA from the R⁻ strain bound only slightly
to the DNA. The extent of hybridization was shown to depend on the
concentration of ^{32}P-tRNA in the reaction mixture (Fig. 1). This hybridization of radioactive tRNA from the R⁺ strain could be reduced
in a competition experiment by adding nonradioactive tRNA from the
resistant strain to the assay mixture. (Data not shown). In contrast,
commercial nonradioactive E.coli tRNA or tRNA isolated from the isogenic R⁻ strain did not effectively compete with the tRNA from the
resistant organism in its hybridization to the plasmid DNA. The small
extent of binding shown by the tRNA from the sensitive organism was
completely eliminated in a similar competition experiment by adding
nonradioactive tRNA from normal E. coli cells (Fig. 2). These experiments clearly show that in the 4S RNA fraction of an E. coli
containing R 1 there are components which in a very specific way
recognize nucleotide sequences on the R-factor DNA and are in all
probability coded for by these segments of the plasmid DNA. The
picture, however, becomes more complex if the hybridization experiments
are done at a higher temperature in the absence of formamide. In this
system the extent of hybridization with the tRNA extracted from the

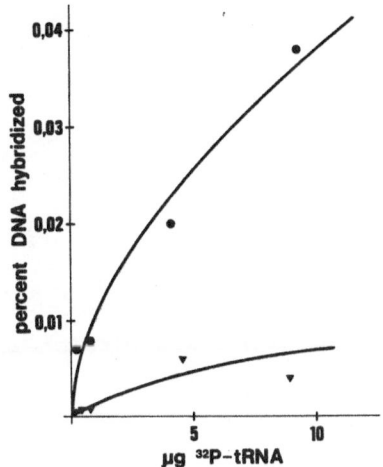

Figure 1: Hybridization of ^{32}P-labeled 4S tRNA from E.coli J5 and E.coli J5/R1 to R1-DNA

The RNA was extracted from cell cultures which were grown in ^{32}P-phosphate containing minimal medium by the standard phenol technique. The RNA was separated into small and large RNA fractions by stepwise elution from a DEAE cellulose column (3). The fraction containing the small RNA was further purified by electrophoresis in 5.5 % polyacrylamide gels according to Loening (4). The location of the RNA species was identified by autoradiography and the appropriate gel portions cut out. Both the 4S RNA and the 5S RNAs were eluted with 6 x SSC[x]. The specific activities of the RNAs obtained in this way ranged from 15000 - 70000 cpm/µg. The plasmid DNA, as obtained by the CsCl-dye gradient centrifugation technique (5) was denatured (6) and applied to Schleicher & Schüll BA 85/1 nitrocellulose filter discs according to Gillespie and Gillespie (1). The filters were baked for 2 hrs at 80°C. The discs were transferred to vials containing 6 x SSC-formamide 1:1 and ^{32}P-tRNA in varying amounts. Hybridization was carried out for 15 hrs at 37°C. The filters were processed by the standard technique. After counting the DNA adhering to the filter discs was quantitatively determined by the diphenylalamine procedure (7). The amount of DNA per filter was 13.5 µg. ▼ tRNA from E.coli J5; • tRNA from E.coli J5/R1

---

[x]
  Abbreviations:

6 x SSC: 0.9 M NaCl, 0.09 M sodium citrate

RPC 5:   Reverse phase chromatography Nr. 5

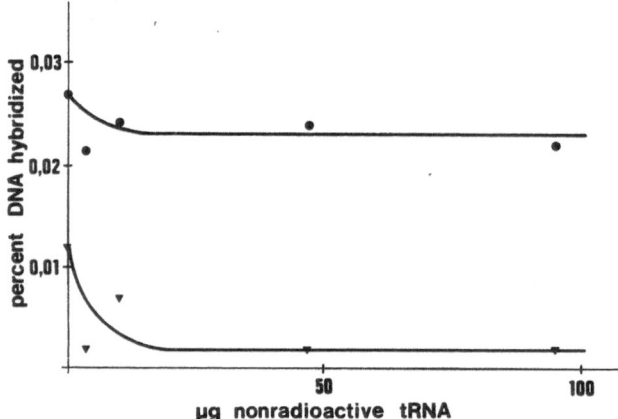

Figure 2: Competition hybridization of ^{32}P-labeled tRNA

The conditions were the same as described in figure 1. 6.3 µg ^{32}P-tRNA
was added to the hybridization mixture. Increasing quantities of nonradioactive tRNA from E. coli J5, which was passed over DEAE-cellulose
but was not further purified, were also included in the hybridization
mixture as indicated on the abscissa. The DNA content per filter was
12.5 µg. ▼ ^{32}P-tRNA from E.coli J5; • ^{32}P-tRNA from E.coli J5/R1

R[+] strain was much higher as compared to the analogous experiment
carried out by the low temperature method. Moreover, under these experimental conditions also some tRNA from the sensitive strain could
be bound to the plasmid DNA (Fig. 3). The interpretation for these
experiments appears to be that some of the 4S RNA are not available
for DNA - RNA hybridization at the low temperature, most probably
because of strong self complementation of uncommon sequences which
are possibly rich in GC. These secondary structures would then open
up at the high temperature and permit the subsequent interaction with
the R1 DNA and thus give positive hybridization results. These sequences in question seem also to be present in one or several components
of the chromosomally coded 4S RNA because the 4S RNA from the sensitive
strain hybridized at 67° but not at the lower temperature to R1 DNA.

Hybridization of ^{35}S-labeled RNA to plasmid DNA was also observed.
The tRNA was labeled with sulfur according to Weiss et al.(8) and

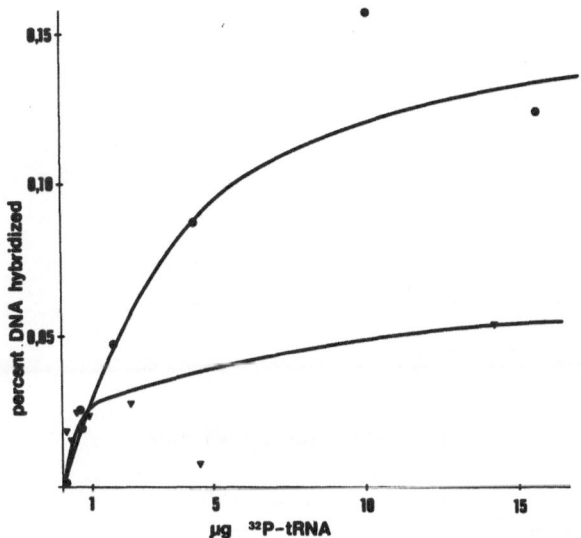

Figure 3: Hybridization of ^{32}P-labeled 4S RNA from E. coli J 5 and
E. coli J5/R1 to R1 DNA at 67° C

The technique is described in figure 1. Instead of the 6 x SSC -for-
mamide mixture 2 x SSC was used. The hybridization was carried out at
67°C for 15 hrs. ▼ ^{32}P 4S RNA from E.coli J5; • ^{32}P 4S RNA from
E.coli J5/R1

purified by DEAE column chromatography as described for the ^{32}P-labeled
RNA. Hybridization with this RNA preparation was performed at 67° in
solution by the method of Nygaard and Hall (9). After adding 10.5 µg
of ^{35}S-labeled RNA from the sensitive or 11 µg from the resistant
organism to 8.2 µg of denatured R1 DNA 0.067 % of the DNA hybridized
to the former and 0.047 % to the latter RNA. This finding supports
the conclusion that at least some of the components of the 4S region
hybridizing to plasmid DNA are indeed tRNAs since only these RNA species
contain thio-nucleotides.

When ^{32}P-labeled 5S RNA, isolated from the electrophoresis gels, was
hybridized against the R-factor DNA, again retention of radioactivity
to the filter discs occurred. The 5S RNA from the isogenic R⁻ strain
did not hybridize at 37° in the formamide system (Fig. 4).

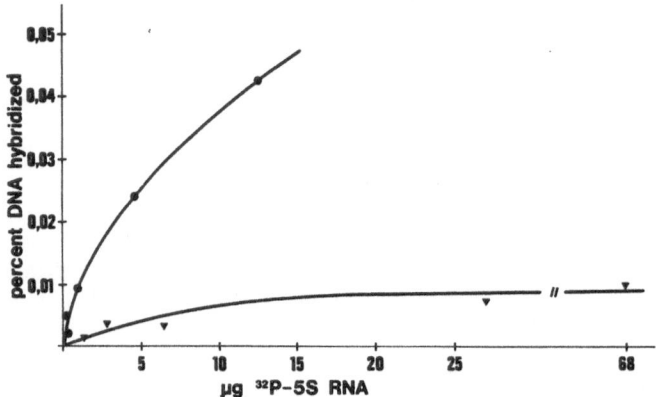

Figure 4: Concentration dependence of 5S RNA binding to R1 DNA

The conditions of the experiment of figure 1 were used. 5S RNA was added in varying amounts as indicated in the graphs. The filter discs contained 14.5 µg R1 DNA. ▼ [32]P 5S RNA from E.coli J5; • [32]P 5S RNA from E.coli J5/R1.

Table 1: Results of a hybridization experiment with the DNA of different R-factors

	per cent DNA hybridized by ^{32}P-tRNA from E.coli J5/R
R 1 - DNA	0.044
R 12 - DNA	0.020

The experiments were carried out as described in figure 1. The amount of R1 DNA was 11.3 µg. The hybridization assay contained 7.7 µg of [32]P tRNA.

These experiments suggest that RNA species which are required for protein synthesis, namely tRNAs and 5S RNA, are coded by the R-factor R1. The question arose whether this phenomenon is unique for this plasmid or occurs also with other R-factors. One first step was made to answer this question by using the DNA from a different R-factor, R 12, which is a multicopy mutant of the resistance factor NR 1 (10). When this DNA was immobilized on filters and ^{32}P-tRNA from the R1 containing strain was hybridized to it, some binding was observed. The hybridization capacity of the R 12 DNA is roughly half of that shown by R 1 DNA as can be seen from table 1. This seems to indicate

that the 4S fraction of E.coli J5/R1 contains more than one tRNA
species coded for by the R 1 DNA and that some of these sequences are
present on the DNA of R 12. From these data it is inferred that the
synthesis of small, stable RNAs is at least not limited to R 1. It
may, therefore, represent a more general genetic phenomenon.

If tRNA from the R1 containing strain is separated by reverse phase
chromatography (11) and compared to the fraction of the tRNA obtained
from sensitive isogenic bacteria no gross differences could be observed either in the optical density profiles or, if ^{35}C-labeled RNA
was used, in the pattern of radioactivity. However, the fractions obtained by chromatography of ^{32}P tRNA from the R1 containing strain
did not show an equal propensity to hybridize R1 DNA. Moreover, the
tRNA which is able to bind to R1 DNA appeared in the late part of the
elution profile and showed at least three peaks of hybridizing activity. The amounts of these specific RNA species appear to be very low
otherwise they would change the optical density profile of the late
part of the tRNA elution pattern (Fig. 5).

Possible implication of this finding:
The function of the R-factor coded tRNA and 5S RNA species is unknown.
Only speculations are possible at the moment. Both of these types of
molecules play an essential part in protein synthesis. As already out-
lined at the beginning the R-factor coded tRNA and 5S RNA molecules
may be causing a modification of the translation machinery of the E.
coli cell by which the expression of R-factor genes is facilitated.
Since tRNAs have been implicated also with regulatory processes (12)
this alternative possibly has to be considered as well. However, since
not only tRNA but also 5S RNA is coded by the R-factor, it appears
more logical that the physiological function of R-factor coded 4S and
5S RNAs is related to the translational process. At the moment it is
impossible to implicate these RNA molecules with a new chemotherapeutic
approach. Yet, the mere fact that the R-factor induces the modification
of an essential biosynthetic process of the cell could make the R-
factor bearing cell more vulnerable. In theory novel types of protein-
synthesis inhibitors might specifically interfere with the R-factor
coded messenger RNA translation. However, until a search for such
compounds is initiated the actual bearing of these R-factor coded
small RNA molecules on the expression of R-factor genes must be established, either by genetic or by biochemical techniques.

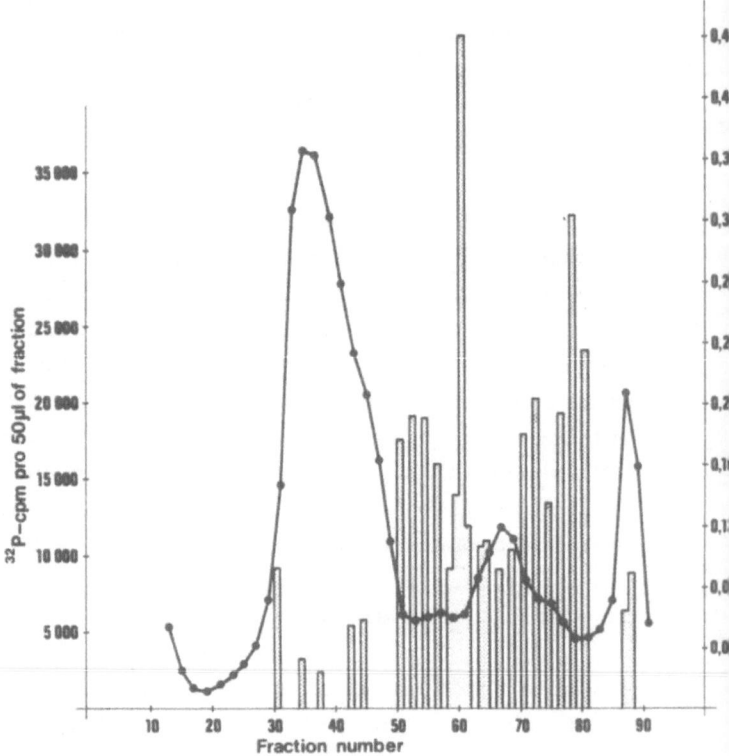

Figure 5: Hybridization of ^{32}P-labeled tRNA from <u>E. coli</u> J5/R1 after
separation by RPC 5

10.5 A_{260} -units of ^{32}P-labeled tRNA was separated on a RPC 5 column.
(0.5 x 47 cm) using a NaCl-gradient with a total volume of 100 ml,
ranging from 0.5 to 0.9 M. Selected fractions were dialyzed against
6 x SSC and hybridized with R1 DNA, immobilized on filters as described
in figure 1. The DNA content per filter was 4.9 μg. The results are
given as percentage hybridization of input RNA and are shown by the
bars. The solid line represents the radioactive elution pattern as
obtained from the column.

Summary

The 4S- and 5S RNA species of <u>E.coli</u> J5/R1 contain components that
could hybridize to R1 DNA as detected by the filter technique. At low
temperature this hybridization was restricted to the 4S or 5S RNA from
the R[+] strain. High temperature (67°C) conditions also prompted the

annealing of sequences of the R⁻ strain with R1 DNA. Moreover, at the high temperature, ^{35}S-labeled RNA also hybridized to the plasmid DNA. This occurred regardless whether the sensitive or the resistant strain was the source of the sulfur labeled RNA.

These data could be explained by the presence of tRNA genes on the DNA of the R-factor R1. Possibly, sequences of the chromosomally coded tRNAs are also present in some of the R-factor specific tRNAs. At the high temperature these sequences anneal to the R1 DNA while other sequences, which are different from the tRNAs of chromosomal origin, contribute to the hybridization at the low temperature.

References

1) Gillespie, S., and Gillespie, D.: Ribonucleic Acid-Deoxyribo-
nucleic Acid Hybridization in Aqueous Solutions and in
Solutions Containing Formamide. Biochem. J. 125, 481-487 (1971).

2) Marmur, J.: Isolation and Characterisation of Low Molecular
Weight Ribonucleic Acid Species From Bacillus subtilis.
J. Mol. Biol. 3, 208-218 (1962).

3) Landy, A., Abelson, J., Goodman, H.M., and Smith, J.D.:
Specific Hybridization of Tyrosine Transfer Ribonucleic Acids
With DNA From a Transducing Bacteriophage Ø 80 Carrying the
Amber Suppressor Gene SM$_{III}$. J. Mol. Biol. 29, 457-471 (1967).

4) Loening, U.E.: The Fractionation of High-Molecular-Weight-
Ribonucleic Acid by Polyacrylamide-Gel Electrophoresis.
Biochem. J. 102, 251-257 (1967).

5) Clewell, D.B., and Helinski, D.R.: Supercoiled Circular DNA-
Protein Complex in Escherichia coli: Purification and Induced
Conversion to an Open Circular DNA Form. Proc. Natl. Acad. Sci.
USA 62, 1159-1166 (1969).

6) Jakovic, S., Casey, J., and Rabinowitz, M.: Sequence Homology
of the Mitochondrial Leucyl tRNA Cistron in Different Organisms.
Biochemistry 14, 2037-2042 (1975).

7) Meijs, W.H., and Schiperoort, R.A.: Determination of the Amount
of DNA on Nitrocellulose Membrane Filters. FEBS Letters 12,
166-168 (1971).

8) Weiss, S.B., Hsu, Wen-Tah, Foft, J.W., and Scherberg, H.:
Transfer RNA Coded by the T4 Bacteriophage Genome. Proc. Natl.
Acad. Sci. USA 61, 114-121 (1968).

9) Nygaard, A.P., and Hall, B.D.: Formation and Properties of RNA-
DNA Complexes. J. Mol. Biol. 9, 125-142 (1964).

10) Morris, C.F., Hashimoto, H., Mickel, S., and Rownd, R.: Round of Replication Mutant of a Drug Resistance Factor. J. Bact. <u>118</u>, 855-866 (1974).

11) Pearson, R.L., Weiss, J.F., and Kelmers, A.D.: Improved Separation of Transfer RNAs on Polychlorotrifluoroethylene-supported Reversed-phase Chromatography Columns. Biochem. Biophys. Acta <u>228</u>, 770-774 (1971).

12) Singer, C.E., Smith, G.R., Cortese, R., and Ames, B.N.: Mutant tRNA[His] Ineffective in Repression and Lacking Two Pseudouridine Modifications. Nature New Biol. <u>238</u>, 72-74 (1972).

Discussion

Levy: I have two questions; the first deals with technique. In the modified Gillespie-Gillespie hybridization technique is there an RNAse step?

Högenauer: Yes.

Levy: So you are RNAse treating. Have you tested to see what effects this has in comparison to not treating? Because there are hybridizations especially, perhaps at the lower temperature, where hybrids will be eluted with the RNase step, although this is not in line with general assumptions. This has been found in eukaryotic DNA/RNA hybridizations and we have seen it ourselves. So you might think about this kind of thing when one uses RNase.

Davies: You are suggesting that he will find more RNA hybridizing to the plasmid.

Levy: That is correct. If you use the right RNase step you are liable to find more hybridizable material and the way that this can be avoided is by eluting and then re-hybridizing. The second is a question in terms of trying to localize the RNA species; have you tried hybridizing against some of the smaller variants of R1? For instance, there is a drd variant which has lost the r-determinants and is just the RTF region.

Högenauer: This is an interesting question. We thought about this experimental approach of localizing the RNA genes but have not yet begun work in this direction.

Saedler: Did you ever then try to hybridize the charged tRNA with R1 DNA?

Högenauer: We had several attempts but failed because of technical difficulties. When you aminoacylate the tRNA there are always trace amounts of protein present and this probably results in a high background against which a small amount of hybridization is difficult to detect.

Davies: Can you estimate the amount of the tRNA that you see by hybridization relative to the content of other tRNAs in the cell?

Högenauer: No. One of the ways of doing it would be to do the reverse hybridization and to increase the DNA concentration.

Starlinger: Could'n you purify these RNA molecules by 2-dimensional gel electrophoresis? This separates tRNA molecules nicely and you could then subject the pure species to T1-RNase fingerprint analysis and get a good characterization and so on.
The other question is along the line of Heinz' question, you could hybridize the tRNA to $EcoR_1$ fragments of the R1 plasmid DNA.

Högenauer: As I said, this is one thing we plan to do, we just wanted to establish the presence of tRNA.

Goebel: This is more or less the same question I wanted to ask; is this a homogeneous species of RNA or is it a mixture of 5S RNA, tRNA and others?

Högenauer: I don't think so, no. In one experiment we were careful to separate the RNA from all contaminants and could see that it is separate from 5S RNA.

Falkow: I was interested if you would try similar experiments with R1 in a more foreign host; for example proteus?

Högenauer: Yes, these experiments are in progress.

Davies: Drs. Michel DeWilde and Francis Schmidt in my laboratory have analyzed small RNA molecules specific to R100 (NR1). We find as many as 10 RNA molecules, specific to R100, that hybridize to different parts of the RTF. Many of these RNAs have been fingerprinted.

Evolutional Process of the Formation of Multiple Resistance Plasmids

S. Mitsuhashi, H. Kawabe, T. Nagate, and K. Inoue

Sulfanilamide(SA) and its derivatives were used in Japan since 1940 against
infections with both gram-positive and gram-negative bacteria and pioneered
a chemotherapy as an effective antibacterial agent. In parallel with the
wide use of the drugs, the isolation frequencies of SA-resistant strains of
bacteria increased and reached a maximum of 90-95% of Shigella and Staphylococcus aureus isolates being resistant to SA(1-4).

The Production of antibiotics such as penicillin(PC), streptomycin(SM), tet-
racycline(TC), and chloramphenicol(CM), started at that time, and they were
quite effective against both gram-positive and gram-negative bacteria. Similarly to SA, however, antibiotic-resistant strains of bacteria rapidly appeared since the introduction of antibiotics. Introduction of new drugs caused
likewise the appearance of strains resistant to them and the emergence of
multiply resistant strains has become one of the most important problems in
practical medicine.

The conjugative resistance(R) plasmid was discovered in Japan from the findings based on epidemiology and genetics of multiple resistance: (1) transmission of resistance by mixed cultivation, (2) interruption of the transmission with a filter to separate the two parental cultures and (3) spontaneous
and artificial loss of drug resistance from resistant cells(5).

Nonconjugative resistance(r) plasmid was discovered later in multiply resistant
S.aureus strains by the irreversible loss of resistance and by genetic analysis
of staphylococcal resistance(3,4,6,7). Thereafter, the range of the host bacteria carrying r plasmids has expanded from gram-positive to gram-negative
bacteria and multiple resistance of clinical isolates has been found to be
mostly due to the presence of R or r plasmids or of both. The findings
of r plasmid and of transfer(T) factor(7,8) give us a useful tool to pursue
the evolutional process of the formation of plasmids encoding multiple resistance.

1. Nonconjugative SA Resistance Plasmid

Since the introduction of SA and its derivatives into practical medicine, bacterial strains rapidly acquired SA resistance and were isolated at a high frequency from clinical specimens(1-4). Thereafter the world-wide use of antibiotics such as TC, CM and SM caused the emergence of multiple-resistant strains in addition to SA resistance. Resistance patterns of Shigella and E.coli strains with reference to TC, CM, SM and SA are shown in Table 1.

Table 1. Isolation frequency of resistant strains

Resistance[a) pattern	Shigella	E.coli
	(%)	(%)
Quadruple	75.7	64.2
Triple	4.7	5.7
Double	2.8	8.9
Single	16.8	21.2

Results based on surveys from 15,903 strains including 12,453 Shigella and 3,450 E.coli strains. [a)]Survey for resistance to TC, CM, SM and SA.

Isolation frequency of quadruple-resistant strains was the highest and followed by single-, triple- and double-resistant ones. Conjugative resistance(R) plasmids were most frequently demonstrated from triple- and quadruple-resistant strains. Among the single-resistant strains, SA-resistant ones were most frequently isolated and those with other single resistance were rather few in number. Demonstration frequency of R plasmids from single-resistant strains was very low except for TC-resistant ones (Table 2).

Table 2. Isolation frequency of R plasmids from single-resistant Shigella and E.coli strains

Bacteria resistant to	Shigella		E. coli	
	Resist. strains (%)	R[+] strains (%)	Resist. strains (%)	R[+] strains (%)
SA	97.8	5.6	82.6	1.8
TC	2.1	34.6	1.4	11.1
SM	0.1	0	2.9	0
CM	0	0	0	0

Results based on surveys from the strains shown in Table 1. Demonstration frequency of R plasmids from the strains with the indicated resistance.

Then we selected <u>Shigella</u> and <u>E.coli</u> strains possessing nonconjugative SA resistance and examined the presence of r(SA) plasmid by spontaneous or artificial elimination of SA resistance. Seventy-two percent of <u>Shigella</u> strains and 56% of <u>E.coli</u> strains lost their SA resistance during storage or by treatment with acriflavine. To know the cytoplasmic inheritance of SA resistance, Rms306(TC) plasmid was conjugally transferred to <u>Shigella</u> and <u>E.coli</u> strains possessing cured SA resistance and examined the mobilization of SA resistance in cooperation with a transmissible Rms306 plasmid, indicating the mobilization of SA resistance to <u>E.coli</u> 58-161 NA^r (resistant to nalidixic acid) at frequencies of 6.8×10^{-6}-7.2×10^{-7}. But the transconjugants that acquired only SA resistance could not transfer their SA resistance by conjugation. The nonconjugative r(SA) plasmids in <u>Shigella</u> and <u>E.coli</u> strains were transformed to <u>E.coli</u> C Rf^r(resistant to rifampicin). Plasmid DNA was prepared for electron microscopy, and micrographs of open circular molecules were enlarged, traced and measured. The contour length of seven r(SA) plasmids ranged from 1.79 to 2.08 μm(Fig. 1).

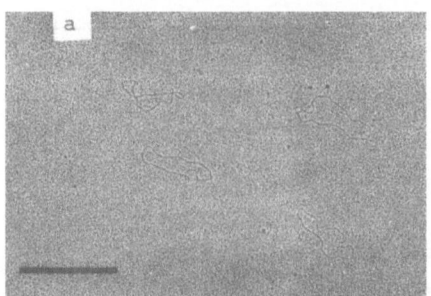 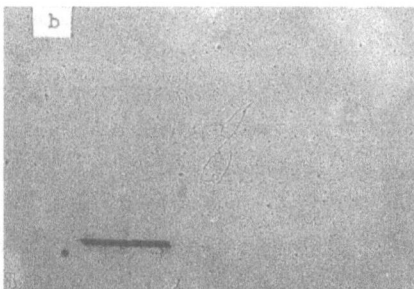

Fig. 1. Electron micrographs from r(SA) and r(SM.SA) plasmids open circular DNA fraction. Bar represents 1 μm. (a) r-ms31(SA) plasmid, (b) r-ms34 plasmid.

2. Mechanisms of SA Resistance

Since <u>p</u>-aminobenzenesulfonamide(sulfanylamide: SA) was established as the active antibacterial moiety of the prontosil molecule, a large number of effective derivatives have been synthesized by the substitution on the amide group. However, all of the sulfonamide and its derivatives have the common mode of action of the inhibitory action being antagonized by <u>p</u>-aminobenzoate (PABA). Sulfonamides are antagonized not only by PABA, but also by a variety of other compounds including folic acid analogs, purines, and unknown constituents of peptone. It is known that sulfonamides inhibit the biosynthesis of tetrahydrofolate by competing at the site for PABA in dihydropteroate syn-

thetase(DHPS, EC 2.5.1.15) and this   DHPS   causes the formation of a
number of raw materials of protein, DNA and RNA biosynthesis. The route of
the synthesis of tetrahydropteroate and the inhibition sites of sulfonamides
as well as trimethoprim(TP) are illustrated in Fig. 2.

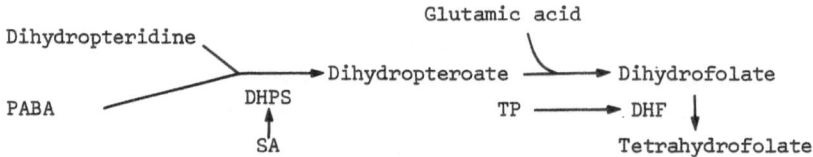

Fig. 2. Enzymatic Synthesis of Tetrahydrofolate

(a) Altered Dihydropteroate Synthetase(DHPS)

Pato and Brown(10) reported that there are two types of mechanism in artificially developed SA-resistant E.coli strains: (i) SA sensitivity of a dihydropteroate synthetase(DHPS), which decreases in accordance with an increase in
SA resistance, and (ii) decrease in permeability of sulfonamides in SA-resistant strains of E.coli. In the latter case the folate synthesizing system in
SA-resistant strains is still inhibited by SA as much as that in SA-sensitive
strains. The former mechanism was found also in in vitro developed SA-resistant
strains of pneumococci(10).

Wise and Abou-Donia(11) studied on the mechanism of SA resistance in several
natural isolates of E.coli strains as well as in Citrobacter and Klebsiella
pneumoniae which were highly resistant to the drugs. These strains were shown
to contain SA-resistant DHPS specified by an R plasmid in addition to the
SA-sensitive enzyme specified by a chromosomal gene of the host cells. The
SA-resistant enzyme in crude extracts of SA-resistant strains was much more
sensitive to heat than that in corresponding strains.

Recently, Sköld(12) demonstrated also that an R plasmid mediating SA resistance
makes a host strain of E.coli diploid for the DHPS. He obtained conditionally
lethal mutants of E.coli C strain which were thermosensitive with no colony
formed at 42°C but with normal growth at 30°C even in the presence of 0.02 mM
sulfathiazole. The parental strain grows normally at 42°C but cannot grow in
the presence of sulfathiazole at 0.02 mM either at 30°C or 42°C. The rescue
of the bacterial mutants with a lesion in the chromosomal DHPS from temperature
sensitivity was achieved by a derepressed R plasmid, R1dr19, encoding SA resistance. Other evidence was obtained by direct measurements of the dihydropteroate synthesizing activity and the degrees of its inhibition by sulfathiazole in partly purified extracts from the parental strain with and without

the plasmid. The result was that the DHPS activity of the extracts from R^+ cells was significantly less inhibited at a concentration of sulfathiazole where the extracts from R^- cells is inhibited more than 95%. This interesting finding indicates that SA resistance mediated by some of R plasmids can be explained by a drug-resistant target enzyme, DHPS, specified by the R plasmids.

We investigated the biochemical mechanisms of SA resistance mediated by conjugative(R) and nonconjugative(r) plasmids by examining the rate of incorporation of ^{14}C-PABA into the dihydropteroate fraction with extracts prepared from E.coli ML1410 carrying various plasmids encoding SA resistance. We selected various R plasmids from our stock cultures and transferred them to E.coli ML1410 NA^r by mixed cultivation. The nonconjugative r plasmids were transferred to ML1410 NA^r by transformation. It was found that there are two types of DHPS activity, i.e., normal SA-sensitive enzyme and an altered enzyme resistant to 100-1000 times the normal inhibitory concentration of SA. A representative result of DHPS inhibition by SA is shown in Fig. 3.

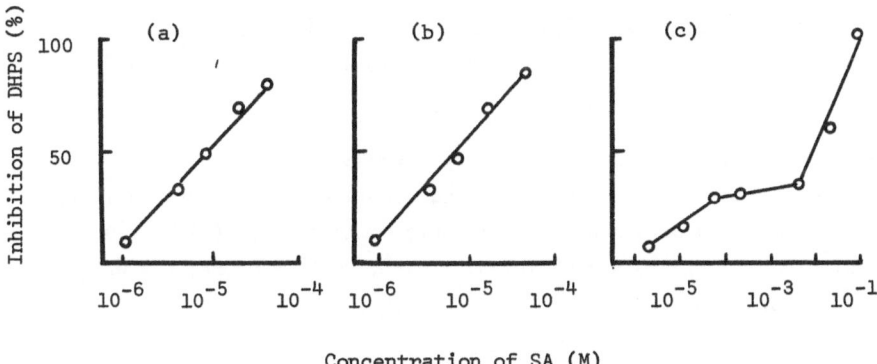

Concentration of SA (M)

Fig. 3. Inhibition of DHPS activities of E.coli ML1410, ML1410 Rms265$^+$ and ML1410 Rms250$^+$. (a) ML1410, (b) ML1410 Rms265(TC.CM.SM.SA)$^+$, (c) ML1410 Rms250(SA)$^+$.

Next we compared the DHPS activities of E.coli ML1410 carrying various plasmids. Fifty percent inhibitory(ID$_{50}$) concentrations of SA for DHPS activity are shown in Table 3. The DHPS activities of ML1410 carrying R(SA), R(TC.SA), r(SA), and some of R(SM.SA) plasmids showed a decreased susceptibility to SA inhibition. By contrast, the DHPS activities of ML1410 carrying R(TC.CM.SM.SA), R(TC.SM.SA), R(CM.SM.SA) and some of R(SM.SA) plasmids were found to be almost the same as that of SA-sensitive ML1410. To confirm the presence of SA-resistant DHPS in addition to the normal sensitive enzyme, we examined the heat sensitivity of DHPS activities of ML1410 carrying various plasmids. The effect

of heating extracts from ML1410, ML1410 Rms265[+] and ML1410 Rms250[+] is shown
in Fig. 4. The loss of total activities in ML1410 and ML1410 Rms265[+] was the
same in spite of the presence or absence of SA, indicating the presence of
a heat-resistant and SA-sensitive DHPS. By contrast, ML1410 Rms250[+] produced
two DHPS activities, i.e., a SA-resistant and heat-sensitive DHPS in addition
to the normal SA-sensitive and heat-resistant DHPS. Therefore, the loss of
total activity in uninhibited extract approximates that of the SA-resistant
activity, as reported by Wise and Abou-Donia(11).

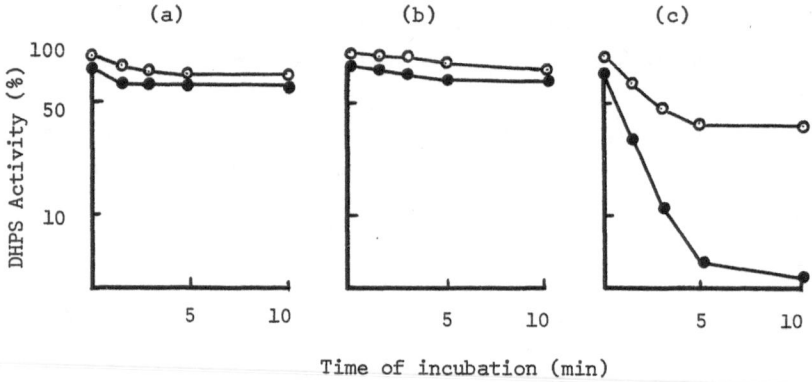

Fig. 4. Heat sensitivity of DHPS activity. Extract was heated at 50° C.
Aliquots were removed at various times and were assayed for DHPS activity
in the presence(●) or absence(○) of sulfisomidine(SA). (a) ML1410,
2×10^{-6}M of SA; (b) ML1410 Rms265(TC.CM.SM.SA)[+], 2×10^{-6}M of SA; (c) ML1410
Rms250(SA)[+], 1×10^{-4}M of SA.

Then we studied the kinetic experiment of SA inhibition for DHPS activity.
When a slope of 1/V against 1/[S] is made, it is known, for competitive
inhibition, that the ordinate intercept, $1/V_{max}$, is the same as the uninhibited reaction, where V is the observed initial velocity and S is the substrate
concentration. As reported by Shiota et al.(13), the DHPSs derived from
ML1410 and ML1410 Rms265(TC.CM.SM.SA)[+] were competitively inhibited by
2×10^{-6}M of SA. By contrast, the ordinate intercept of the slopes of 1/V
against 1/[s] (1×10^{-4}, 6×10^{-3} and 1×10^{-2}M of SA) for ML1410 Rms250(SA)[+] DHPS
was the same but different from the uninhibited reaction. According to the
studies of kinetcs of enzyme reaction and of heat stability of DHPS, it was
concluded that there are two types of DHPS in ML1410 carrying plasmids encoding resistances to SA, (TC.SA), and (SM.SA), i.e., SA-resistant but heat-
sensitive DHPS and normal SA-sensitive DHPS.

(b) Mechanism of SA resistance mediated by R Plasmids

Akiba and Yokota(14) reported SA resistance mediated by E.coli R$^+$ due to an increase in permeability barrier to SA. We also observed that the permeation of SA into the cells carrying R plasmid encoding multiple resistance was decreased and the antibacterial activity of SA increased by treatment of the cells with EDTA. Hence, this decreased permeability may be one of the mechanisms of SA resistance mediated by R plasmids with multiple resistance. The comparison of DHPS activities in E.coli ML1410 carrying plasmids encoding SA resistance is shown in Table 3.

Table 3. Comparison of the dihydropteroate synthetase(DHPS) activities in ML1410 strains carrying plasmids encoding SA resistance

Enzyme source		MIC of SA(μg/ml)	Specific DHPS activity $\times 10^2$ u/mg protein	50% Inhibitory concentration of SA($\times 10^{-3}$M)
ML1410 R$^-$		25	1.1	8.5×10^{-3}
ML1410	Rms248(SA)$^+$	6400	1.5	15.2
	Rms249(SA)$^+$	6400	1.8	10.1
ML1410	Rms272(SA.TC)$^+$	6400	1.6	0.4
ML1410	rms38(SA)$^+$	6400	1.8	8.5
	rms39(SA)$^+$	6400	2.0	11.2
ML1410	Rms254(SM.SA)$^+$	6400	2.3	11.0
	Rms255(SM.SA)$^+$	6400	1.7	9.4
	Rms256(SM.SA)$^+$	3200	0.76	7.6×10^{-3}
	Rms257(SM.SA)$^+$	3200	1.4	6.2×10^{-3}
ML1410	Rms260(TC.SM.SA)$^+$	1600	0.95	8.9×10^{-3}
	Rms261(TC.SM.SA)$^+$	3200	1.0	7.1×10^{-3}
	Rms262(CM.SM.SA)$^+$	800	1.1	4.5×10^{-3}
	Rms263(CM.SM.SA)$^+$	800	0.76	7.2×10^{-3}
ML1410	Rms265(TC.CM.SM.SA)$^+$	3200	0.92	8.0×10^{-3}
	Rms266(TC.CM.SM.SA)$^+$	3200	1.0	10.0×10^{-3}

3. SM Resistance Plasmid

Following the practical use of SA, we used many antibiotics such as PC, SM, TC, CM, etc. as effective agents against bacterial infection. However, we noticed the appearence of antibiotic-resistant bacteria, developing from single to multiple resistance. In relation to resistance to TC, CM, SM and SA, the singly SM-resistant strains were scarecely isolated(Table 2). Among the double-resistant strains, the strains with (SM.SA) resistance were most frequently isolated and followed by those with (TC.SA) resistance. But the

strains with other combinations of double resistance were scarecely isolated. The demonstration frequency of conjugative R plasmids from doubly resistant strains was low, except for the strains with (TC.SA) resistance
(Table 4).

Table 4. Types of resistance among double-resistant E.coli and Shigella
strains

Type of [a] resistance	Shigella		E.coli	
	No. (%)	R[+] strains (%)	No. (%)	R[+] strains (%)
SM.SA	73.2	18.0	75.2	19.2
TC.SA	21.2	88.9	20.3	86.3
CM.SA	2.5	– [b]	2.5	– [b]
TC.CM	1.9	–	1.0	–
TC.SM	0.9	–	0.8	–
CM.SM	0.3	–	0.2	–

Results based on surveys of 348 Shigella and 307 E.coli strains with double
resistance. [a] Survey for resistance to TC,CM,SM and SA. [b] Percentage was not
computed when the number of strains was fewer than 10.

Then, we examined the presence of nonconjugative resistance(r) plasmid encoding (SM.SA) resistance. According to genetic analyses, i.e., curing experiment, mobilization of r by conjugative plasmid, transduction and transformation, it was found that about 70 to 80 percent of the strains with
nonconjugative (SM.SA) resistance carried r(SM.SA) plasmid. The contour
length of r(SM.SA) plasmids ranged from 2.6 to 2.8 μm(Fig. 1).

a). Biochemical Mechanisms of SM Resistance

The mechanisms of resistance to aminoglycoside antibiotics have been extensively characterized by many research workers. Okamoto and Suzuki(15)
observed that Escherichia coli carrying an R factor could inactivate dihydro-
streptomycin(DH-SM), kanamycin(KM) and chloramphenicol(CM) using adenosine
triphosphate(ATP) or acetyl CoA as a cofactor. Thus, studies on the biochemical mechanisms of aminoglycoside resistance were initiated, and many
types of drug inactivation were reported. Streptomycin is also inactivated
by phosphorylation of the drug by SM-resistant strains in the presence of ATP.

(1) SM 3"-Phosphotransferase; APH(3")

Ozanne et al.(16) reported that E.coli strains carrying an R factor which
are SM-resistant and spectinomycin(SP)-sensitive, have been found to phospho-

rylate the 3"-hydroxyl group of SM. Although the phosphorylating enzyme as
well as the adenylylating enzyme reacts with the same hydroxyl group on the
N-methyl-L-glucosamine, the chemical structure of the inactivated product
of SP was not fully investigated. SM-resistant but SP-sensitive strains
produce the SM-phosphorylating enzyme, and the strains resistant to both SM
and SP produce the adenylylating enzyme. Dihydrostreptomycin(DH-SM) was also
phosphorylated by P.aeruginosa, and the phosphorylated product was determined to be the 3"-hydroxyl group of DH-SM.

(2) SM 6-Phosphotransferase; APH(6)

Kida et al.(17) reported that the crude extracts from P.aeruginosa phosphorylated DH-SM and the phosphorylated product showed the same R_f value as
that of dihydrostreptomycin 6-phosphate, which was formed by an extract
prepared from a SM-producing strain of Streptomyces, as reported by Walker
et al.(18).

(3) SM 3"-Adenylyltransferase; AAD(3")

Umezawa et al.(19) reported on an E.coli strain with R-mediated SM resistance
whose resistance resulting from adenylylation of the drug. The inactivated
product of the drug was determined to be 3"-adenylylstreptomycin.

(4) SM 6-Adenylyltransferase; AAD(6)

We described intermediate SM-resistance in S.aureus strains, which inactivate
the drug by adenylylation(20). Epidemiological surveys disclosed that there
are three types of resistance to SM and SP in staphylococci; (SM^sSP^r), (SM^r
SP^s) and (SM^rSP^r). The (SM^sSP^r) and (SM^rSP^s) mutants of S.aureus could be
obtained from a (SM^rSP^r) strain by transduction or by elimination of resistance. S.aureus (SM^rSP^r) was found to inactivate both SM and SP by adenylylation. Genetic analysis disclosed that the genes governing resistance to
SM and SP are located separately and on different nonconjugative(r) plasmids.
We purified an inactivated product of SM by S.aureus (SM^rSP^r) which was shown
to be different from 3"-adenylylstreptomycin using electrophoresis. Adenylyl-
streptidine was obtained from the methanolysis product of adenylylstreptomycin
and was determined to be 6-adenylylstreptidine by elemental analysis and by
periodate consumption. The adenylylated product of SM was, therefore, determined to be 6-adenylylstreptomycin. These facts indicate that there is a
type of SM resistance in staphylococci resulting from the production of 6-
adenylylstreptomycin which is different from R-mediated (SM.SP)-resistance

resulting from adenylylation of the 3"-hydroxyl group of SM. The inactivated sites of SM are shown in Fig. 5.

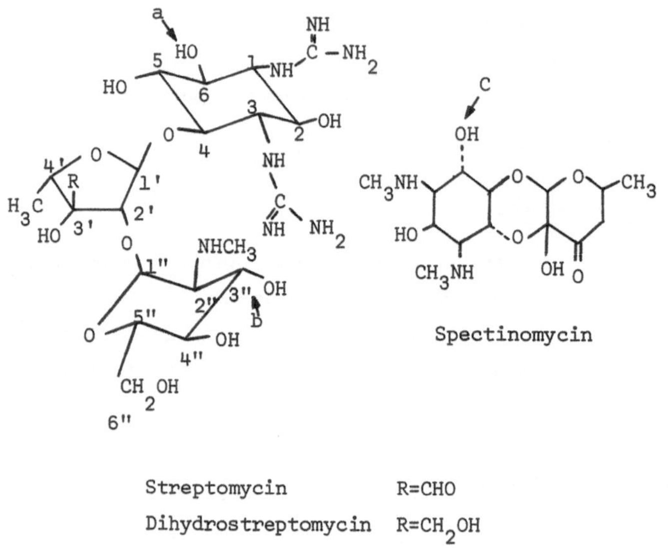

Streptomycin	R=CHO
Dihydrostreptomycin	R=CH$_2$OH

Fig. 5. Inactivated Sites of Streptomycin

4. Two Types of SM Resistance Plasmid

We selected conjugative and nonconjugative plasmids encoding various types of resistances including SM and examined the biochemical mechanisms of SM resistance by the incorporation of (γ^{32}P) or ($8-^{14}$C) from the isotope labelled ATP into SM. We selected 50 r(SM.SA) plasmids and found that they inactivated SM by phosphorylation regardless of the presence or absence of the gene governing spectinomycin(SP) resistance. About half the number of R(SM.SA) plasmids carry a gene governing SP resistance and inactivated SM by adenylylation, but the remaining R(SM.SA) plasmids without SP resistance inactivated SM by phosphorylation. Similarly, about half the number of R(TC.SM.SA) plasmids carried SP resistance and inactivated SM by adenylylation and the remaining R(TC.SM.SA) plasmids without SP resistance inactivated SM by phosphorylation. By contrast, we could not demonstrate so far R(CM.SM.SA) and R(TC.CM.SM.SA) plasmids without SP resistance and all of them inactivated SM by adenylylation. The results are shown in Table 5.

Table 5. Inactivation of SM by conjugative or nonconjugative plasmids

S-30 fraction from ML1410 carrying	Resistance pattern	Inactivation of SM by	
		Adenylylation	Phosphorylation
r-ms24	SM.SA		+
r-ms26	SM.SA		+
r-ms28	SM.SA.SP		+
r-ms29	SM.SA.SP		+
r-ms42	SM.SA		+
r-ms45	SM.SA		+
r-ms46	SM.SA.SP		+
r-ms47	SM.SA.SP		+
Rms302[a]	SM.SA		+
Rms303	SM.SA		+
Rms340	SM.SA.SP	+	
Rms345	SM.SA.SP	+	
Rms298[a]	CM.SM.SA.SP	+	
Rms299	CM.SM.SA.SP	+	
Rms358[a]	TC.SM.SA		+
Rms363	TC.SM.SA		+
Rms331	TC.SM.SA.SP	+	
Rms340	TC.SM.SA.SP	+	
Rms304[a]	TC.CM.SM.SA.SP	+	
Rms305	TC.CM.SM.SA.SP	+	
ML1410	-	-	-

[a] About 100 R plasmids were selected from our stock cultures and examined the presence or absence of SP resistance.

Discussion

According to the epidemiological studies of R plasmids in clinical isolates, it was found that R plasmids were demonstrated at high frequencies from triple- and quadruple-resistant strains in relation to resistance to TC, CM, SM and SA. But the demonstration frequency of R plasmids was rather low from double- and single-resistant strains. By contrast, the nonconjugative re-sistance(r) plasmid was demonstrated at a high frequency from the strains with double or single resistance. It can be said therefore that drug re-sistance of clinical isolates is mostly due to the presence of R or r or of both plasmids . As is seen in staphylococcal r plasmids (2-4), most of the r plasmids carry only single resistance and the r plasmid with double resist-ance is rather few except for r(SM.SA) and r(PC.Mac)(Mac, macrolide resis-tance). Among the conjugative R plasmids carrying triple resistance in relation to resistance to TC, CM, SM and SA, R(CM.SM.SA) and R(TC.SM.SA) plasmids are most frequently isolated and R plasmids with other combinations of triple resistance are scarecely demonstrated. Among the R plasmids possessing double resistance, R(SM.SA) plasmid is most frequently isolated and R plasmid with other combinations of double resistance is scarecely demonstrated. We could isolate R(SA), r(SA), R(TC) and r(TC) plasmids but the number of plasmids with single resistance is rather few. We have not demonstrated plasmid carrying only single CM or single SM resistance. From these results, we can conclude that there are easily joinable resistance determinants such as SA and SM, resulting in the formation of (SM.SA) resistance. Hence, the (SM.SA) resistance unit can be easily associated with TC or CM resistance determinant, resulting in the formation of (CM.SM.SA) or (TC.SM.SA) resistance unit. Finally, R(TC.CM.SM.SA) plasmid is formed by translocation of resistance determinant from other genetic elements and is increased by selective force of drugs.

According to the studies of biochemical mechanisms of SM- and SA-resistance mediated by plasmids, it was found that SM is inactivated by phosphorylation or adenylylation of the drug. Plasmid mediated SA resistance is due to the formation of SA-resistant DHPS and probably due to increase in the permeability barrier. It should be noted that SM resistance mediated by R(TC.CM.SM.SA) and R(CM.SM.SA) plasmids is mostly due to adenylylation of the drug. Sulfanilamide resistance mediated by these plasmids is mostly due to increase in the permeability barrier to SA. By contrast, the mechanism of SA resistance mediated by r(SA) and r(SM.SA) plasmids is mostly due to the formation of SA-resistant DHPS. The mechanism of SM resistance mediated by r(SM.SA) plasmid is mostly due to phosphorylation of the drug. Two types of SM- and SA-resistance exist in half in R(SM.SA) plasmids. From these results we present the evolutional process to the formation of multiple resistance plasmids: (SA)→(SM.SA)→(TC.SM.SA) and (CM.SM.SA), and finally (TC.CM.SM.SA) (Fig.6),

```
r(SA)  ⟹  r(SM.SA)  ⟹  R(TC.SM.SA)   ⟹  R(TC.CM.SM.SA)
R(SA)      R(SM.SA)      R(CM.SM.SA)

r(sa)  ⟶  r(sm.sa)
R(sa)      R(sm.sa)

           r(sm.SA) ⟶  R(TC.sm.SA) ⟶  R(TC.CM.sm.SA)    ?
           R(sm.SA)     R(CM.sm.SA)

           r(SM.sa) ⟶  R(TC.SM.sa) ⟶  R(TC.CM.SM.sa)    ?
           R(SM.sa)     R(CM.SM.sa)
```

Fig. 6. Evolutional process to the formation of multiple resistance plasmids. r, nonconjugative; R, conjugative plasmid. SM, adenylylation of SM; SA,

probably increase in the permeability barrier. sm, phosphorylation of SM; sa, formation of SA-resistant DHPS.

Summary

Epidemiological studies have disclosed that conjugative(R) and nonconjugative (r) resistance plasmids are demonstrated at high frequencies from clinical isolates. From triple- and quadruple-resistant strains in relation to resistance to TC, CM, SM and SA, R(TC.CM.SM.SA), R(TC.SM.SA) and R(CM.SM.SA) plasmids are demonstrated at high frequencies. By contrast, nonconjugative r plasmids are frequently isolated from single- and double-resistant strains. According to the epidemiological studies of plasmid resistance patterns, there are some resistance patterns which are frequently demonstrated, i.e., (SM.SA), (TC.SM.SA), (CM.SM.SA) and (TC.CM.SM.SA). According to the facts, i.e., the presence of easily demonstrable resistance types, easily joinable resistance determinants and two types of mechanism of resistance to SM and SA, the evolutional process to the formation of multiple resistance plasmids is presented.

Literature

1. Mitsuhashi, S.: Epidemiology of bacterial drug resistance. In:Transferable drug resistance factor R(S.Mitsuhashi), p.1-16. University of Tokyo Press; University Park Press, Tokyo, Baltimore and London. 1971.
2. Mitsuhashi, S.: Epidemiology and genetical study of drug resistance in Staphylococcus aureus. Japan.J.Microbiol. 11, 49-68 (1967).
3. Mitsuhashi, S., Inoue, M., Kawabe, H., Oshima, H., Okubo, T.: Genetic and biochemical studies of drug resistance in staphylococci. In: Staphylococci and Staphylococcal Infections(J.Jeljaszewicz), p.144-165. Karger, Basel. 1973.
4. Mitsuhashi, S., Inoue, M., Oshima, H., Okubo, T., Saito, T.: Epidemiologic and genetic studies of drug resistance in staphylococci. In:Staphylococci and Staphylococcal Infections(J.Jeljaszewicz), p.255-274. Gustav Fischer Verlag, Stuttgart and New York. 1976.
5. Mitsuhashi, S.: Epidemiology of R factors. In:Transferable drug resistance factor R(S.Mitsuhashi), p.25-38. University of Tokyo Press; University Park Press, Tokyo, Baltimore and London. 1971.
6. Anderson, E. S., Lewis, M. J.: Characterization of a transfer factor associated with drug resistance in Salmonella typhimurium. Nature 208, 843-849 (1965)

7. Mitsuhashi, S., Kameda, M., Harada, K., Suzuki, M.: Formation of recombinants between nontransferable drug-resistance determinants and
transfer factor. J. Bacteriol. 97, 1520-1521 (1969).

8. Mitsuhashi, S., Morimura, M., Kono, M., Oshima, H.: Elimination of drug
resistance in Staphylococcus aureus by treatment with acriflavine.
J. Bacteriol. 86, 162-163 (1963).

9. Novick, R. P.: Analysis by transduction of mutations affecting penicillinase formation in Staphylococcus aureus. J.gen.Microbiol. 33, 121-136 (1963).

10. Pato, M. L., Brown, G. M.: Mechanisms of resistance of Escherichia coli
to sulfonamides. Arch. Biochem. Biophys. 103, 443-448 (1963).

11. Wise, E. M. Jr., Abou-Donia, M. M.: Sulfonamide resistance mechanism in
Escherichia coli: R plasmids can determine sulfonamide-resistant dihydropteroate synthases. Proc. Natl. Acad. Sci. U.S.A. 72, 2621-2625 (1975).

12. Sköld, O.: R-factor-mediated resistance to sulfonamides by a plasmid-
borne, drug-resistant dihydropteroate synthetase. Antimicrob. Agent
Chemother. 9, 49-54 (1976).

13. Shiota, T., Disraely, M. N., McCann, M. P.: The enzymatic synthesis of
folate-like compounds from hydroxy-methyl-dihydro-pteridine pyrophos-
phate. J. Biol. Chem., 239, 2259-2266 (1964).

14. Akiba, T. Yokota, T.: Studies on the mechanism of transfer of drug resistance in bacteria. 18. Incorporation of ^{35}S-sulfathiazole into cells
of the multiple resistant strain and the artificial sulfonamid-resistant
strain of E. coli. Medicine and Biology. 63, 155-159 (1962).

15. Okamoto, S., Suzuki, Y.: Chloramphenicol-, dihydrostreptomycin- and
kanamycin-inactivating enzymes from multiple drug-resistant E. coli
carrying episome "R". Nature 208, 1301-1303 (1965).

16. Ozanne, B., Benveniste, R., Tipper, D., Davies, J.: Aminoglycoside antibiotics: inactivation by phosphorylation in Escherichia coli carrying R
factor. J. Bacteriol. 100, 1144-1146 (1969).

17. Kida, M., Asako, T., Yoneda, M., Mitsuhashi, S.: Phosphorylation of
dihydrostreptomycin by Pseudomonas aeruginosa. In: Microbial Drug Re-
sistance(S.Mitsuhashi and H.Hashimoto), p.441-448. University of Tokyo
Press; University Park Press, Tokyo, Baltimore and London. 1975.

18. Walker, J. B., Skorvaga, M.: Phosphorylation of streptomycin and dihydrostreptomycin by Streptomyces. J. Biol. Chem. 248, 2435-2440 (1973).

19. Umezawa, H., Takasawa, S., Okanishi, M., Utahara, R.: Adenylylstreptomycin,
a product of streptomycin inactivated by E. coli strain carrying R factor.
J. Antibiotics 21, 81-82 (1968).

20. Kawabe, H., Kobayashi, F., Yamaguchi, M., Utahara, R., Mitsuhashi, S.:
3"-Phosphoryldihydrostreptomycin produced by the inactivating enzyme
of Pseudomonas aeruginosa. J. Antibiot. 24, 651-652 (1971).

Discussion

Davies: In the strains that have a streptomycin phosphorylating enzyme and are also spectinomycin resistant, what is the mechanism of spectinomycin resistance?

Mitsuhashi: I don't know.

Falkow: What is the level of spectinomycin resistance?

Mitsuhashi: Very high.

Davies: In our experience we have not seen any examples of non-enzymatic spectinomycin resistance.

Falkow: You have the non-conjugative sulfonamide plasmids and then you found the non-conjugative sulfonamide-streptomycin plasmids. Have you done any homology studies to see if one is the progenitor of the other?

Mitsuhashi: We are just starting that.

Falkow: It is interesting because in the Su Sm plasmids which Barth and Grinter have shown to be a family, our studies indicate that Su Sm is part of a single operon.

Starlinger: Did you imply that your enzyme is made temperature sensitive by the addition of subinhibitory concentrations of sulfonamide?

Mitsuhashi: Yes.

Anderson: Stanley said that Sm Su plasmids are members of the same family. Many are but some are compatible with each other and show a differential pattern of mobilization. Thus, although they are carrying the same sort of resistance genes they are members of a different compatibility family. Whether in fact the resistance operons are the same is something that has to be tested.

Richmond: I think these may be exceptional plasmids in Japan, I don't think they are exceptional plasmids in Europe.

Anderson: I think this is a very important point. The pressure of antibiotics in different parts of the world may have the same end results so far as spectra of resistance is concerned, but we may be dealing with a variety of mechanisms, genes and operons. To resolve this would be a mammoth task that I don't think anyone would undertake; it is a mistake to generalize from a particular part of the world and say in absolute terms how something originated. All one can say is, we think, in our part of the world.

Nordström: There is one exception to the rule that a conjugative plasmid does not contain a sulfonamide resistant dihydropteroate synthetase and that is R1 which definitely produces a sulfonamide resistant enzyme. Your assay is very indirect for the presence of two enzymes. Your observation could, therefore, be produced by a copy effect. Conjugative plasmids are often present in small copy numbers and small plasmids in high copy numbers. In such a case you simply wouldn't detect the other enzyme.

Mitsuhashi: I cannot say.

Richmond: This point is very relevant. When you have single copy plasmids the amount of a resistant form of an enzyme can be very low indeed and so when you have multicopy plasmids, in fact you can see an enzyme and are led to believe that the enzyme is not produced when there is one copy, whereas in fact it is just there in very small amounts.

Anderson: I can give you a beautiful example of that, we have a multicopy, non-transmissible plasmid in which the ampicillin resistance level is 2000 μg and cephaloridine is 34.

Richmond: In my laboratory we see a lot of single ampicillin resistance plasmids that are transmissible.

Falkow: The incidence of ampicillin resistance in Japan has always been reported to be rather low, is this still the case?

Mitsuhashi: Yes, very low.

Plasmid-Mediated Tetracycline Resistance in E. coli

Stuart B. Levy, Laura McMurry, Philip Onigman, and Richard M. Saunders

The tetracyclines are effective bacteriostatic drugs for a wide variety of microbial infections. They inhibit the binding of aminoacyl transfer RNA to the 30S ribosomal subunit (1). More specifically they appear to interfere with the codon-anticodon interaction (2). The drug has worldwide usage therapeutically as well as prophylactically in humans, domestic and farm animals, and plants. It is, therefore, not surprising that the emergence of resistance to this drug has also occurred worldwide and in epidemic proportions. In fact, in most organisms tested, if resistances to antibiotics have been found, tetracycline resistance is among them. The list includes all Enterobacteriaceae, Pseudomonas, Hemophilus influenza, Streptococcus fecalis, Clostridia perfringins, and Staphylococcus aureus (3,4). The most common mode of resistance is by plasmids on which are found the genes for resistance. A clear understanding of the mechanism of resistance in these different species has not yet been reached. Some information has been obtained, however, in studies of Enterobacteriaceae (5,6,7) and Staphylococcus aureus (8,9). In most Enterobacteriaceae studied and in Staphylococcus, expression of resistance is regulated (6,7,9). We have identified a tetracycline-inducible protein, TET, associated with tetracycline resistance (7,10) in E. coli and we have partially purified a "repressor" which regulates synthesis of this protein (11). Our results suggest that, as is TET protein, so is the whole tetracycline resistance operon under negative control releasable by tetracycline.

We shall present some recent results we have obtained in three areas of study of tetracycline resistance in E. coli: 1) the uptake and relative accumulation of tetracycline in sensitive and resistant cells, 2) the internal location and biologic activity of tetracycline taken up by E. coli, and 3) the regulatory event controlling phenotypic expression of tetracycline resistance and the synthesis of the inner membrane protein TET.

The bacterial strains we have used in these studies are listed in Table 1. We have examined particularly the characteristics of R factor 222 which codes for resistance to four drugs including tetracycline. For comparisons we have looked at other plasmids including RP1 and pSC101 which have lower tetracycline resistance levels. Our general approach has been to compare the metabolism and activity of tetracycline in sensitive and resistant cells.

Table 1. E. coli Strains

Strain	Relevant Cellular Characteristics	Plasmid	Source
DO-1	(CSH-2) pro⁻ met⁻	--	T. Watanabe
D1-1	DO-1	R222[1]	this laboratory
χ984	minicell⁺, Sm^R	--	R. Curtiss, III
DO-7	Nal^R derivative of χ984	--	this laboratory
D1-7	χ984	R222	this laboratory
DO-21	wild type (AN 180)	--	J. Davies (ref.26)
DO-22	unc A (AN 120)	--	J. Davies (ref.26)
D1-186	DO-21	R222	this laboratory
D1-187	DO-22	R222	this laboratory
D15-3	χ984	RP1[2]	this laboratory
D19-3	χ984	pSC101[3]	M. Malamy

[1]Codes for resistance to chloramphenicol, streptomycin, sulfonamides, tetracycline. Plasmid originally received from T. Watanabe.

[2]Codes for resistance to ampicillin-carbenicillin, neomycin and tetracycline.

[3]Codes for tetracycline resistance.

Accumulation of Tetracycline

Since previous studies have used a radioactively labeled tetracycline as probe in which some drug appears to bind non-specifically to cells at $0^{\circ}C$ (6,10,12), we re-examined our labeled tetracycline preparation before it was given to the cell. A preparation which had been in solution for two months at $4^{\circ}C$ contained several labeled substances which were not tetracycline. More importantly, in uptake studies, over half of the ^3H-material bound to the cell at $0^{\circ}C$ was shown not to be tetracycline, but one of the contaminating breakdown products (Figure 1). In fact, cells could be used to absorb out this contaminant since it appeared to bind preferentially to the cells. These findings may help explain some of the quantitative differences in uptake studies reported by different groups. As a result of these findings, we use only freshly dissolved ^3H-tetracycline (New England Nuclear) for studying tetracycline metabolism in E. coli.

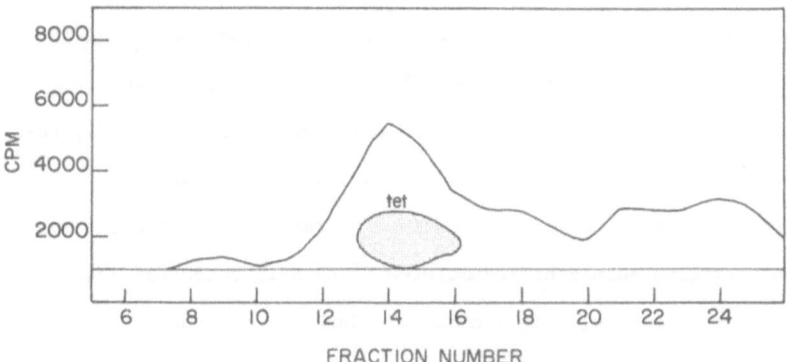

Figure 1. Chromatography of Aged Tetracycline Taken up by R^+ Cells

Dl-7 cells were incubated at 1.2 X 10^9 cells/ml in a potassium phosphate buffered minimal medium (including 4mM $MgSO_4$) for 30 minutes at $0^{\circ}C$ with 1.2 X 10^7 cpm/ml ^3H-tetracycline (1 X 10^6 cpm/µg) which had been stored at $4^{\circ}C$ in water for 2 months. The cells were pelleted, washed four times in 12 volumes of cold medium, and the tetracycline extracted with butanol:methanol:10% citric acid (4:1:2) at $37^{\circ}C$ for 30 minutes. All labeled material was extracted. The extract, which represented 3% of the total cpm added, was chromatographed (ascending) on Whatman #1 pretreated with .1M EDTA. The solvent was the top layer of a butanol:acetic acid:water mixture (4:1:5). The chromatogram was cut into equal sized pieces (the origin being zero) and counted in a liquid scintillation counter. The spot represents undegraded tetracycline.

Early studies of tetracycline resistance demonstrated that the resistant E. coli took up less tetracycline than did the sensitive cell (5,6). It is noteworthy, however, that the amounts of tetracycline presumably taken up by the cells, did not correlate with the levels of resistance expressed by the cells (12,13,14,15). We have made similar observations. For instance, although the minimal inhibitory concentration (MIC) for tetracycline of DO-1 is 1 µg/ml, that for D1-1, its R222-containing derivative, is more than 200 µg/ml, a difference of over 200 fold. And yet, the difference in total uptake of tetracycline between these two strains is only 3-5 fold (16) (see Tables 3,4). Thus, the difference in uptake does not explain resistance to this drug. We were interested, therefore, in determining whether the biologic activity of the drug or its chemical composition had been altered. It had been reported previously that tetracycline extracted from resistant cells did not show any detectable structural change (8,17). We also found no paper chromatographic evidence for any structural change of drug as extracted from sensitive or resistant cells (data not shown). Furthermore, we found no difference in antibacterial activity between tetracycline extracted from resistant cells and a standard tetracycline solution (Table 2). Thus, resistance could not be explained by an inactivation of the antibiotic.

If permeability were the only mechanism for resistance, then the same amount of tetracycline should be accumulated by sensitive and resistant cells when protein synthesis is equally inhibited. Such was not the case. About 20-30 fold more tetracycline was taken up by the resistant cell than the sensitive cell before similar inhibition of protein synthesis was obtained (Table 5) (16).

The lack of correlation between accumulation of tetracycline and resistance might be explained if tetracycline were transported to a different location in the resistant as compared with the sensitive cell. Since TET protein is in the inner membrane, it was possible that all the tetracycline in the resistant cell was held back in the periplasmic space. However, in

Table 2. Antibacterial Activity of Tetracycline Extracted from Cells

µg/ml tetracycline	source of extract	growth of sensitive cells: $\frac{1}{\text{doubling time}}$	% inhibition
0		.036	0
1.5	uninduced (- tet)	.013	65
1.5	induced (+ tet)	.010	71
2.6	uninduced (- tet)	.005	82
2.6	induced (+ tet)	.007	80
1.0	standard tet solution	.019	47
1.5	standard tet solution	.011	69
2.6	standard tet solution	.009	75

Preinduced D1-1 cells (+ tet) at 6.5 X 10^9 cells/ml were incubated at 37°C in L broth with ^{3}H-tetracycline (25 µg/ml; 3 X 10^4 cpm/µg) for 1 hour. Cells were washed twice in 1 volume of L broth at 4°C. All radioactivity was extracted from the pellets into butanol:10% acetic acid:methanol (4:2:1) at 37°C. The extracts were dried under N_2 and redissolved in L broth. To control for any inhibitory effects of cellular extracts, extracts were similarly prepared from uninduced D1-1 cells (- tet) which were incubated without ^{3}H-tetracycline. The effect of the tetracycline in the (+ tet) extract on the growth rate of tetracycline-sensitive DO-1 cells was compared to that of a standard tetracycline solution as well as to standard tetracycline added to the (- tet) extract from uninduced cells. The concentration of tetracycline in the (+ tet) extract was determined by specific radioactivity.

analyzing the sensitive and resistant cells, there was little if any difference between the relative amount of tetracycline released from the periplasm of either (Table 3). Furthermore, the proportion of the released tetracycline bound to a high molecular weight component in the periplasm was about 20% in both cells. Subsequently, other studies examined the location of tetracycline within the cell. Resistant and sensitive cells incubated in the presence of ^{3}H-tetracycline were washed and lysed by two different procedures (7,34). Once again, there was little difference between the sensitive and resistant cells in the proportion of tetracycline in the cytoplasmic and membrane fractions (Table 4). Under these lysis conditions, the same amount of tetracycline was bound to membranes of sensitive or resistant cells. Separation of the membrane fraction into inner and outer membranes demonstrated most of the tetracycline bound to the outer membrane (Figure 2).

None was found associated with the inner membrane of resistant cells where
TET protein is located.

Since the site of activity of tetracycline is the ribosome, we determined the amount of drug associated with the ribosomes of resistant and sensitive cells when protein synthesis was inhibited equally (Table 5). Both
sensitive and resistant cells had similar relative proportions of tetracycline in the cytosol. By this lysis procedure the resistant cells had a
greater relative amount attached to the membranes and a 3-fold less relative
amount with ribosomes. However, the total amount of tetracycline associated
with ribosomes in resistant cells was 10 times that found in sensitive cells.

Table 3.   Release of Tetracycline from Periplasmic Space

A.   EDTA – Lysozyme Treatment

	R^- tetracycline mμg	%	R^+ tetracycline mμg	%	R^-/R^+
TOTAL UPTAKE	630	100	128	100	4.9
Released from periplasm	110	17	30	23	3.7
Excluded from Sephadex G50	21	3.3	5.7	4.5	3.7
% of periplasmic material excluded from G50		19		19	1.0

B.   Osmotic Shock

	R^- tetracycline mμg	%	R^+ tetracycline mμg	%	R^-/R^+
TOTAL UPTAKE	1570	100	530	100	3.0
Released during sucrose incubation	440	28	174	33	2.5
Released from peri- plasm into water shockate (corrected)	220	14	36	6.8	6.1

Cells were incubated at 4 X 10^9 cells/ml with ^{3}H-tetracycline (1.9 X 10^6
cpm/μg) at 1.8 μg/ml (A) or 4.5 μg/ml (B) in L broth at 37°C for 40 minutes.
Periplasmic material was released from cells by EDTA-lysozyme treatment (A)
or osmotic shock (B) using the methods of Heppel (18). In (B) a significant
amount of radioactivity was solubilized from cells during sucrose incubation.
Also in (B), the shockage was corrected for leakage from the cytoplasm by
assuming such leakage was proportional to that measured for the cytoplasmic
protein β-galactosidase. The periplasmic material was chromatographed (A)
on Sephadex G50 in .01M Tris pH 8 at 4°C.

Table 4. Distribution of Tetracycline in Cell

	Tetracycline (mμg/A$_{530}$)					
	total		membrane		cytosol	
Expt. 1						
R$^-$	20.1	(100%)	2.2	(11%)	17.9	(89%)
R$^+$	5.6	(100%)	1.8	(32%)	3.8	(68%)
R$^-$/R$^+$	3.6		1.1		4.8	
Expt. 2						
R$^-$	56.0	(100%)	2.1	(3.8%)	53.8	(96.1%)
R$^+$	19.0	(100%)	2.0	(10.5%)	16.8	(88.6%)
R$^-$/R$^+$	2.9		1.0		3.2	

The data in Expt. 1 were taken from the experiment described in Figure 2. Labeling was at 2 μg/ml tetracycline. Cells for Expt. 2 were labeled as described for Table 3 B (at 4.5 μg/ml tetracycline). They were lysed by incubating 15 minutes in .01M Tris pH 8, .001M EDTA, 100 μg/ml lysozyme, followed by two 30 second sonications. Membranes were pelleted at 29,000 X g for 20 minutes. After centrifugation for 3 hours at 260,000 X g the amount of radioactivity in the supernatant was determined.

These studies, therefore, could not implicate compartmentalization of the drug as a distinguishing feature of resistance although our methods may have failed to detect this difference. We considered, however, that resistance could be linked to control of tetracycline activity intracellularly. In previous studies using an in vitro "coupled" DNA-dependent protein synthesis system, we had noted an increased resistance to tetracycline in the system prepared from the resistant cell as compared to the sensitive cell(11).

We have subsequently examined the effect of tetracycline on translation (RNA-dependent) systems in vitro. With endogenous mRNA to code for protein, the system prepared from sensitive cells was more sensitive to tetracycline than that from resistant cells (Table 6). These findings were also found when a synthetic mRNA, polyuridylic acid was used (Table 7). In both instances, repeatedly a 2-3 fold difference in resistance to the inhibitory effect of tetracycline was found. Similar findings have been

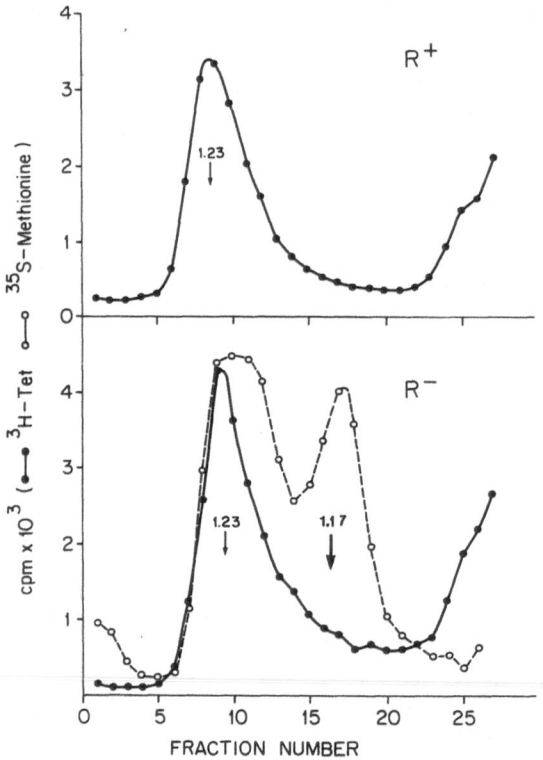

Figure 2.   Binding of ^{3}H-Tetracycline Incorporated <u>In Vivo</u> to Outer Membranes
of Sensitive and Resistant Cells

Freshly grown DO-1 and preinduced D1-1 cells at 2.5 X 10^9 cells/ml
were incubated in L broth (33) at 37°C with 2 ug/ml of ^{3}H-tetracycline
(5 X 10^5 cpm/µg) for 45 minutes. An aliquot of cells was labeled separately with .075 mC/ml ^{35}S-methionine. Cells were washed three times in
12 volumes L broth, lysed and fractionated to give inner and outer membranes
by the method of Osborn <u>et al.</u> (34) except that 15mM EDTA was used during
spheroblast formation, the membranes were not washed, the gradient was
25-58% w/w sucrose in 0.5mM EDTA, and centrifugation was in a Beckman SW
50.1 rotor at 47,000 rpm for 14 hours. Gradient fractions with ^{3}H-tetra-
cycline were counted in Aquasol (New England Nuclear Corporation). ^{35}S
protein fractions were hot TCA precipitated on paper discs and counted in
Liquifluor (N.E.N.). Sucrose density was determined by refractive index.
Outer membrane = ρ1.23; inner membrane = ρ1.17.

reported in comparisons between other sensitive and resistant <u>E. coli</u> in

<u>in vitro</u> translation systems (20).

In summary, the resistant cell accumulates large amounts of tetracy-

cline without inhibition of its protein synthesis. The distribution of

tetracycline seems to be similar in both sensitive and resistant cells ex-

Table 5. Distribution of Accumulated Tetracycline in Cells

	tet in media μg/ml	% inhibition of protein synthesis	Tetracycline (mμg/A$_{530}$)						
			total uptake	membranes	%	cytosol	%	ribosomes	%
DO-1	0.2	46	7.2	0.52	7.2	5.46	75.8	0.66	9.2
D1-1	71	32	215	54	25.1	136	63.3	6.7	3.1
R$^+$/R$^-$	350		30	104		25		10.2	

Cells were labeled in L broth at 37°C with ^{3}H-tetracycline (5 X 10^5 cpm/ml) for 90 minutes, diluted 1/5 into cold L broth, centrifuged, washed in 1 volume .05M Tris pH 8, and lysed in a French pressure cell as described (32). Unlysed cells were removed by centrifugation for 5 minutes at 1,000 X g. The membranes were pelleted by centrifugation for 35 minutes at 30,000 X g and the ribosomes pelleted in 2 hours at 170,000 X g. The rate of protein synthesis was determined from 60 to 90 minutes of labeling in L broth by measuring ^{35}S-methionine incorporation into TCA-precipitable material. In another experiment the ribosome fractions were further separated on 15-30% w/v sucrose gradients made with extraction buffer (.01M in magnesium). About half the ^{3}H-tetracycline in the gradients was bound to the 70S ribosomes for both DO-1 and D1-1; the rest was on top of the gradients.

Table 6. Inhibiton of Protein Synthesis In Vitro by Tetracycline

Expt.	tetracycline μg/ml	% inhibition R$^-$	R$^+$	Δ% (R$^-$ - R$^+$)
1A	20	80	63	17
B[a]	20	77	69	8
2A	15	57	27	30
B	45	87	82	5
C	100	94	100	-6
3A	1	13	-4	17
B	3	32	18	14
C	10	49	37	12
D	20	76	67	9

Extracts were prepared from DO-1 or preinduced D1-1 cells as described (32), except that for these experiments the crude pressure cell lysate freed only of unlysed cells was used. Protein synthesis was performed as described (32) using ^{3}H-phenylalanine or ^{3}H-lysine. The reaction was initiated by adding radioactivity (Expt. 1,2) or by placing at 30°C (3). Every 10 minutes samples of the in vitro reaction were removed to assay for rate of protein synthesis. Final concentration of crude lysate in assay was 3.2 mg/ml; it was the sole source of mRNA, ribosomes, and soluble factors.

[a]Mg^{++} 12.0mM (all others 6.8mM)

cept for an apparent proportionate increase in the membrane fraction of re-sistant cells at high concentrations of the drug. Ten-fold more drug is associated with the resistant cell ribosomes under conditions where protein synthesis in sensitive and resistant cells is equally inhibited. These data along with the results in in vitro translation systems imply that there is an internal inhibition of the activity of tetracycline. Current atten-tion is being given to isolating and characterizing this "inhibitor".

Table 7. Effect of Tetracycline on In Vitro Translation with Poly-uridylic Acid

A. 205 µg/ml poly-U

% inhibition

tet	0.2 µg/ml	1.0 µg/ml	10 µg/ml
DO-1	0	4.5	28
D1-1	0.5	3.0	18

B. 5 µg/ml poly-U

% inhibition

tet	0	10 µg/ml	50 µg/ml
DO-1	0	58	72
D1-1	0	40	59

In vitro protein synthesis assay performed as in Table 6, except syn-thetic mRNA (poly-U) was used in .015M Mg^{++}, and the purified S30 (after Sephadex G25) (32) was used as a source of ribosomes and soluble factors. In part A the reaction was stopped with .1 N NaOH at 37°C for 10 minutes; protein was precipitated with 10% TCA. Part A: 35 minute assay; Part B: 20 minute assay.

Kinetics of Tetracycline Uptake

The decreased entry of tetracycline into the resistant cell was still an unexplained phenomenon. From previous studies, uptake in both sensitive and resistant cells appeared to occur by active transport (21,22). It was not clear how the plasmid was suppressing uptake in the sensitive host cell.

We studied uptake in DO-1 and D1-1 cells with different concentrations of tetracycline from 1-100 µg/ml. At all concentrations the uptake was biphasic, characterized by an initial rapid uptake which appeared to terminate by 4-6 minutes, followed by a slower uptake which would continue indefinitely (Figures 3,4) (16,23). The rapid uptake system was unsaturatable with concentrations of tetracycline up to 400 μg/ml of tetracycline. These findings may indicate that affinity for the "tet carrier" is very low, so that free carrier is still far in excess at these concentrations of tetracycline, or that there is no rate-limiting step involving a tet carrier. We were concerned, however, that the initial uptake, which amounted to about 3% of the labeled material per 10^9 cells, represented an impurity in the ^{3}H-tetracycline, undetected biologically or by paper chromatography. Studies proved that this was not so: 1) the amount of ^{3}H-tetracycline in this rapid uptake phase increased proportionally with the number of cells up to at least 20% of the total labeled material in the preparation (23), and 2) when the tetracycline which had accumulated in 6 minutes by sensitive cells from a dense culture (6 X 10^9 cells/ml) and which represented about 16% of the total radioactivity in the preparation was extracted and given to a fresh culture of cells, the same biphasic kinetics of uptake were seen and the same proportion of drug was transported by the rapid uptake system (23). Similar results were also found for the ^{3}H-tetracycline remaining in the supernatant above this dense culture of cells. These particular studies in addition to previous ones confirmed that 1) all the labeled material was tetracycline, 2) the rapid uptake and slow uptake represented two transport systems for tetracycline in the cell, and 3) the tetracycline was not altered in its biologic activity, its structure or its transport kinetics when accumulated by the resistant cell.

Studies were undertaken to determine whether both uptake systems were subject to active transport. Initially the effect of arsenate, a general inhibitor of the synthesis of high energy phosphate compounds was tried (24,25). As seen in Figure 3, pre-incubation of the cells with arsenate inhibited uptake in both sensitive and resistant cells, but the kinetics of inhibition were somewhat different. In the resistant cell, there appeared to be an increase in the level of uptake of the drug by the rapid uptake system, although the slow uptake system was blocked. In the sensitive cell, arsenate blocked the slow uptake system, and did not change the kinetics of the rapid uptake system.

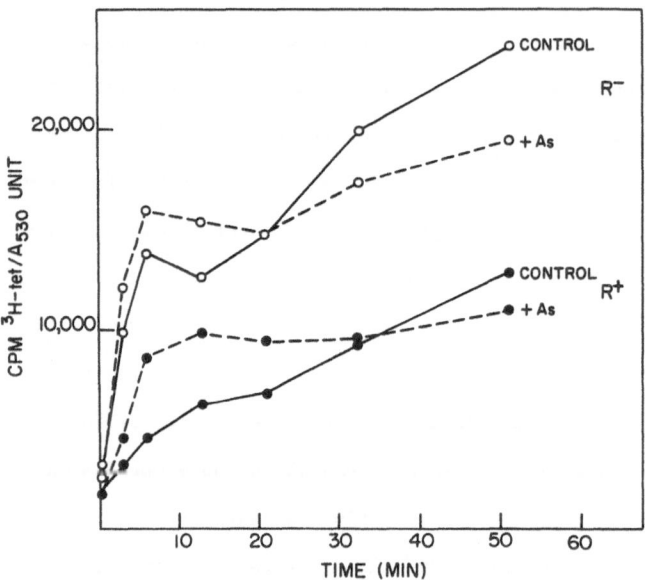

Figure 3. Effect of Arsenate on ^{3}H–tetracycline Uptake

Freshly grown DO-1 and preinduced Dl-1 cells (2.3 X 10^9 cells/ml) were incubated in the presence or absence of .01M sodium arsenate in L broth at 37°C for 19 minutes. ^{3}H–tetracycline (2 μg/ml; 7 X 10^5 cpm/μg) was added. Culture samples were diluted 1/17 in cold buffered saline (per liter: NaCl 8.5 g, Na_2HPO_4 .6 g, KH_2PO_4 .3 g, gelatin .1 g) and centrifuged within 5 minutes at 4°C. Cells were resuspended and samples were taken for A_{530} and radioactivity (100 μl).

The results with the resistant cell suggested that arsenate was also inhibiting an active efflux system in the cell. We are currently examining this possibility. Subsequent studies were designed to determine whether oxidative phosphorylation was required for tetracycline transport. In these studies we used both cyanide (CN) and 2, 4–dinitrophenol (DNP) which are inhibitors of oxidative phosphorylation (24). A rather dramatic difference was seen between the effect of either of these drugs on uptake in the sensitive and the resistant cell (23). Only the sensitive cell was inhibited. There was turn off of the slow uptake system with no effect on the rapid uptake system (Figure 4).

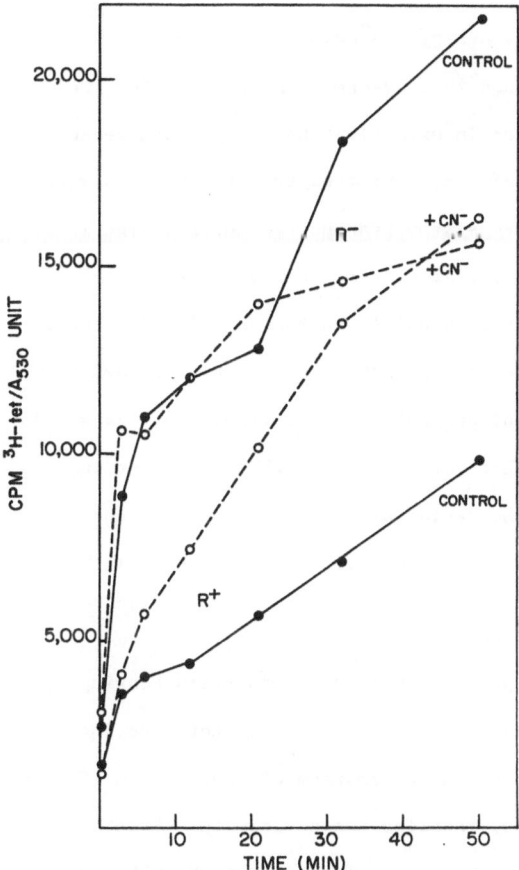

Figure 4. Effect of Cyanide on ^{3}H-tetracycline Uptake

Methods were the same as in Figure 3. Cells were preincubated with or without .52mM NaCN for 20 minutes before addition of ^{3}H-tetracycline.

In the resistant cell, both CN and DNP produced an initial increase in uptake presumably by the rapid uptake system. In these cells, the slow uptake system, however, was not affected by DNP (16) and was actually increased by CN. The results with these inhibitors clearly demonstrated that the uptake systems for tetracycline in the sensitive and the resistant cell were different. Active transport of the drug into the sensitive cell appeared to occur by oxidative phosphorylation. This inherent uptake system was blocked in the resistant cell and was replaced by another uptake system, presumably plasmid encoded, which showed less affinity for tetracycline and which was generated from a different energy source.

In order to confirm these findings in a system without inhibitors we examined an "unc A" mutant (uncoupled in oxidative phosphorylation because the $Mg^{++}Ca^{++}$ATPase is missing (23,26)). As predicted from the results with the inhibitors, only the rapid uptake system transported tetracycline into this unc mutant. There was no slow uptake system. However, when an R^+ tetracycline resistant derivative of this unc A was tested (D1-187), there was now uptake of the drug via a slow uptake system presumably encoded by the plasmid (23). The sensitivity of unc mutants to tetracycline was similar to that of the wild type parent. Therefore, even though the present inhibitor studies have not shown that the rapid uptake system requires energy, this system still places tetracycline into an active site in the cell.

Role of TET Protein in Tetracycline Resistance

A new inducible inner membrane protein appears in minicells bearing tetracycline resistant plasmids labeled in the presence of tetracycline (7). It has also been detected in the inner membrane of whole cells (Figure 5). Its detection was facilitated by labeling the cells with ^{35}S-methionine in the presence of rifamycin. We had noted previously that the mRNA for TET protein was sufficiently stable to be active after removal of the inducer, tetracycline, from minicells (10). Using rifamycin, we decreased the synthesis of inner membrane proteins from less stable mRNAs and were able to detect TET protein in induced, but not in uninduced, resistant cells.

The role of TET protein in tetracycline resistance is yet unknown. Some insight into the complexity of its relationship to tetracycline resistance has come from studies in minicells. Minicells purified from tetracycline-resistant but uninduced host cells are not inducible to high level tetracycline resistance (10,27). In these minicells, however, synthesis of TET in is induced (7). These studies indicated that the presence of TET

in in the cells was not sufficient for complete expression of tetra-

ne resistance. Uptake studies showed that induction of TET protein

ese minicells was not accompanied by decreased uptake of tetracycline

re 6). Coincident with the lack of a change in tetracycline uptake,

he absence of increased resistance to tetracycline in the minicells

ed after purification as compared with uninduced minicells (Figure 6).

owever, the minicells were purified from a culture of cells which had

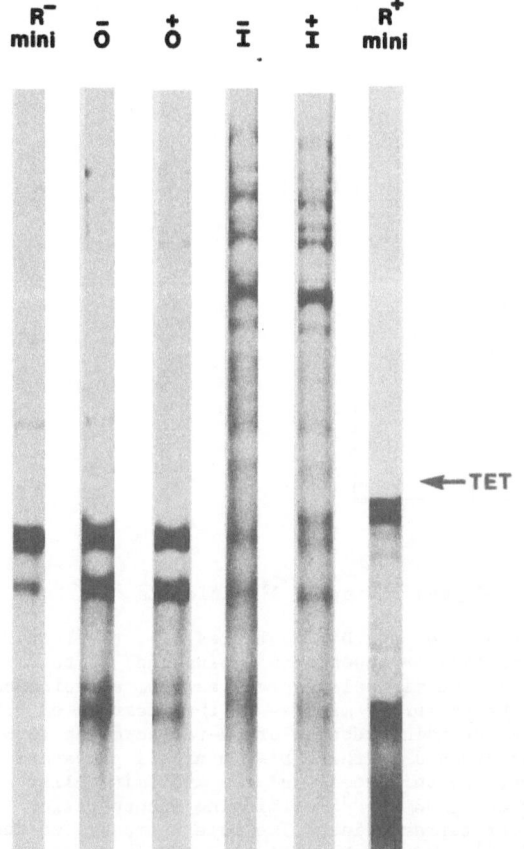

e 5. SDS Gel Electrophoresis Showing TET Protein in Inner Membrane of
Resistant Cells

D1-7 cells were grown in the presence (+) or absence (-) of 2 µg/ml
cycline. They were purified away from their minicells and incubated
0 minutes in methionine assay medium with methionine (1 µg/ml) and
g/ml rifamycin. The cells were centrifuged and resuspended at 4 X 10^8

cells/ml in methionine assay medium without methionine but with rifamycin (200 µg/ml) and labeled with ^{35}S-methionine (.017 mC/ml) for 30 minutes at 37°C. The cells were washed in .01M Tris pH 8, lysed, and inner and outer membranes separated as described in Figure 2. The inner (ρ = 1.17) and outer (ρ = 1.26) membrane fractions were pooled separately, precipitated with 5% TCA at 4°C, and SDS polyacrylamide gel electrophoresis performed as described (7) except that the gel was treated with dimethylsulfoxide and PPO to enhance sensitivity of autoradiography (35). Arrow points to TET protein identified by its induction in R222 minicells. It was found only in inner membrane of induced cells. O = outer membrane. I = inner membrane. Outer membrane proteins synthesized in R⁻ minicells were used as standards (37).

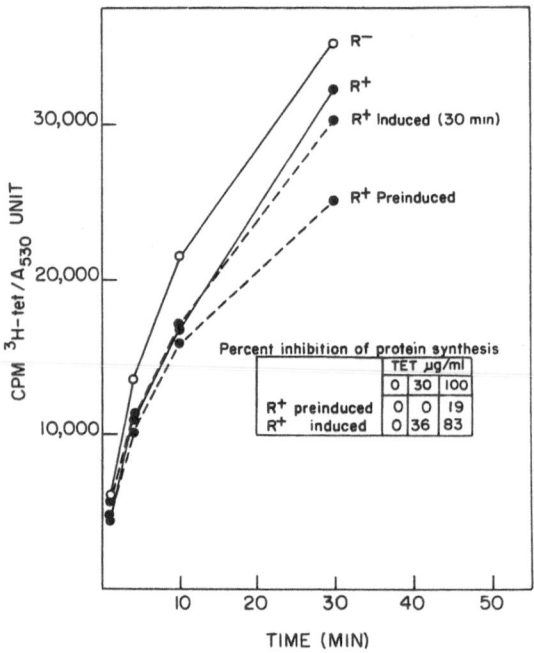

Figure 6. Tetracycline Uptake and Sensitivity of R⁺ Minicells

    Minicells were harvested from χ984 and D1-7 cultures (7), the latter grown in the presence (R⁺ preinduced) or absence (R⁺ uninduced) of tetra-cycline (0.5 µg/ml). A sample of the minicells harvested from an uninduced R⁺ culture were incubated in L broth for 30 minutes in the presence of 0.6 µg/ml tetracycline to induce TET protein. Uptake of ^{3}H-tetracycline (0.67 µg/ml, 1.7 X 10⁶ cpm/µg) was determined in these D1-7 minicell preparations (preinduced, induced 30 minutes, and uninduced) and the χ984 minicells: Minicell protein synthesis was measured by ^{35}S-methionine incorporation (7) in the presence and/or absence of tetracycline. The same tetracycline sen-sitivity was found for induced or uninduced R⁺ minicells. Only the mini-cells harvested from the pre-induced cell culture showed increased resistance.

been induced with tetracycline, these minicells demonstrated high levels of

resistance to the drug, similar to that found in the induced resistant cell

(Figure 6). As seen with whole cells, the difference in uptake did not correlate with difference in resistance: The uptake in induced minicells was only one-half that of the uninduced minicells. Furthermore, there was less than a 2-fold difference in tetracycline uptake between minicells purified from an induced R^+ cell culture and those from a sensitive R^- cell culture (Figure 6). This minimal difference in uptake is even less than the 3-5 fold difference seen in tetracycline uptake by resistant and sensitive cells. The lack of induced resistance in R^+ minicells may result from 1) malpositioning or malfunctioning of the TET protein placed in the already formed minicell membrane, 2) lack of sufficient TET protein synthesis in the minicell, 3) inability of the induction process in minicells to completely turn off the inherent host uptake system, or 4) absence in the minicell of a chromosomal product needed for complete expression of this resistance. These possibilities are under experimentation. These present findings suggest, however, that TET protein cannot act alone in determining tetracycline resistance although it most likely is involved in the reduced uptake of tetracycline by the resistant cell.

Despite the yet unknown role of TET protein in tetracycline resistance, the amount synthesized in minicells appears to correlate with the level of tetracycline resistance expressed in whole cells. For instance, we find that the amount of TET protein synthesized in minicells containing pSC101 (cellular MIC 25 µg/ml) is much less than that found in minicells containing R222 (cellular MIC 200 µg/ml). Results with other plasmids and mutants of R222 (see below) have also demonstrated this correlation. We have also observed that the tetracycline determinants on different plasmids may not be identical. We see two proteins induced by tetracycline in pSC101-containing minicells, only one of which is seen in induced minicells containing R222. One pSC101 protein is of similar molecular weight as the TET protein. The other is of smaller molecular weight (about 25-30,000) and appears to be releasable into the supernatant upon lysis of the minicells (Figure 7). This second protein has not been seen in preparations of R222 minicells, but its size, similar to another R222-encoded membrane protein

MRB (28), may obscure its presence in these preparations especially if it is synthesized in small amounts. This second inducible protein may be related to the intracellular inhibitor which we detect in our in vitro assay systems from R222 cells.

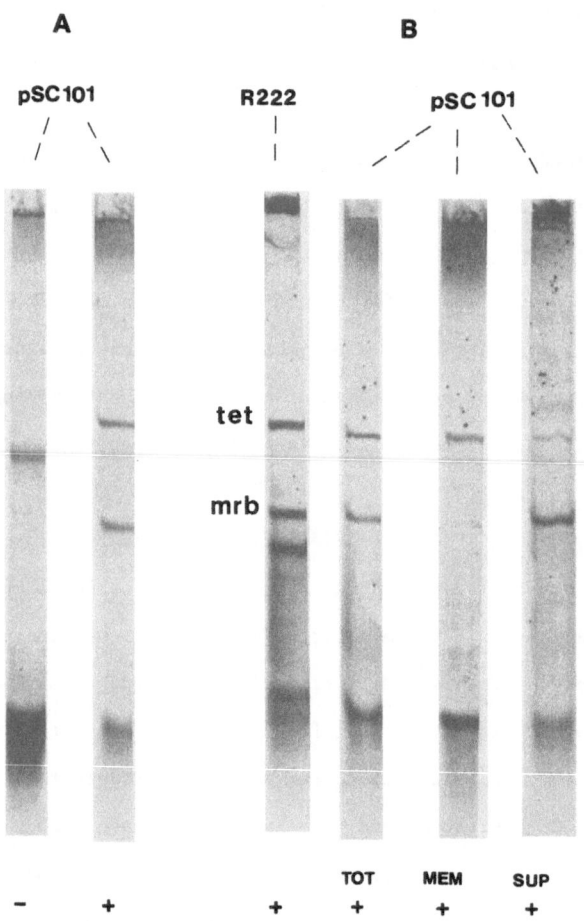

Figure 7. SDS Polyacrylamide Gel Electrophoresis of R222- and pSC101-containing Minicells

Minicells were purified and labeled as described (7). The pSC101 minicells were lysed (7) and separated into membrane and supernatant fractions by centrifugation for 20 minutes at 29,000 X g. The total and supernatant were precipitated with 5% TCA, the fractions dissolved in SDS and analyzed by gel electrophoresis (7,19). A. Total pSC101 minicells labeled in the absence or presence of tetracycline. B. R222 and pSC101 minicells labeled in the presence of tetracycline. Total (TOT), supernatant (SUP) and membrane

(MEM) fractions from pSC101. Most of TET protein sediments with the membrane fraction whereas most of the second inducible pSC101 protein remains in the supernatant fraction. mrb = major R plasmid protein band (28). Second pSC101 inducible protein has same molecular weight.

Tetracycline Resistance Mutants of R222

In order to determine the number of loci functioning in the expression of tetracycline resistance, we have isolated various types of mutants in the tetracycline determinant on R222. Among these mutants are tetracycline sensitive, low level constitutive, intermediate constitutive and high level constitutive mutants.

1) **Tetracycline sensitive.** These mutants were derived by mutagenesis with ethyl methane sulfonate which should produce primarily point mutations. Thus far, we have been unable to demonstrate complementation between a large number of tetracycline sensitive plasmids examined. This failure in complementation between sensitive mutants has been reported by other investigators (29), and may reflect loss of the complete determinant (see below). Of ten tetracycline sensitive mutants studied in the minicell, none coded for TET protein.

2) **Low level constitutives.** Resistance levels of the low level constitutives were expressed at 2-10 μg/ml, about 1-5% of normal. Studies of these mutants in the minicell system demonstrated constitutive synthesis of the TET protein, but at low amounts. These mutants frequently reverted to sensitivity with no back mutation to resistance. These findings suggested complete deletion of the tetracycline determinant. With loss of resistance there was loss of synthesis of TET protein in minicells. Complementation studies with these mutants were unsuccessful since the resistance determinant was lost so rapidly.

3) **Intermediate level constitutives.** These mutants showed a constitutive level of resistance to 50 μg/ml (about 25% of wild type). They were isolated after multiple penicillin screening tests following mutagenesis. They frequently reverted to the wild type (inducible resistance to 200 μg/ml).

4) **High level constitutives**. Up to the present we have been studying high level constitutive mutants whose resistance level is 100 µg/ml which is only half of the induced wild type. These mutants are, therefore, unlike the completely derepressed constitutive mutants described by Reeve for R57 (30). Furthermore, two of these mutants have shown a transition to constitutive low level resistance (i.e. 10 µg/ml). Constitutive synthesis of TET protein in minicells was noted with these plasmids as well, in amounts about half of the induced wild type.

The multiplicity of regulatory mutants which we have isolated do not allow their placement into a classic gene regulatory category. They resemble certain mutants described for the negatively regulated galactose operon (31). In these cell mutants IS2 elements have been inserted into the operon. In one orientation the effect is a polar mutation within the galactose operon. In this case there is about 1% constitutive synthesis of the galactokinase. One property of these low level constitutive mutants is the complete loss of the galactokinase activity in what appears to be a deletion of the operon. Intermediate level constitutives are also described in this operon with levels of activity 25-30%. Some of these show a fast reversion to the original phenotype (H. Saedler, personal communication). The analogy of our tetracycline resistance mutants with these galactose mutants is obvious. Studies are in progress to elucidate the molecular mechanism responsible for these multiple regulatory types and the possible role of insertion elements in producing the different phenotypes.

Conclusions

Tetracycline resistance appears to result from two separate but coordinated mechanisms: decreased uptake and internal inhibition. An alternate tetracycline transport system encoded by resistance plasmids is introduced into the host cell with apparent turn-off of the inherent host transport system. Although this uptake system may place tetracycline in a different compartment of the cell, studies have so far not been able to

demonstrate this to be the case. In fact, there appeared to be no difference
in the distribution of the drug in sensitive and resistant cells. The 30-
fold accumulation of tetracycline (still biologically active) in the tetracycline resistant cell as compared to the sensitive cell at equal inhibitory
levels implies an internal inhibition of tetracycline activity within the
resistant cell. Whether decreased uptake and internal inhibition result
from the product of one or more genes is the subject of present study using
mutants in the tetracycline resistance determinant. Regulatory mutants
expressing different levels of resistance may help in defining the quantitative role of these two mechanisms in the complete phenotypic expression
of resistance. The rapid loss of the resistance determinants from some of
these mutants suggests insertions and deletions of genetic material. This
laboratory-observed phenomenon may explain the common spontaneous loss of
tetracycline resistance determinants from wild type plasmids.

Acknowledgment

This work has been supported by American Cancer Society grant #VC-202
and a NIAID Research Career Development Award to S.B.L. We thank Sandra
Keeney for her assistance.

References

1. Suzuki, I., Kaji, H. and Kaji, A.: Binding of specific sRNA to 30s
    ribosomal subunits: effects of 50s ribosomal subunits. Proc. Nat.
    Acad. Sci., USA 55:1483-1490, 1966.

2. Högenauer, G. and Turnowsky, F.: The effects of streptomycin and
    tetracycline on codon-anticodon interactions. FEBS Lett. 26:185-188,
    1972.

3. Falkow, S.: Infectious Multiple Drug Resistance. Pion. Limited, 1975.

4. Davies, J. and Novick, R. (edit.): Proceedings of the 2nd ASM Conference
    on Extrachromosomal Elements. Microbiology, 1977.

5. Izaki, K., Kiuchi, K. and Arima, K.: Specificity and mechanism of te-
    tracycline resistance in a multiple drug resistant strain of Escherichia
    coli. J. Bact. 91:628-633, 1966.

6. Franklin, T.J.: Resistance to Escherichia coli to tetracycline. Changes
    in permeability to tetracyclines in Escherichia coli bearing transferable
    resistance factors. Biochem. J. 105:371-378, 1967.

7. Levy, S.B. and McMurry, L.: Detection of an inducible membrane protein associated with R factor mediated tetracycline resistance. Biochem. Biophys. Res. Comm. 56:1060–1068, 1974.

8. Sompolinsky, D., Krawitz, T., Zaidenzaig, Y. and Abramova, N.: Inducible resistance to tetracycline in Staphylococcus aureus. J. Gen. Microbiol. 62:341–349, 1970.

9. Sompolinsky, D., Zaidenzaig, Y., Ziegler-Schlomowitz, R. and Abramova, N.: Mechanism of tetracycline resistance in Staphylococcus aureus. J. Gen. Microbiol. 62:351–362, 1970.

10. Levy, S.B.: The relation of a tetracycline-induced R factor membrane protein to tetracycline resistance, in Drug-Inactivating Enzymes and Antibiotic Resistances. (Editors: Mitsuhashi, S., Rosival, L., Krčméry, V.) Berlin, Springer-Verlag, 1975.

11. Yang, H-L., Zubay, G. and Levy, S.B.: Synthesis of an R plasmid protein associated with tetracycline resistance is negatively regulated. Proc. Nat. Acad. Sci., USA 73:1509–1512, 1976.

12. Shipley, P.L. and Olsen, R.H.: Characteristics and expression of tetracycline resistance in gram negative bacteria carrying the Pseudomonas R factor RP1. Antimicrob. Agents and Chem. 6:183–188, 1974.

13. Unowsky, J. and Rachmeler, M.: Mechanisms of antibiotic resistance determined by resistance transfer factors. J. Bact. 92:358–365, 1966.

14. Reynard, A.M., Nellis, L.F. and Beck, M.E.: Uptake of ^{3}H-tetracycline by resistant and sensitive Escherichia coli. Applied Microbiol. 21:71–75, 1971.

15. Del Bene, V.E. and Rogers, M.: Comparison of tetracycline and minocycline transport in Escherichia coli. Antimicrob. Agents and Chem. 7:801–806, 1975.

16. Levy, S.B. and McMurry, L.: Probing the expression of plasmid-mediated tetracycline resistance in E. coli. Microbiology, 1977 (in press).

17. DeZeeuw, J.R.: Accumulation of tetracyclines by Escherichia coli. J. Bact. 95:498–506, 1968.

18. Heppel, L.A.: The concept of periplasmic enzymes in Structure and Function of Biological Membranes. (Editor: Rothfield, L.I.) Academic Press, New York and London, pp. 223–247, 1971.

19. Levy, S.B.: R factor proteins synthesized in Escherichia coli minicells: Incorporation studies with different R factors and detection of deoxyribonucleic acid-binding proteins. J. Bact. 120:1451–1463, 1974.

20. Novashin, S.M., Beliavskaya, I.V., Sazykin, Y.O. and Gryaznora, N.S.: Tetracycline resistance unassociated with a change of cell wall permeability in Escherichia coli in Drug-Inactivating Enzymes and Antibiotic Resistances. (Editors: Mitsuhashi, S., Rosival, L., Krčméry, V.) Berlin, Springer-Verlag, pp. 227–230, 1975.

21. Arima, K. and Izaki, K.: Accumulation of oxytetracycline relevant to its bacterial action in the cells of Escherichia coli. Nature 200:192–193, 1963.

22. Franklin, T.J. and Godfrey, A.: Resistance of _Escherichia coli_ to tetracyclines. Biochem. J. 94:54-60, 1965.

23. Levy, S.B. and McMurry, L.: Plasmid-mediated tetracycline resistance involves an alternative transport system for tetracycline. (To be submitted.)

24. Klein, W.L. and Boyer, P.D.: Energization of active transport by _Escherichia coli_. J. Biol. Chem. 247:7257-7265, 1972.

25. Lehninger, A.L.: _Biochemistry_. North Pub., New York, p. 429, 1975.

26. Cox, G.B. and Gibson, F.: Studies on electron transport and energy-linked reactions using mutants of _Escherichia coli_. B.B.A. 346:1-25, 1974.

27. Franklin, T.J. and Foster, S.J.: Expression of R factor-mediated resistance to tetracycline in _Escherichia coli_ minicells. Antimicrob. Agents and Chem. 5:194-195, 1974.

28. Levy, S.B., McMurry, L. and Palmer, E.: R factor proteins synthesized in _Escherichia coli_ minicells. II. Membrane-associated R factor proteins. J. Bact. 120:1464-1471, 1974.

29. Foster, T.J.: Tetracycline-sensitive mutants of the F-like R factors R100 and R100-1. Molec. Gen. Genet. 137:85-88, 1975.

30. Reeve, E.C.R. and Robertson, J.M.: The characteristics of eleven mutants of R factor R57 constitutive for tetracycline resistance, selected and tested in _Escherichia coli_ K12. Genet. Res. Cant. 25:297-312, 1975.

31. Starlinger, P. and Saedler, H.: Insertion elements in micro-organisms in _Current Topics in Microbiology and Immunology_ 75:111, 1976.

32. Blumberg, D.D. and Malamy, M.H.: Evidence for the presence of non-translated T7 late mRNA in infected F' (PIF$^+$) episome-containing cells. J. Virol. 13:378-385, 1975.

33. Lennox, E.S.: Transduction of linked genetic characters of the host by bacteriophage P1. Virology 1:190-206, 1955.

34. Osborn, M.J., Gander, J.E., Parisi, E. and Carson, J.: Mechanism of assembly of outer membrane of _Salmonella typhimurium_: isolation and characterization of cytoplasmic and outer membrane. J. Biol. Chem. 247:3962-3972, 1972.

35. Bonner, W.N. and Laskey, R.A.: A film detection method for tritium-labeled proteins and nucleic acids in polyacrylamide gels. Eur. J. Biochem. 46:83-88, 1974.

36. Studier, F.W.: Analysis of bacteriophage T7 early RNAs and proteins on slab gels. J. Mol. Biol. 79:237-248, 1973.

37. Levy, S.B.: Very stable prokaryotic messenger RNA in chromosomeless _Escherichia coli_ minicells. Proc. Nat. Acad. Sci. USA 72:2900-2904, 1975.

Discussion

Högenauer: Does tet protein bind to the ribosomes?

Levy: We have not done those experiments. We are not sure whether
we can isolate tet protein from the membrane. We are planning
to do these experiments and tetracycline binding, but have no
information.

Högenauer: Did you do two dimensional gels of the proteins of
tet resistant ribosomes?

Levy: No. I might say that if you use washed ribosomes you don't
see the effect so we believe that this is not a ribosome change
but that it is a cytoplasmic soluble factor present in the cell;
it is not related to a change in the ribosome.

Drews: Can you say anything about the mechanism involved in the
inhibition of protein synthesis; is it something that relates
to initiation or elongation? Can this be said from experiments
you have done? You showed that resistant protein synthesis is
somewhat less sensitive to tetracycline than the system from
sensitive cells -- is that due to a higher resistance of the
process of initiation?

Levy: I don't know. The differences are not large at the moment,
I think we will achieve a better in vitro system than we presently
have; when we succeed we can answer these questions.

Nordström: When you introduce a new transport system, do you get
rid of the old one?

Levy: Yes, the fact that the old system is shockable and the new
transport is not shockable would indicate that something is
occurring to whatever would appear to be the carrier protein
which is required. Alternatively, the carrier protein could be
there but another protein which takes it to the inner membrane
for transport in the cell is now missing or replaced by what we
call the tet protein. We are now studying isolated membrane
vesicles to answer that very question to see, when we get the

vesicles from sensitive and resistant cells, whether we can demonstrate the presence or absence of both uptake systems and how it is blocked.

Nordström: Bob Rownd has a copy mutant of R100 and if you compare tet resistance it is lower in the copy mutant than in the wild type, although gene dosage is 3-4 times higher. He speculates about the presence of an inhibitor of resistance.

Levy: There are two possibilities. We have not looked at that mutant but the question is whether it is inducible or non-inducible and that question is not answered. It could be that there is a higher level of repressor being expressed and the cell is never induced.

Nordström: Do you see anything like this in your second protein band?

Levy: We see (I didn't get to that slide) for certain r-determinants for tet, for example pSC101, two proteins which are induced. One is isolated from the membrane fractions and one is actually released when we lyse the cells. Eighty percent is in the soluble fraction and it is a smaller protein. Whether or not this is the soluble protein that we are looking for is unclear. One problem is that its migration is hidden by the major membrane protein that we see in our normal plasmids, which we call MRB. The other point is that pSC101 makes much less of the protein than R222; when you take pSC101 you have 10-fold less resistance than with R222. You make a tet protein in both, the amount of tet protein is less in pSC101 than in R222 and you also get a soluble protein being made.

We only see one protein with R222, the membrane protein, produced in large amounts. We would assume that we have been using the presence of this tet protein to analyze the whole operon since we have now shown that with many different plasmids the amount of tet protein expressed does correlate very nicely with the phenotypic expression of the whole "resistance operon".

We do have mutants that have different levels, Kurt, but we don't have copy mutants. We received one mutant from Tim Foster which makes the tet protein but it's actually sensitive, and we have temperature sensitivities for the tet protein. The question is not only: is the tet protein being made but is it being correctly positioned in the inner membrane itself. I hope to get an answer by using the minicell inner membrane, induced and uninduced, to see whether the transport systems are the same.

Starlinger: Since your uptake system is probably not designed
by E. coli for tetracycline, do you know of any compounds that
are more or less physiological and which compete with tet for
uptake?

Levy: No, not yet but we have tried. We are very much interested
in this and have tested amino acids but they also have alternate uptake systems.

Davies: Is there a medium effect on tet uptake?

Levy: Part of the problem lies in the fact that tetracycline
is a chelator and we have to be concerned about the divalent
cation concentration. Other than this we see both uptake systems
and similar levels of resistance in all media.

Bennett: I would like to comment on the suggestion that there
may, in fact, be different types of tetracycline resistance and
different mechanisms.

Levy: I am quite convinced that there are different tetracycline
determinants. We can now categorize four different types differ-
entiated by either the relative sensitivity or resistance to
tetracycline and to minocycline and by the level of the resistance and by the number of proteins that they make in the minicell system. All we have looked at are naturally inducible
operons; I haven't found any in E. coli that are constitutive.
We see them in streptococci where they are constitutive, but
proteus and staph are inducible.

Bennett: Some of the Chabbert strains are reputed to be constitutives.

Levy: Those are mutant strains that were isolated by using a
derivative of tetracycline. The constitutive mutants that are
high-level constitutive make a large amount of tet protein,
low-level constitutives make a small amount.

What Is the Mechanism of Plasmid-Determined
Resistance to Aminoglycoside Antibiotics?*

Julian Davies and Sarah A. Kagan

In considerations of the mechanisms of antibiotic resistance in bacteria
that contain plasmids, four mechanisms are generally possible. In one,
the plasmid encodes an enzyme (or enzymes) that alters the target site
for the antibiotic such that the binding of the antibiotic is greatly
reduced. There are very few examples of this mechanism but such is known
to be the case with macrolide-lincosaminide resistance in Staphylococcus
aureus; plasmids mediate specific methylation of the 23S ribosomal RNA
and destroy the binding site for the drug (1). In a second mechanism,
plasmids encode a replacement function that is insensitive to the drug,
allowing the inhibited form of the enzyme to be bypassed. For example,
in sulfonamide resistance where the resistant cell contains two dihydropteroate synthetases, one chromosomally determined and inhibited by sulfa
drugs, the other plasmid determined and refractory to this inhibition
(2). A similar situation exists for trimethoprim resistance (3).

A well-established mechanism is that in which the plasmid-containing cell
produces an enzyme that completely detoxifies the drug in the medium; β-
lactamases catalyze the hydrolysis of the β-lactam ring of penicillins
and cephalosporins (4). Tetracycline resistance exemplifies the fourth
mechanism: a plasmid encoded system perturbs the normal entry or exit
mechanism of the drug. The net result is that of a permeability block
and no drug is accumulated inside the cell (5).

In the case of the aminoglycoside-aminocyclitol antibiotics, resistance
in clinical isolates is usually associated with the presence of enzymes

---

* This work was supported by grants from the National Institutes of Health
and Cell and Molecular Biology Training Grant, University of Wisconsin.

Table 1. Enzymes Modifying Aminoglycoside-Aminocyclitol Antibiotics in
          Plasmid-Containing Strains.

Modification	Site, abbreviated enzyme names	Substrates*
O-nucleotidylation (adenylylation) Aminoglycoside adenylyl-transferases	3",[AAD(3")]	Streptomycin, Spectinomycin
	4',[AAD(4')]	Kanamycin, Amikacin, Tobramycin, Neomycin
	2",[AAD(2")]	Gentamicins, Tobramycin, Kanamycin
	6,[AAD(6)]	Streptomycin
O-phosphorylation Aminoglycoside phospho-transferases	3",(APH(3")]	Streptomycin
	3', [APH(3')]	Neomycin, Kanamycin, Lividomycin, Butirosin, Amikacin
	2",[APH(2")]	Gentamicins
	6,[APH(6)]	Streptomycin
N-acetylation Aminoglycoside acetyl-transferases	6',[AAC(6')]	Kanamycin, Neomycin Amikacin
	2',[AAC(2')]	Gentamicins, Tobramycin
	3,[AAC(3)]	Gentamicins, Kanamycin, Tobramycin, Neomycin

*It is important to note a) that not all substrates are included in the
resistance phenotype associated with the enzyme; as is explained in the text,
certain APH(3') enzymes can modify amikacin but do not determine resistance
to this drug; and b) for each enzyme type there are several different forms
that differ in substrate range, e.g., APH(3')-I modifies neomycin and
lividomycin but not butirosin; APH(3')-II modifies neomycin and lividomycin
but not butirosin.

that catalyze N-acetylation, O-phosphorylation, or O-adenylylation of
amino- or hydroxyl-groups on the drug molecule (6). Several such modifications
have been characterized (Table 1) and in the majority of cases, the
modified drugs are devoid of biological activity. They are ineffective
in preventing bacterial growth, and have greatly reduced inhibitory
effects on protein synthesis in cell-free extracts; this includes error
induction and inhibition of translation (7). It has been assumed that
the aminoglycoside modifying enzymes establish resistance by detoxification,
but it is clear that things are not as simple as this. There are several
modified aminoglycosides (7) that retain substantial biological activity;
when an R^+ strain is grown in the presence of drug no modified aminoglycoside
can be detected free in the culture medium; finally, in a number of
instances, bacterial strains are extremely sensitive to a drug even
though the strain produces a potent modifying enzyme for that drug (8, 9)!

Although the presence of a modifying enzyme does not necessarily determine
the expected resistance phenotype, the majority of R^+ resistant strains
do possess a modifying enzyme. There is little doubt that, in many
cases, the presence of an aminoglycoside modifying enzyme is alone necessary
and sufficient to establish the resistance phenotype. This has been
confirmed from studies of the properties of certain transducing phages,
in which a single resistance determinant has been transposed from a
plasmid on to the phage genome, to produce a specialized transducing
phage (10). However, many bacteria lack any detectable modifying enzyme
but are resistant to a variety of aminoglycosides; these strains have
been classified under the vague heading of "permeability" mutants (11)
and are becoming more common among clinical isolates of Pseudomonas
aeruginosa.

Another surprising fact concerns the relationship between levels of
aminoglycoside modifying enzymes and the degree of resistance. When
genes for some of these enzymes [e.g. AAC(6') or AAD(3")] are cloned on
to colicin E_1, a small plasmid that exists in about twenty copies per
cell, the minimal inhibitory concentration does not change even though
the modifying enzyme content of the cell may be increased some 10-fold.
If detoxification alone were the resistance mechanism, one would expect
proportionality between the amount of enzyme and the level of resistance,
especially since the M.I.C. values are relatively low in these cases.

At the present time there are three reasonable possibilities for a
mechanism of resistance to aminoglycosides that requires a modification

of the antibiotic: a) the modification takes place on the inner membrane
and is associated with a system for transport of the antibiotic into the
cell; modification of a small amount of drug blocks the transport system;
b) the modification is associated with the transport system and, instead
of blocking transport, stimulates a pump-out mechanism, as has been
suggested for tetracycline;c) the modification takes place inside the
cell and the drug is essentially inactivated; a large quantity of drug
derivative remains in the cell and this concentration impedes further
entry of the antibiotic.

None of these models is entirely satisfactory! They cannot account
for all of the observations and cannot be tested easily. One stumbling
block concerns the specificity of the resistance phenotype, even when
the modifying enzyme lacks specificity. For example, one of the 3'-N-acetyl-
transferases [AAC(3)], determines resistance to gentamicin without
influencing the cell's sensitivity to tobramycin; however, the enzyme
is capable of acetylating both gentamicin and tobramycin in vitro
(13). The same holds true for certain 3'-phosphotransferases [APH(3')]
that are capable of modifying amikacin but do not determine resistance
to the drug (9). In these cases, the presence of an enzyme and (apparent)
modification of the drug in the cell is not sufficient to explain the
observed resistance pattern. Another paradoxical situation occurs
when a plasmid encoding a 6'-acetyltransferase [AAC(6')] is transferred
from E. coli to P. aeruginosa. In the latter strain, such an enzyme
determines resistance to kanamycin, amikacin, neomycin and tobramycin,
etc.; however, the same enzyme in E. coli determines kanamycin resistance
only, the organism retaining sensitivity to the other drugs (8, 14).

These results imply that the plasmid determined resistance enzymes
interact with transport systems and the cell membrane and in addition,
that rates of modification of the antibiotics must be important. In
the case of the 3-N-acetyltransferase, the Km for gentamicin differs
by a factor of ten from that for tobramycin as substrate (13). The
difference in sensitivity might also be explained by the existence of
two separate transport mechanisms, one for gentamicin and one for
tobramycin. However, the two drugs are so similar in structure that
this is unlikely. Interestingly, the clinical use of tobramycin has
led to the appearance of bacterial strains resistant to both tobramycin
and gentamicin that contain a 3-N-acetyltransferase that catalyzes
modification of both gentamicin and tobramycin to an equal extent
(15).

The plasmid-encoded adenylyltransferase that is responsible for resistance
to streptomycin is a (relatively) inefficient enzyme and does not
determine high levels of resistance. In order to explain the mechanism
of this resistance, Nordström (personal communication) has suggested
that streptomycin is taken up by cells slowly, and that the inefficient
inactivation mechanism provided by the adenylyltransferase is sufficient
to counteract this uptake. Thus there is a "balance" between entry
and inactivation. If this were true, one would expect to find an
accumulation of streptomycin adenylylate inside or outside the cell.

In order to understand the mechanisms of resistance, it is essential that
we understand how the aminoglycosides enter sensitive cells. Are there
transport systems? What are the roles of the cell membrane and the
ribosomes in this uptake? Many attempts have been made to analyze these
questions, and, like the studies of mode of action of aminoglycoside
antibiotics, the conclusions remain unsatisfactory in a biochemical
sense. The most instructive studies have been those of Bryan and his co-
workers (11). Three phases of uptake of gentamicin (and related antibiotics) can be detected (Fig. 1). The first is an energy independent
rapid binding, followed by two separate energy dependent phases of binding.
It is presumed that the first phase is an ionic association with the
external surface of the cell since this can be reduced by washing with
sodium chloride. What is not known is how much of this rapidly bound
material may be subsequently transported into the cell, and what effect
it has on the sensitive cell. The three phases are only seen at low drug
concentration.

There is evidence that aminoglycoside entry into sensitive cells is an
energy dependent-active process. A number of bacterial mutants, resistant
to aminoglycoside antibiotics, have been found that are either unc locus
mutants (i.e., ATPase-negative) or deficient in energy dependent functions
(16). Such mutants can arise spontaneously at high frequency and the
resistance spectrum appears to include structurally unrelated aminoglycoside
antibiotics. Further analysis of mutants of this type is warranted, to
examine the possibility that specific resistances may be established in
some cases; this would indicate the existence of specific transport
mechanisms for structurally different antibiotics. In addition, uptake
of aminoglycosides into the cell can be arrested by uncouplers, such as
CCCP, or by inhibitors of oxidative phosphorylation, such as KCN (Fig. 2).
Chloramphenicol and other inhibitors of protein synthesis also prevent
uptake and killing; this may indicate a role for active ribosomes in the
uptake of the drug for the continuous production of a specific protein (17).

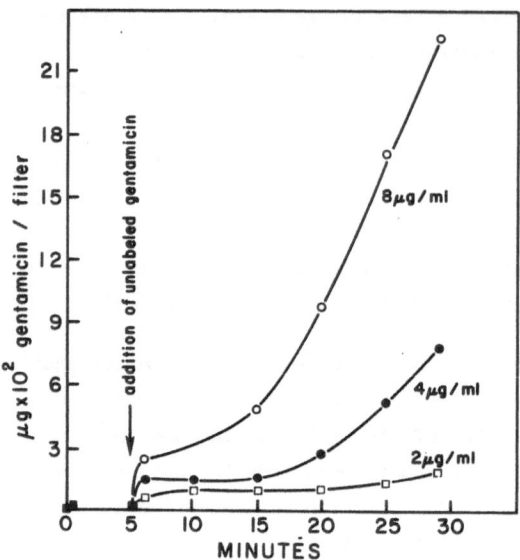

Fig. 1. Concentration dependent uptake of ^{3}H-labelled gentamicin by a
sensitive strain of E. coli. ^{3}H-gentamicin (1 µg/ml) was added to
actively growing cells at time zero, at 5 minutes unlabelled drug was
added to give the final concentrations indicated. Samples (0.5 ml) were
collected, and washed on nitrocellulose filters at the times indicated
and radioactivity determined by scintillation counting.

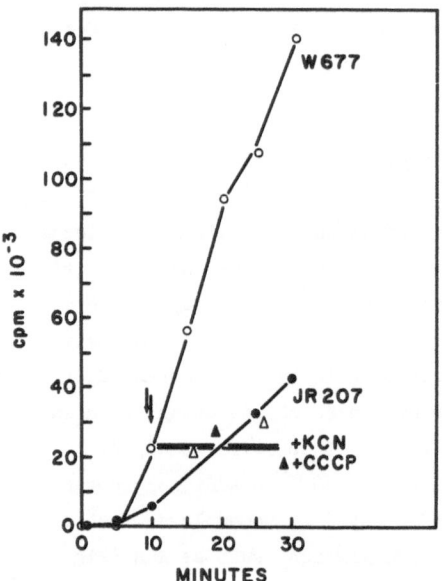

Fig. 2. Uptake of radioactive gentamicin by sensitive (W677) and resistant
(JR207) strains of E. coli and the effect of an uncoupler of oxidative

phosphorylation (CCCP) and an inhibitor of oxidative phosphorylation (KCN). The resistant strain JR207 possesses aminoglycoside adenyltransferase (2").

Regardless of the exact mechanism of influx, we can ask questions concerning the difference in uptake of aminoglycoside antibiotics by resistant and sensitive strains. For those strains that are resistant by virtue of a plasmid-coded modifying enzyme, no modified drug can be detected in the culture medium. When uptake is measured, as is shown in Fig. 2, the resistant cells incorporate less drug than sensitive strains, but there is still significant uptake of labelled drug. This finding is not consistent with a mechanism of resistance involving complete exclusion of the drug, i.e., there is not a total block to transport. It seems likely that the drug is entering the cell and being modified, and that modified drug remains in the cell.

Let us return to the "rate" phenomenon described for some of the aminoglycoside modifying enzymes. There is an active system for transport of aminoglycoside antibiotics into cells that transports drug at a finite rate. We can imagine that if the rate of modification of the drug in resistant strains is not sufficient to prevent unmodified, active drug from reaching its target (the ribosomes), then the cell will be inhibited. In the case of the 3-N-acetyltransferase we assume that the modification of tobramycin is not fast enough to prevent the active drug from binding to ribosomes. On the other hand, gentamicin is modified rapidly, and could block further transport, so that the active molecule never reaches the target ribosomes. What we don't know is how modification actually prevents the active drug from reaching ribosomes. Why doesn't preloading the resistant cell with gentamicin protect it from bacteriocidal effects of tobramycin (12)?

Conclusion

Transport of aminoglycoside antibiotics into bacterial cells is an energy requiring process; it is unlikely to be specific and probably involves a system that transports structurally related molecules into the cell (aminosugars?), although this has not been demonstrated. Tight binding to ribosomes probably assists transport by acting as a "sink"; once the aminoglycoside enters a sensitive cell it is retained in the cell. Bacterial mutants with "resistant" ribosomes have been reported to be unable to transport aminoglycoside antibiotics into the cell, thus attachment of the drug to ribosomes may play a role in unloading the transport system (11).

214

In strains that are resistant by virtue of plasmid-encoded modifying
enzymes, the resistance is apparently due to a lack of sufficient active
drug passing through inner membrane and reaching ribosomes. This could
be due to a failure of modified drug to bind to ribosomes and so "unsaturate"
the transport system, or to the establishment of a block in the active
transport mechanism by some complex of the modifying enzyme and the
modified drug. The rate of modification of the aminoglycoside in the
cell is of paramount importance; if the modification is not efficient or
rapid, ummodified drug can reach its target site and inhibition of protein
synthesis and cell death ensue.

Any model of aminoglycoside transport and resistance must take into
account several observations. These include: varying phenotypic expression
of the same antibiotic resistance determinant in different strains; the fact
that the phosphotransferases always determine much higher levels of
resistance than the other modifying enzymes; and the effects of cations and
anions on the efficacy of the aminoglycoside antibiotics (18).

Literature
1. Lai, C. J., Weisblum, B.: Altered methylation of ribosomal RNA in an
    erythromycin-resistant strain of Staphylococcus aureus. Proc. Natl.
    Acad. Sci. U.S.A. 68, 856-860 (1971).
2. Wise, E. M. Jr., Abou-Donia, M. M.: Sulfonamide resistance mechanism
    in Escherichia coli: R plasmids can determine sulfonamide-resistant
    dihydropteroate synthases. Proc. Natl. Acad. Sci. U.S.A. 72, 2621-
    2625 (1975).
3. Amyes, S. G. B., Smith, J. T.: R-factor trimethoprim resistance
    mechanism: An insusceptible target site. Biochem. Biophys. Res.
    Commun. 58, 412-418 (1974); Sköld, O., Widh, A.: A new dihydrofolate
    reductase with low trimethoprim sensitivity induced by an R factor
    mediating high resistance to trimethoprim. J. Biol. Chem. 249, 4324-
    4325 (1974).
4. Richmond, M. H., Jack, G. W., Sykes, R. B.: The β-lactamases of gram-
    negative bacteria including pseudomonads. Ann. N. Y. Acad. Sci., 182,
    243-257 (1971).
5. Franklin, T. J.: Resistance of Escherichia coli to tetracyclines:
    Changes in permeability to tetracyclines in Escherichia coli bearing
    transferable resistance factors. Biochem. J. 105, 371-378 (1967).
6. Benveniste, R., Davies, J.: Mechanisms of antibiotic resistance in
    bacteria. Ann. Rev. Biochem. 42, 471-506 (1973).

7. Benveniste, R., Davies, J.: Structure-activity relationships among the aminoglycoside antibiotics: Role of hydroxyl and amino groups. Anti. Ag. Chemoth. 4, 402-409 (1973).

8. Benveniste, R., Davies, J.: Enzymatic acetylation of aminoglycoside antibiotics by Escherichia coli carrying an R factor. Biochemistry 10, 1787-1796 (1971).

9. Courvalin, P., Davies, J.: Plasmid-mediated aminoglycoside phospho-transferase of broad substrate range that phosphorylates amikacin. Antimicrob. Ag. Chemoth. 11, 619-624 (1977).

10. Davies, J., Berg, D., Jorgensen, R., Fiandt, M., Courvalin, P., Sehloff, J.: Transposable neomycin phosphotransferases. This volume.

11. Bryan, L. E., van den Elzen, H. M., Shahrabadi, M. S.: The relationship of aminoglycoside permeability to streptomycin and gentamicin suscepti-bility of Pseudomonas aeruginosa in "Microbial Drug Resistance" (eds. Mitsuhashi, S., Hashimoto, H.), University Park Press, Baltimore, Md, 1975, pp. 475-490.

12. Davies, J.: unpublished observations.

13. Williams, J. W., Northrop, D. B.: Purification and properties of gentamicin acetyltransferase I. Biochemistry 15, 125-131 (1975).

14. Jacoby, G. A.: Properties of an R plasmid in Pseudomonas aeruginosa producing amikacin (BBK-8), butirosin, kanamycin, tobramycin and sisomicin resistance. Antimicrob. Ag. Chemother. 6, 807-810 (1974).

15. Biddlecome, S., Haas, M., Davies, J., Miller, G. H., Rane, D. F., Daniels, P. J. L.: Enzymatic modification of aminoglycoside antibiotics: A new 3-N-acetylating enzyme from a Pseudomonas aeruginosa isolate. Antimicrob. Ag. Chemother. 9, 951-955 (1976).

16. Kanner, B. I., Gutnick, D. L.: Use of neomycin in the isolation of mutants blocked in energy conservation in Escherichia coli. Bacteriol. 111, 287-289 (1972).; Lieberman, M. A., Hong, J.-S.: A mutant of Escherichia coli defective in the coupling of metabolic energy to active transport. Proc. Natl. Acad. Sci. U.S.A. 71, 4395-4399 (1974).

17. Bryan, L. E., van den Elzen, H. M.: Gentamicin accumulation by sensitive strains of Escherichia coli and Pseudomonas aeruginosa. J. Antibiot. 28, 696-703 (1975).

18. Zimelis, V. M., Jackson, G. G.: Activity of aminoglycoside antibiotics against Pseudomonas aeruginosa: Specificity and site of calcium and magnesium antagonism. J. Infect. Dis. 127, 663-669 (1973).

Discussion

Davies: It is unlikely that the modified aminoglycosides compete for binding sites on the ribosome with unmodified drug. The binding of streptomycin to ribosomes is a simple one site affair. The binding of a gentamicin to ribosomes is very complex. At least five molecules bind and both subunits are involved; the binding sites appear to have different affinities and this explains why one cannot obtain ribosome mutants resistant to high levels of gentamicin.

Anderson: I was wondering if you could not test the viability of cells by direct examination in a phase contrast microscope.

Davies: We haven't done any experiments of that type but other workers (e.g. Margot Kogut) have, and at early times you can certainly see which cells are dead because DNA begins to agglomerate within the cell, but that takes place a long time after addition of the drug.

Falkow: Do you mean acridine staining?

Davies: No, you begin to see the chromosome come together.

Falkow: There is a method for distinguishing viable from dead cells by their ability to take up acridine and the kind of fluorescence that you get.

Davies: Yes, but the trouble may be that cells treated with aminoglycosides continue to take up molecules.

Falkow: But is there a change in fluorescence?

Davies: I don't know.

Falkow: Nor do I.

Richmond: Another question I wanted to ask concerns the Bryan experiment. If at the end of phase one you add an excess of enzyme to inactivate external antibiotic and then plate for viability, have the cells suicided at that point?

Davies: That is a good experiment but it hasn't been done.

Richmond: In other words, you can help yourself with these viability studies if you inactivate external drug.

Davies: Right. One thing that has been tried is to take sensitive cells, feed them modified drugs, and then ask if the modified drug gets into the cells to set up some kind of resistance mechanisms. The answer, so far, is no.

Richmond: But it gets in.

Davies: We don't know.

Saedler: Do you find a substantial amount of the modifying enzyme in the membrane fraction? I'm asking if the modification is occurring while the drug is taken up?

Davies: The modifying enzyme is (apparently) not free in the periplasmic space and we believe that they are associated with the inner membrane where they are accessible to their substrates, acetyl coenzyme A and adenosine triphosphate. This is clearly where the transport mechanism is taking place.

Saedler: Do the modified products actually inhibit the enzyme in this action?

Davies: Some of them may do, as I mentioned, the enzymes are quite susceptible to product inhibition. One thing that I failed to mention concerns studies that we have done on the effect of copy number e.g. how does the amount of enzyme affect resistance? We have cloned several of the modifying enzyme genes on to the small multicopy colicin E_1 plasmid and asked if the M.I.C. changes. In most cases with acetylating, phosphorylating and adenylylating enzymes the M.I.C. is the same whether one has one or twenty copies of the gene for the modifying enzyme.

Falkow: This is a difficulty about cloning on colicin E_1 because you make the cells sick and the multicopy plasmid puts an enormous burden on the cell, often leading them into amino acid starvation so that you get lots of DNA made and little protein.

Davies: Even under normal growth conditions?

Falkow: Particularly under normal growth conditions! We have had a problem cloning some determinants since the cells become really ill and we have to supplement with large amounts of amino acid or glucose. If the gene product is glucose repressible, we have had dreadful difficulties with cloned toxin strains.

Anderson: The point about Julian's argument which seems a reasonably logical one, is that if resistance is dependent on the presence of the intracellular modified drug and if no normal drug gets into the cell, it is a different situation from a thing like,

for example, the destruction of a ß-lactam antibiotic which
greatly diminishes the amount accessible to the cell so that
to me it makes sense that the M.I.C. is less sensitive to the
gene dosage in the case of aminoglycosides.

Davies: Yes, I agree. We can show that more enzyme is made and
this doesn't affect the level of resistance. I can't eliminate
the possibility that the cell is sicker because of the additional
load and therefore it doesn't matter how much enzyme is being
made, it's still going to be sensitive.

Falkow: I would like to ask one practical question, I don't
know if anyone has the answer. In how many instances in clinical
isolates has it been determined that the cell carries both
chromosomal resistance mutations as well as plasmid resistance?

Davies: In the clinical isolates we have seen, it is very rare.
It does definitely occur though, in pseudomonas for example.
There are several examples where there is a chromosome mutation
for aminoglycoside resistance and a plasmid determining resistance
to a variety of other drugs.

Falkow: Our experience at a burn unit has been that the first
thing that occurs are chromosome mutants followed by a plasmid
and not vice versa.

Davies: I don't know. What may have considerable clinical significance is the fact that in a lot of pseudomonads we have a plasmid
determining gentamicin and tobramycin resistance, in fact, to
all aminoglycosides except amikacin. Amikacin resistant derivatives of these strains appear as clinical isolates that are
probably mutants. The plasmid determines resistance by enzymatic
mechanisms to some of the aminoglycosides and the mutation sets
up resistance to amikacin and incidentally to the whole spectrum
of aminoglycosides. Probably by a nonspecific transport defect.
So even though the spontaneous mutation frequency to aminoglycosides is supposed to be low, the presence of a plasmid may increase this, so that one can get "unlikely" mutants in clinical
situations.

Richmond: The explanation is probably that if some sort of
penetration process is involved, by modifying the barrier you
could add that extra factor that would make enzymatic inactivation more efficient.

Levy: Speaking of the first possibility: transport could be
inhibited by modification of the drug, since you have two drugs
which are differentially active, gentamicin and tobramycin.

Can you ask the question whether there is a difference in uptake
of the two drugs in the same cell, since if one is modified
rapidly then the uptake should be slowed down rapidly, whereas
in the other case it should continue to go in?

Davies: Right. We would like to do that experiment. The problem
is that we have radioactive gentamicin but not tobramycin; we
have tried to do it by looking at inhibition levels and the
results have been unsatisfactory, because if you have a sensitive
cell and add radioactive gentamicin, and nonlabeled tobramycin,
there is an augmentation of the rate of gentamicin transport --
because it is concentration dependent. It doesn't seem to matter
what aminoglycoside you add, gentamicin uptake is increased.

Drews: Did I understand you correctly, were you implying that
alterations of the transport system, of any transport system
bringing aminoglycosides into the cell, are always chromosomally
located?

Davies: There are chromosomal mutations that affect aminoglycoside
uptake, for example the unc mutations. But I wouldn't want to
imply that plasmids cannot affect transport.

Drews: I wonder if you could do an experiment or perhaps you
have done it, where you have a mutation in a plasmid gene, in a
gene specifying the synthesis of one of these modifying enzymes.
Does that affect the rate of transport for that particular antibiotic?

Davies: We have found that mutations in plasmid coded modifying
genes restore the cell to wild-type sensitivity to the drug. We
don't know if transport per se is affected but the sensitivity
is now like a plasmid-free strain. We have not examined transport
characteristics of the drug under these conditions.

Effect of Plasmids on Cell Division and on the Cell Envelope of Escherichia coli

Kurt Nordström, Birgitta Engberg[1], Petter Gustafsson, Søren Molin,
and Bernt Eric Uhlin

Plasmids are replicating DNA molecules that are present in a stable number of copies per cell in an exponentially growing population of bacteria (1,2). They directly affect the phenotype of their host bacteria by carrying genes mediating antibiotic resistance, bacteriocin production, catabolic functions, etc. (1,3). However, apart from these direct effects, the presence of plasmids in a cell may also indirectly affect the phenotype of the host bacterium.

Some years ago we discovered that it was possible by mutation in the plasmid genome to increase the copy number of plasmid R1 severalfold (4,5). Such mutants have been denoted copy mutants and have been isolated from a number of plasmids (6,7,8,9). There are also chromosomal mutations that affect the copy number of some plasmids (10,11). The existence of plasmid copy mutants makes it possible to study the effect of plasmid gene dosage on the phenotype of the host bacterium. This communication will discuss some of the direct and indirect phenotypic consequences of the presence of plasmid R1 in Escherichia coli. The copy mutants allow quantitative changes to be made without qualitatively affecting the genotype of the system.

1. The System Used

Escherichia coli K-12 was used throughout this work. The plasmids used were R1a (R1 of Meynell and Datta (12) in which kanamycin resistance has been spontaneously lost (4)), R1drd-19 (a mutant of

---

[1] Department of Microbiology, University of Umeå, Sweden.

plasmid R1 derepressed with respect to transfer (13)), and a series
of copy mutants of these plasmids (see (14)). The properties of these
plasmids have been summarized in Tables 1,2, and 3.

Table 1. General properties of plasmid R1

Molecular weight	65×10^6	(15)
Transfer system	F-like	(16)
Compatibility group	$IncF_{II}$	(17)

Table 2. Antibiotic resistance mediated by plasmid R1

Resistance	Genotype[1]	Enzyme
Ampicillin	bla⁺	ß-lactamase
Chloramphenicol	cat⁺	Acetyltransferase
Kanamycin	aphA⁺	Phosphotransferase
Streptomycin	aadA⁺	Adenylyltransferase
Sulphonamide	sul⁺	Dihydropteroate synthase (18)

[1]For symbols see Novick et al. (19).

2. Effect of Gene Dosage on Antibiotic Resistance

Plasmid R1 mediates resistance to five different antibiotics. In all
cases the enzymatic mechanism of resistance is known (Table 2). We
have measured the specific activity of three of these enzymes in cells
carrying plasmid R1drd-19 and a number of its copy mutants. The specifi
activity of these enzymes (ß-lactamase, chloramphenicol acetyltransferase, and streptomycin adenylyltransferase) was found to be proportional to the gene dosage (or copy effect, Table 4) (5, 20). It
should be noted that the specific activity of the three enzymes are
very different; in particular, the activity of the streptomycin-inactivating enzyme is very low.

The presence of the R plasmid caused a drastic increase in antibiotic
resistance (Table 5). This also applies to streptomycin. Ampicillin
and chloramphenicol resistance can be explained by detoxification of

the drugs (22). Streptomycin, on the other hand, is not metabolized to any measurable extent (22).

Table 3. Copy mutants of plasmid R1 (4, 20)

Plasmid	Parent	Copy effect[1]	Transfer frequency[2]
R1drd-19	R1	1.0	Derepressed
pKN103	R1drd-19	1.9	Derepressed
pKN213	"	2.5	Low
pKN102	"	3.6	Derepressed
pKN224	"	4.5	Low
pKN211	"	5.3	Derepressed
pKN210	"	7.2	Derepressed
pKN104	"	8.2	Low
pKN205	"	9.7	Derepressed
R1a	R1	1.0	Repressed
pKN101	R1a	2.0	Repressed

[1]The copy number of plasmid R1drd-19 has been given the value 1.0 of 1.0.

[2]Those labelled "low" transfer with about the same frequency as the repressed plasmid R1a, i.e. 10^{-3} - 10^{-4} times as efficient as the derepressed ones (21).

Table 4. Effect of plasmid R1 gene dosage on specific activity of drug-metabolizing enzymes (5)[1]

Enzyme	Specific activity (units/mg protein)
ß-lactamase	1.0 x (copy effect)
Chloramphenicol acetyltransferase	9.0 x "
Streptomycin adenylyltransferase	0.015 x "

[1]Activities were measured in cultures grown in steady state in LB medium at 37°C, and are expressed as units (µmoles of substrate metabolized per min at 37°C). The copy effect of the wild type plasmid has been given the value of 1.0.

Table 5. Antibiotic resistance of E. coli carrying the plasmid R1<u>drd-19</u>

Antibiotic	Single-cell resistance (μg/ml)[1]	
	R[−]	R[+]
D-Ampicillin	1	100
Chloramphenicol	3	300
Streptomycin	1	15

[1]Measured by growing the bacteria exponentially in LB medium and then spreading about 200 cells per LA plate containing an antibiotic (23). The resistance level is given as the highest concentration of the drug at which all cells plated formed colonies.

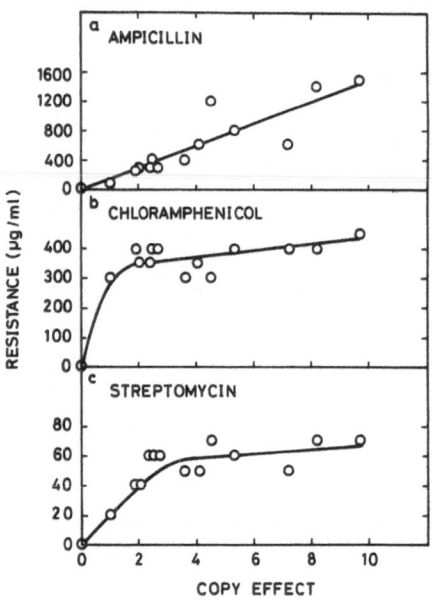

Fig. 1. Effect of copy number of the R plasmid R1<u>drd-19</u> in resistance to ampicillin, chloramphenicol, and streptomycin.

Resistance to all three antibiotics increased with increasing gene dosage (Fig.1). Ampicillin resistance was proportional to the gene dosage over the whole range tested (20). Experiments with copy mutants having a copy effect 50 times that of the wild type plasmid demonstrated that this linea relation is valid with much higher gene dosages than those shown in Fig. (unpublished). The situation was clearly different for the two other

antibiotics tested, chloramphenicol and streptomycin, for which resistance increased with increasing gene dosage only at low copy effects
and then levelled off at higher ones. Therefore, above a certain value
an increasing specific activity of the enzyme that metabolizes chloramphenicol and streptomycin has no effect on resistance to the corresponding antibiotics. For chloramphenicol, the upper resistance limit
is clearly due to energy limitation (22); all ATP made available by
catabolism is consumed by chloramphenicol acetyltransferase, an enzyme
that uses acetyl coenzyme A as cosubstrate. In liquid culture chloramphenicol inactivation by a population of cells carrying plasmid R1 is
initially very rapid, but then slows down and ceases completely after
a few hours (22). This may be a secondary consequence due to lack of
maintenance energy; periplasmic material (22) as well as outer membrane
components are lost during incubation in the presence of chloramphenicol (24).

Energy limitation cannot explain the levelling off of streptomycin
resistance at higher copy number. The enzyme that inactivates streptomycin resistance at higher copy number. The enzyme that inactivates
streptomycin uses ATP as cosubstrate, but the low specific activity
of the enzyme precludes that the pressure on energy metabolism can
be more than marginal (22). We will discuss streptomycin resistance
later in this paper.

3. Effect of Gene Dosage on Conjugal Transfer

Plasmid R1 carries genes for conjugal transfer (Table 1). The first
copy mutant described, pKN101 (earlier denotation R1B1 (4)), was found
to cause a 2-3-fold increase in the ability to form mating pairs (4)
(Table 6). Thus, there seems to be a gene dosage effect also on transfer. Plasmid pKN101 is a copy mutant of plasmid R1a, which is repressed
with respect to conjugal transfer (Table 3). It is not possible to
note any effect of plasmid copy number on the frequency of conjugal
transfer of the derepressed plasmid R1drd-19, since this plasmid transfers very efficiently already at the wild type copy number. However,
we should like to stress that a considerable fraction (about 30 %, cf.
Table 3) of the copy mutants of plasmid R1drd-19 transfer with a reduced
frequency (21). Cells carrying these plasmids do not form sex pili as
judged by the inability of male specific phage Qβ to grow on these
bacteria. The reason for these plasmids showing a heavily reduced

frequency of transfer compared to the wild type plasmid is not known. The high frequency of copy mutants showing a low transfer frequency excludes a pure coincidence, but it is uncertain whether the result indicates that transfer and control of replication share an element or that some copy mutants are caused by deletions also covering genes involved in (control of) conjugal transfer.

Table 6. Effect of plasmid copy number on cunjugal transfer

Plasmid	Copy effect	Transfer frequency (% of donor)[1]
R1a	1.0	0.2
pKN101	2.0	0.5

[1]Exponentially growing cultures of donor and recipient bacteria were mixed to a concentration of 10^7 and 10^8 per ml, respectively. Mating was allowed for 30 min before plating on selective medium.

4. Effect of Plasmid Gene Dosage on the Bacterial Cell Division Cycle

Cells carrying plasmid R1drd-19, particularly copy mutants of the plasmid, are larger than plasmid-free cells, as judged by the optical density (25) or protein content (26) per cell (Table 7). The effect was the more pronounced the slower the growth rate; no effect was observed in broth media (Fig. 2). The effect on cell size increased with increasing copy number (Fig. 3). It should also be mentioned that the number of plasmid R1 copies per chromosome equivalent increases with decreasing growth rate (Fig. 4).

The increased size of plasmid-carrying cells compared to plasmid-free cells was found to be due to two effects (25) (Table 7); the average cell length as well as the average cell diameter was increased in the plasmid carrying population. The effect on cell length was found to be due to the fact that a fraction of the cells formed elongated cells. There was no effect on the length of newborn cells (L) and the majority of the cells divided at a normal cell length (2L). However, in plasmid containing cells there was a tendency for omitting cell division at the normal cell length (2L); this tendency increased with increasing plasmid copy number. If cell division was omitted in a cell, no cell

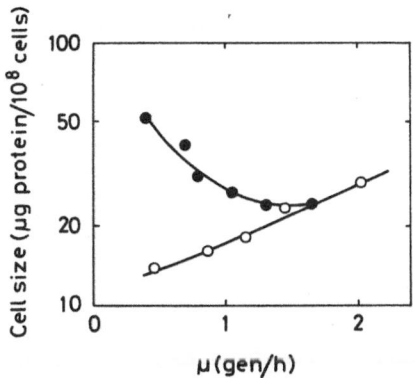

Fig. 2. Cell size of plasmid-free E. coli (o) and of E. coli carrying the plasmid copy mutant pKN102 (•). The populations were analyzed in the exponential growth phase. The growth rate was varied by using different carbon sources (25).

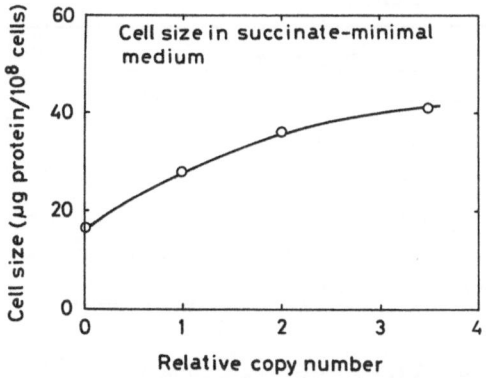

Fig. 3. Effect of plasmid copy number on cell size of exponentially growing populations of E. coli; the plasmids used were R1drd-19, pKN103, and pKN102 with the copy effects 1.0, 1.9 and 3.6, respectively.

division took place until another doubling in cell length had occurred (to a length of 4L). In the majority of those cells where divisions occurred to a cell length of 4L, cell division was asymmetric, yielding one cell of normal baby length (L); only one cell division occurred in these cells. Consecutive cell division could be omitted, leading to a minority of the cells being very long (at least 20 L). Hence, the omission of cell division was reversible and the phenomenon observed may prove useful in understanding the mechanism that governs the bacterial cell division cycle (see (26)). The effect of plasmid R1 on

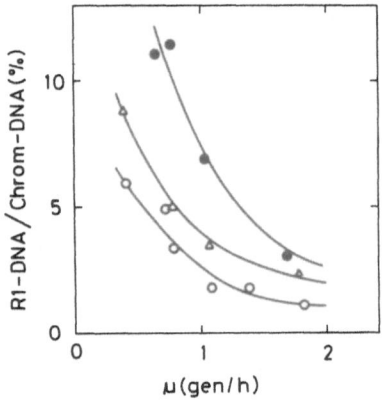

Fig. 4 Relative content of Plasmid R1 DNA in <u>E.coli</u> growing exponentially in different media; plasmid used: R1<u>drd-19</u> (o), pKN103 (△) and pKN102 (●) (26).

Table 7. Effect of plasmid R1 on cell dimensions[1]

Cell parameter	Plasmid		
	None	R1<u>drd-19</u>	pKN103
Plasmid copies per genome	0.0	1.3	2.2
Length of newborn cell (µm)	1.3	1.6	1.6
Length of average cell (µm)	2.0	2.1	3.1
Diameter of average cell (µm)	0.57	0.57	0.76
Frequency of cells longer than 3L (%)	3	6	20

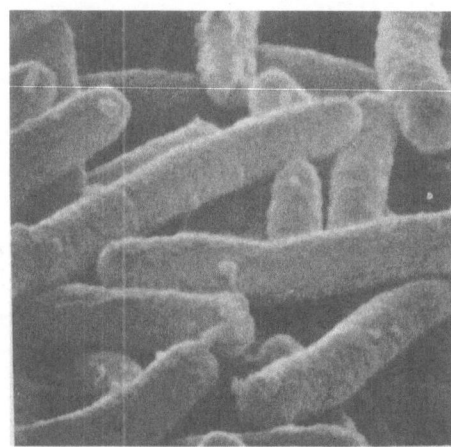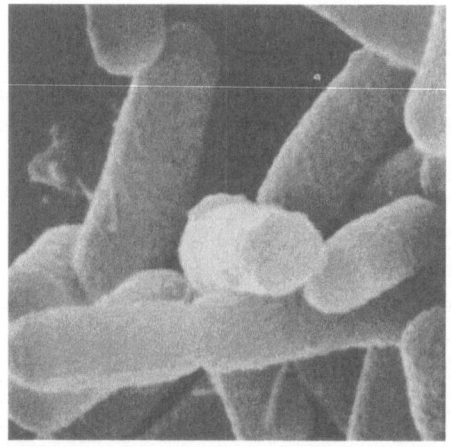

Fig. 5. Scanning electron micrographs showing <u>E.coli</u> carrying the plasmid R1<u>drd-19</u> (left) and the plasmid pKN103 (right) (Engberg, Hörstedt, and Winblad, unpublished).

the diameter of the cells was measured in a scanning electron microscope (Fig. 5). The effects of plasmid R1 on the bacterial morphology
have been summarized in Table 8.

Table 8. Effect of plasmid R1 on the bacterial cell cycle.

---

1. The mean cell size is increased
2. The cell diameter is increased.
3. The average cell length is increased.
4. There is no effect on the length of newborn cells.
5. There is a tendency for omitting (reversibly) cell division.
6. A minority of the population forms very long cells.

The formation of elongated cells in populations carrying plasmid R1
does not involve the recA$^+$ gene product (cf. (27)) and does not seem
to be related to the induction of prophage lambda (see (26)). The process, therefore, seems to be distinct from other described cases of
filamentation.

The effect of plasmid R1 on cell division may be due to competition
between the plasmid and the bacterial chromosome for some essential
replication factor or to cross-reaction between repressors of initiation of replication. The plasmid uses essentially the same replication
factors as the bacterial chromosome (28,29,30). Filaments are known to
be induced by a number of factors that slow down or inhibit chromosome
replication (31). The increased diameter of plasmid-carrying cells may
be caused by a reduced rate of chromosome elongation; an increased
cell diameter and a reduced fork rate have been reported for thymine-
requiring E. coli grown at suboptimal concentrations of thymine (32)
and for rep mutants of E. coli (33). We have so far not measured the
rate of chromosome elongation in our system.

5. Effect of Gene Dosage on the Outer Penetration Barrier

There are indications that plasmid-carrying Gram-negative cells
have a less efficient outer penetration barrier than plasmid-less
cells (see (34)). One way to demonstrate this is to measure rifampicin resistance. This drug is at least 100-fold less toxic to
Gram-negative cells than to cell-free RNA polymerase (35). Sphe-

roplasts, produced by treatment of Gram-negative cells with lysozyme EDTA, are 100-fold more rifampicin-sensitive than intact
cells (36). Many plasmids seem to reduce the rifampicin resistance
of their host cells (37). Therefore, we measured rifampicin resistance as a function of the plasmid R1 copy number by plating
exponentially growing bacteria on plates containing graded concentrations of rifampicin. The efficiency of plating of the
plasmid-less bacteria was 100 % at rifampicin concentrations of up
to 3 μg/ml. However, this threshold concentration decreased to
about 1 μg/ml for cells carrying the plasmid R1drd-19 and to
still lower values for cells carrying copy mutants of the plasmid.
In Fig. 6 we have plotted colony formation on plates containing
2 μg of rifampicin per ml as a function of the plasmid copy number. The resistance to rifampicin decreased with increasing plasmid
copy number and was more than 100-fold less at the highest copy
number tested than in the absence of any plasmid. Hence, the
bacteria containing high-copy-number plasmids were about as rifampicin-sensitive as bacterial spheroplasts. This indicates
that the penetration barrier against rifampicin had been severely
impaired - this barrier is assumed to be located in the bacterial
outer membrane. Rifampicin has a molecular weight well above that
which precludes free penetration through the outer membrane (38).

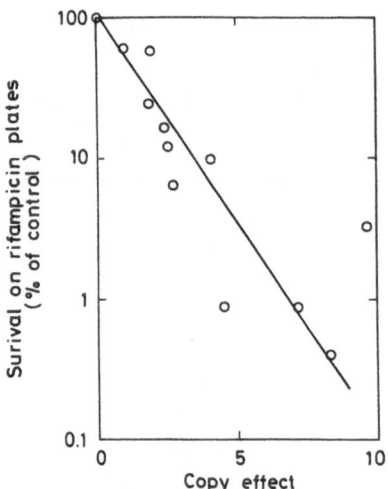

Fig. 6. Survival of exponentially growing bacteria on LA plates
containing 2 μg of rifampicin per ml. The bacteria carried the
plasmids listed in Table 3.

It is well-known that by changing the chemical composition of the outer membrane, the rate of influx of various substances may be greatly affected (34,39,40). We have tested a few such test substances, such as gentian violet (39) and sodium cholate (40), but we did not find any change in sensitivity to them for bacteria that carry plasmids or plasmid copy mutants.

We have so far not measured whether there are any chemical differences in the composition of the outer membrane of plasmid-carrying bacteria compared to plasmid-less ones. The effects observed may be due to one or several plasmid gene products that may be present in the outer membrane; several of the plasmid gene products are cell-bound but located outside the cytoplasmic membrane. However, the reduced rifampicin resistance cannot be due to sex pili since there was no difference with respect to rifampicin resistance between cells carrying plasmids mediating normal derepressed piliation and those that did not mediate any piliation (cf. Table 3).

ß-lactamase is a periplasmic enzyme (42) and it forms about 0.05 % of the total protein of a cell carrying the plasmid R1 (42). Hence, this enzyme should constitute about 0.5 % of the total protein of a cell carrying the copy mutant pKN205; this quantity of protein amounts to a considerable part of the protein which is located outside the cytoplasmic membrane. Whether this can have any effect on the effectivity of the outer penetration barrier is not known.

Mickel and Bauer (41) have reported that a copy mutant of plasmid R100 (this plasmid carries the tet gene mediating tetracycline resistance) confers a lower resistance to tetracycline than that mediated by the parent plasmid R100. This does not seem to be due to an effect of the plasmids on the penetration barrier since we did not find any difference with respect to tetracycline resistance in cells carrying copy mutants of plasmid R1drd-19 and those not carrying any plasmid (plasmid R1 does not carry any tet gene).

6. Streptomycin Resistance

Streptomycin has a molecular weight above that which allows free penetration through the outer membrane (38). Therefore, penetra-

tion of streptomycin into the cell is a slow process, at least
at concentrations up to the resistance level (43). It is possible
by mutation affecting the outer membrane to decrease the rate of
influx of streptomycin severalfold; this results in a severalfold
increase in streptomycin resistance (43). The presence of a minute
streptomycin-inactivating activity drastically increases streptomycin resistance (Table 5). We strongly believe that this is due
to a synergistic effect of a strong penetration barrier and a
low drug-metabolizing activity that inactivates the few molecules
of streptomycin that penetrate into the cell. By decreasing the
activity of streptomycin inactivation, resistance to this drug
increases, since the enzyme now can cope with an increasing rate
of influx of the drug; this rate is presumably proportional to
the concentration of streptomycin in the medium. Hence, streptomycin resistance is likely to be proportional to the plasmid copy
number. However, the presence of plasmid R1 impairs the barrier
against rifampicin (see above) and it is tempting to suggest that
the same is true for streptomycin. If this is correct, the result
will be that an increasing plasmid copy number will increase the
specific activity of streptomycin adenylylase, but also increase
the rate of influx of streptomycin into the cells. The net effect
of these counteracting tendencies may explain why streptomycin
resistance reaches a constant level at all plasmid R1 copy numbers
above three times that of the wild type (Fig. 1).

A preliminary experiment that seems to support the idea presented
above was performed as follows: A plasmid (pKN230) in which the
streptomycin region was deleted was constructed by the phage lamb-
da-cointegration technique described by Willetts (44). Copy mutants of plasmid pKN230 were isolated on ampicillin plates. The
sensitivity to streptomycin of cells carrying these copy mutants
increased gradually with increasing copy number. Cells carrying
copy mutants of plasmid pKN230 with a copy effect of ten were
sensitive to a fivefold lower streptomycin concentration than
were plasmid-less bacteria.

7. Concluding Remarks

Plasmid R1 has a molecular weight of 65×10^6 and may therefore
carry more than 100 genes. Only few of these are known

at present. The phenotype of the host bacterium is affected in
many ways by the presence of plasmid R1. Some of these effects
can easily be traced to known plasmid genes, e. g. antibiotic
resistance, conjugal transfer, sensitivity to male specific phages.
However, there are other phenotypic effects of plasmid R1, effects that seem to be more indirect. There is an effect on cell
division, which perhaps is due to competition between the plasmid and the chromosome of the host for factors involved in initiation and/or elongation of chromosome replication. Cell division
has a tendency to be omitted in plasmid-carrying cells. Resistance
to rifampicin is reduced in cells carrying plasmid R1; this implies that the penetration barrier of the host has been impaired.
Indirect evidence suggests that the uptake of streptomycin, which
is very slow in E. coli, is facilitated in cells carrying plasmid
R1. All these phenotypic effects of plasmid R1, the direct as
well as the indirect ones, are the more pronounced the higher the
plasmid content of the host bacteria; this was concluded from
experiments involving a series of plasmid copy mutants.

Acknowledgments

Our work was supported by the Swedish Medical Research Council
(Project No. 4236), the Danish Medical Research Council (Project
No. 6866), and the Danish Natural Science Research Council (Pro-
ject No. 6532 and 7077).

References

1. Falkow, S.: Infectious Multiple Drug Resistance. Pion Ltd.
   1975.
2. Clowes, R. C.: Molecular Structure of Bacterial Plasmids.
   Bacteriol. Rev. 36, 361-405 (1972).
3. Reanny, D.: Extrachromosomal Elements as Possible Agents
   of Adaption and Development. Bacteriol. Rev. 40, 552-590
   (1976).
4. Nordström, K.: Increased Resistance to Several Antibiotics
   by One Mutation in an R-factor. J. Gen. Microbiol. 66, 205-
   214 (1971).

5. Nordström K., Ingram, L. C., Lundbäck, A.: Mutations in R-Factors of Escherichia coli Causing an Increased Number of R-Factor Copies per Chromosome. J. Bacteriol. 110, 562-569 (1972).

6. Kool, A. J., Nijkamp, H. J. J.: Isolation and Characterization of a Copy Mutant of the Bacteriocinogenic Plasmid Clo DF13. J. Bacteriol. 120, 569-578 (1974).

7. Matsubura, K., Takeda, Y.: Role of the tof Gene in the Production of the λ dv Plasmid. Mol. Gen. Genet. 142, 225-230 (1975).

8. Morris, S. F., Hashimoto, H., Mickel, S., Rownd, R.: Round of Replication Mutant of a Drug Resistance Factor. J. Bacteriol. 118, 855-866 (1974).

9. Timmis, K., Winkler, U.: Gene Dosage Studies With Pleiotropic Mutants of Serratia marcescens Superactive in the Synthesis of Marcescin A and Certain Other Exocellular Proteins. Mol. Gen. Genet. 124, 207-217 (1973).

10. Cress, D. E., Kline B. C.: Isolation and Characterization of Escherichia coli Chromosomal Mutants Affecting Plasmid Copy Number. J. Bacteriol. 125, 635-642 (1946).

11. Macrina, F.L., Weatherly, G. G., Curtiss III, R.: R6K Plasmid Replication: Influence of Chromosomal Genotype in Minicell-Producing Strains of Escherichia coli. J. Bacteriol. 120, 1387-1400 (1974).

12. Meynell, E., Datta, N.: The Relation of Resistance Transfer Factors to the F-Factor (Sex Factor) of Escherichia coli K-12. Genet. Res. 7, 134-140 (1966).

13. Meynell, E., Datta, N.: Mutant Drug-Resistant Factors of High Transmissibility. Nature (London) 214, 885-887 (1967).

14. Nordström, K., Engberg, B., Gustafsson, P., Molin, S., Uhlin, B. E.: Copy Mutants of the Plasmid R1 as a Tool in Studies of Control of Plasmid Replication. This volume.

15. Cohen, S. N., Miller, C. A.: Non-Chromosomal Antibiotic Resistance in Bacteria. II. Molecular Nature of R-Factors Isolated From Proteus mirabilis and Escherichia coli. J. Mol. Biol. 50, 671-687 (1970).

16. Meynell, E., Meynell, G. G., Datta, N.: Phylogenetic Relationship of Drug-Resistance Factors and Other Transmissible Bacterial Plasmids. Bacteriol. Rev. 32, 55-83 (1968).

17. Hedges, R. W., Datta, N.: R124, a fi[+] R-Factor of a New Compatibility Class. J. Gen. Microbiol. 71, 403-405 (1972).

18. Sköld, O.: R-Factor-Mediated Resistance to Sulphonamides by a Drug-Resistant Dihydropteroate Synthase. Antimicrob. Ag. Chemother. 9, 49-54 (1976).

19. Novick, R. P., Clowes, R. C., Cohen, S. N., Curtiss III, R., Datta, N., Falkow, S.: Uniform Nomenclature for Bacterial Plasmids: A Proposal. Bacteriol. Rev. 40, 168-198 (1976).

20. Uhlin, B. E., Nordström, K.: R-Plasmid Gene Dosage Effects in Escherichia coli K-12: Copy Mutants of the R-Plasmid R1drd-19. Plasmid, 1, in press (1977).

21. Uhlin, B. E., Nordström, K.: Plasmid Incompatibility and Control of Replication: Copy Mutants of the R-Factor R1 in Escherichia coli K-12. J. Bacteriol. 124, 641-649 (1975).

22. Lundbäck, A. K., Nordström, K.: Effect of R-Factor-Mediated Drug-Metabolizing Enzymes on Survival of Escherichia coli K-12 in Presence of Ampicillin, Chloramphenicol, or Streptomycin. Antimicrob. Ag. Chemother. 5, 492-499 (1974).

23. Nordström, K., Eriksson-Grennberg, K. G., Boman, H. G.: Resistance of Escherichia coli to Penicillins. III. AmpB, a Locus Affecting Episomally and Chromosomally Mediated Resistance to Ampicillin and Chloramphenicol. Genet. Res. 12, 157-168 (1968).

24. Rothfield, L., Pearlman-Kothencz, M.: Synthesis and Assembly of Bacterial Membrane Components. A Lipopolysaccharide-Phospholipid-Protein Complex Excreted by Living Bacteria. J. Mol. Biol. 44, 477-492 (1969).

25. Engberg, B., Nordström, K.: Replication of the R-Factor R1 in Escherichia coli K-12 at Different Growth Rates. J. Bacteriol. 123, 179-186 (1975).

26. Engberg, B., Hjalmarsson, K., Nordström, K.: Inhibition of Cell Division in Escherichia coli K-12 by the R-Factor R1 and Copy Mutants of R1. J. Bacteriol. 124, 633-640 (1975).

27. Inouye, M.: Pleiotropic Effect of the recA Gene of Escherichia coli: Uncoupling of Cell Division From Deoxyribonucleic Acid Replication. J. Bacteriol. 106, 539-542 (1971).

28. Goebel, W.: The Influence of dnaA and dnaC Mutations on the Initiation of Plasmid DNA Replication. Biochem. Biophys. Res. Commun. 51, 1000-1007 (1973).

29. Goebel, W.: Replication of Plasmid DNA in Escherichia coli. Proc. Soc. Gen. Microbiol. 1, 1-2 (1973).

30. Nordström, U. M., Engberg, B., Nordström, K.: Competition for DNA Polymerase III Between the Chromosome and the R-Factor R1. Mol. Gen. Genet. 135, 185-190 (1974).

31. Slater, M., Schaechter, M.: Control of Cell Division in Bacteria. Bacteriol. Rev. 38, 199-221 (1974).

32. Zaritsky, A., Pritchard, R. H.: Changes in Cell Size and Shape Associated With Changes in the Replication Time of the Chromosome of Escherichia coli. J. Bacteriol. 114, 824-837 (1973).

33. Lane, H. E. D., Denhardt, D. T.: The rep Mutation. III. Altered Structure of the Replication Escherichia coli Chromosome. J. Bacteriol. 120, 805-814 (1974).

34. Boman, H. G., Nordström, K., Normark, S.: Penicillin Resistance in Escherichia coli K-12: Synergism Between Penicillinases and a Barrier in the Outer Part of the Envelope. Ann. N. Y. Acad. Sci. 235, 569-586 (1974).

35. Hartman, G., Honikel, K. O., Knüsel, F., Nüesch, J.: The Specific Inhibition of the DNA-Directed RNA Synthesis by Rifampicin. Biochem. Biophys. Acta 145, 843-844 (1967).

36. Reid, P., Speyer, J.: Rifampicin Inhibition of Ribonucleic Acid and Protein Synthesis in Normal and Ethylenediaminetetra Acetic Acid-Treated Escherichia coli. J. Bacteriol. 104, 376-389 (1970).

37. Riva, S., Fietta, A. M., Silvestri, L. G.: R-Factors Determined Changes in Permeability of E. coli Towards Rifampicin and Other Antibiotics. (Bacterial Plasmids and Antibiotic Resistance, pp.343-348). Berlin-Heidelberg-New York: Springer 1972.

38. Payne, J. W. Gilvarg, C.: Size Restriction on Peptide Utilization in Escherichia coli. J. Biol. Chem. 243, 6291-6299 (1968).

39. Gustafsson, P., Nordström, K., Normark, S.: Outer Penetration Barrier of Escherichia coli K-12: Kinetics of the Uptake of Gentian Violet by Wild Type and Envelope Mutants. J. Bacteriol. 116, 893-900 (1973).

40. Eriksson-Grennberg, K. G., Nordström, K., Englund, P.: Resistance of Escherichia coli to Penicillins. IX. Genetics and Physiology of Class II Ampicillin-Resistant Mutants That Are Galactose Negative or Sensitive to Bacteriophage C21, or Both. J. Bacteriol. 108, 1210-1223 (1971).

41. Mickel, S., Bauer, W.: Isolation, by Tetracycline Selection, of Small Plasmids Derived From R-Factor R12 in Escherichia coli K-12. J. Bacteriol. 127, 644-655 (1976).

42. Lindquvist, R. C., Nordström, K.: Resistance of Escherichia
    coli to Penicillins. VII. Purification and Characterization
    of a Penicillinase Mediated by the R-Factor R1. J. Bacteriol.
    101, 232-239 (1970).

43. Lundbäck, A. K., Nordström, K.: Mutations in Escherichia
    coli K-12 Decreasing the Rate of Streptomycin Uptake: Syner-
    gism With R-Factor-Mediated Capacity to Inactivate Strepto-
    mycin. Antimicrob. Ag. Chemother. 5, 500-507 (1974).

44. Dempsey, W. B., Willetts, N. S.: Plasmid Co-Integrates of
    Prophage Lambda and R-Factor R100. J. Bacteriol. 126, 166-
    176 (1976).

Discussion

Anderson: Can you select the long cells, when I say select I mean perhaps by micromanipulation? If you select long cells, do you then get a random distribution of sizes when you grow them or can you get a trend towards reproduction of the long cell?

Nordström: We get a random population.

Anderson: Have you done any acridine orange studies of nuclear bodies in the long cell?

Nordström: We used a Giemsa staining technique to see whether they have a nuclear body; they seem to exist with about the same length frequency.

Anderson: Well, this is the point because you may in effect have a number of independent physiological units.

Nordström: They do not resemble normal filaments.

Anderson: This would fit in perfectly with your so-called "new-born cell of normal length" because they begin to form their cell septa.

Nordström: And it's not from one end.

Richmond: Yes, if your hypothesis is right, and I think it is attractive, if you put R1 into NV, then resistance to streptomycin should be decreased.

Nordström: And it is. We would like to do the obvious control and delete the streptomycin region and see if streptomycin resistance actually goes down.

Richmond: And I'd also predict that if you look at ß-lactamase resistance the effect on ampicillin resistance will be very marked and negligible on cephalosporin resistance.

Davies: That kind of experiment is nice; I think it is difficult to look at a single gene function in terms of an absolute phenotype. You can change the influence of the cell envelope by changing the cell line. If you cross certain R factors from E. coli to pseudomonas you can see a thousandfold difference in expression of gentamicin resistance.

Levy: I have two questions. One, have you looked at small plasmids for their effect on permeability?

Nordström: No, I haven't.

Levy: And second, do you think that the permeability effect of rifamycin is a general effect for all R plasmids or do you think that it is linked to particular genes?

Nordström: I haven't any results of my own, I believe it was generally observed in the Italian workers' studies.

Falkow: Mostly F-like plasmids.

Levy: I can make one comment concerning tetracycline uptake. If you take R222 or R222 without the tet-determinant, the uptake of tetracycline is the same as the sensitive strain. The presence of the plasmid hasn't altered anything in terms of tetracycline uptake.

Anderson: What is the maximum copy number that you havè got so far?

Nordström: 50 copies.

Anderson: Are these normal size?

Nordström: Yes.

Anderson: This ought to be about the size of the chromosome. Have you tried to see whether there is any apparent difference in the appearance of cells carrying these very large numbers? I am thinking in terms of acridine staining.

Nordström: No, we haven't.

Anderson: You are getting the point where you ought to be able to detect it visually.

Nordström: No, we haven't done this. These mutants are fairly new, it should be done.

Falkow: I was interested in the stability of the mutations in the absence of selection pressure.

Nordström: They seem to be perfectly stable, with one exception: when you increase the copy number you get an increase in the probability of forming minicircles and they may eventually dominate the population. So particularly if you let the cultures go to stationary phase you arrive at the situation where you do not find the original large size plasmid, but only small size (7-8 x 10^6 and upwards) plasmids.

Falkow: With all genes represented?

Anderson: With what properties?

Falkow: I was just interested in the competition of these versus an F$^-$.

Nordström: We haven't done this yet.

Anderson: Have you done ultrathin sections?

Nordström: No.

Starlinger: I have a point that I didn't understand, with respect to copy effect on transfer properties. You have more copies and should transfer more, but you should also make twice the amount of repressor and this should reduce the frequency of transfer. These two effects should compensate to give approximately the wild-type behaviour. Why doesn't this happen?

Nordström: I don't know whether repressor is formed constitutively or not.

Anderson: You may need only a reversion of one copy for the repressor to be produced in sufficient amounts to drop the frequency to the wild-type level.

Starlinger: Do you think there is the possibility of autogenous repression or something of that sort?

Högenauer: Did you look at the lipid A content in relation to copy number?

Nordström: No, we didn't.

Anderson: Is the property stable in transfer?

Nordström: Yes.

Anderson: Have you put it into a host such as S. typhimurium?

Nordström: We get the same effect.

Drews: Could you enhance the effect by co-cultivating R$^+$ and R$^-$ strains in such a way that transfer would be excluded? Is it amplified?

Nordström: Yes, but it might fail.

Drews: Is the effect or are these multicopy effects very much dependent on the medium that you use?

Nordström: Yes, definitely they are.

Anderson: What about cell mass product in a given time. Is it slow, is there a retardation?

Drews: Is the total mass of cells the same as in R$^-$ strains?

Nordström: You mean in the median cell?

Anderson: No, in the total population.

Nordström: We have measured that and there is no difference.

Metabolism of R-Factor DNA

Molecular Cloning of DNA from the R-Plasmid R6K

Jorge H. Crosa, Linda K. Luttropp, and Stanley Falkow

1. Introduction

Bacterial plasmids are non-essential in the sense that they may be lost
from a cell under most circumstances without affecting cell viability. As
adequately documented elsewhere in this volume, the presence of a plasmid
may confer upon a host cell the capacity to survive in an adverse environment or to better compete with organisms of the same or related species.
Plasmids have a range of molecular mass from 0.5×10^6 daltons to greater
than 150×10^6 daltons and vary in their mol fraction guanine and cytocine
content from 0.39 to 0.72. Consequently it is as difficult to make gen-
eralizations about the basic biology of plasmids as it is about the micro-
organisms in which their life cycle takes place. Nonetheless at the
molecular level one can make the generalization that plasmids are double-
stranded covalently closed molecules of DNA. In addition plasmids generally
fall into two molecular classes. One class, best typified by ColE1, is of
relatively small size (generally less than 10×10^6 daltons in mass), nonconjugative and is generally found as a multi-copy pool within its host
cells. The other class, best typified by the classical sex factor, F, is of
relatively large molecular mass (generally greater than 30×10^6 daltons),
usually conjugative and present in a limited number of copies per host cell.
One (but certainly not the only) exception to these general molecular
properties of plasmids is R6K. The R plasmid R6K is conjugative, confers
resistance to ampicillin (Ap^r) and streptomycin (Sm^r), is of relatively

small molecular mass, 26×10^6 daltons, but replicates as a multicopy pool, /20/. Because of these rather unusual molecular properties R6K has been an attractive focus of attention to study R plasmid maintenance and replication.

2. The Topology of R-Plasmid DNA Replication

All bacterial plasmids may be readily isolated from bacterial cells as double-stranded covalently closed DNA molecules. R6K and RSF1040, a deletion mutant of R6K /11/, like other plasmids and the small animal viruses, polyoma and SV40, appear to replicate semiconservatively according to the Cairns model. That is, replicative intermediates of R6K have two branch points, three branches and no free ends (the so-called theta structure). DNA synthesis occurs on a covalently closed circular (CCC) superhelical template (Form I) /12/. Kinetic studies as well as the direct visualization of replicating molecules in the electron microscope are compatible with the model that replication proceeds by the progressive unwinding of a CCC molecule accompanied by replication in which two open circular branches of equal size containing the nascent DNA are generated (Fig. 1). Because the parental strands are maintained as covalently closed structures, it is postulated that a transient nick serves as a swivel as the parental strands unwind; such a transient nick could be produced by a nuclease acting in conjunction with polynucleotide ligase or it could be produced by the DNA untwisting enzyme /9/, /31/. The DNA untwisting enzyme appears to be the most likely candidate. In vitro, this enzyme acts to relax superhelical DNA by first introducing a single stranded break into the DNA and then sealing the same nick /8/. During the lifetime of this nick, at least one end of the broken DNA appears to be free to rotate about the other strand. In any event as replication proceeds the DNA unwinds until two daughter molecules are generated. The daughter molecules then separate with at least one of the progeny molecules containing a nick (or gap). Such a nicked (or gapped) progeny molecule (Form II) must be subsequently closed and converted to a Form I molecule, the end product of replication.

Recent experiments by us and others have established Form II as an intermediate in replication /12/, /27/, /29/. A postulated intermediate stage
between Form II and Form I DNA as a terminal replication event envisions a
covalently closed species with no superhelical turns (Form Io). These
postulated transient forms have, in fact, been identified during the life
cycles of the plasmids RSF1040 /13/ and pSC101 /30/, viruses SV40 /14/ and
polyoma replicating in the presence of protein synthesis inhibitors /6/,
/32/, PM2 /15/, and mitochondrial DNA /1/, /2/.

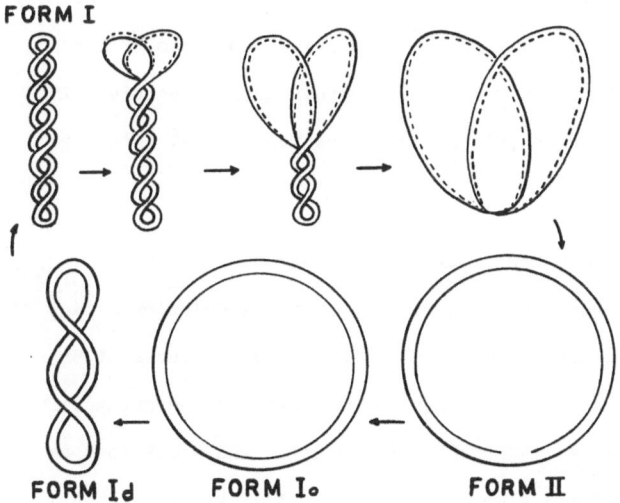

FORM I

FORM Id   FORM Io   FORM II

Fig. 1. The topology of R-Plasmid DNA Replication

Our data and those of other groups suggest an intermediate stage between
Form II and Form I DNA as one of the terminal events of replication. Form
II DNA is presumably sealed to a covalently closed species with no superhelical turns (Form Io). These transient forms, which appear as heavy DNA
in dye-CsCl gradients, are in turn modified by the progressive introduction
of negative superhelical turns (the forms deficient in superhelical density
are identified as Id) until the superhelical density of Form I DNA is
achieved (Fig. 1).

This maturation process is carried out through a series of nicking and sealing events, or by a protein or protein system which can introduce super-helical turns. A good candidate for this activity is the recently described E. coli DNA gyrase which can introduce negative superhelical turns into Form Io DNA /17/. DNA gyrase is certainly involved in in vitro plasmid replication and appears to be required for DNA synthesis because the anti-biotics novobiocin and coumermycin inhibit E. coli DNA synthesis in vivo and DNA gyrase activity in vitro /18/.

All of the topological features of R6K and RSF1040 replication have been also described for animal viruses as well as the ColEl plasmid. Presumably these common features reflect an analogous sequential process of DNA repli-cation. Although replicating R6K DNA shares certain common features with several other diverse DNA species, it nevertheless has several unique repli-cative properties.

3. The Mode of R6K and RSF1040 Replication in E. coli

We have recently reported the isolation of a spontaneous deletion mutant of R6K, RSF1040, which has retained most of the distinctive features of the parental R6K plasmid but which now possess several distinct advantages for the study of replication /11/. RSF1040 is conjugative and maintained as a multicopy pool, yet RSF1040 has a molecular mass of 17.3×10^6 daltons in contrast to 26.5×10^6 daltons for R6K. The deletion of 9×10^6 daltons from R6K is associated with the loss of the gene determining streptomycin resistance and as a shift in mol fraction guanine + cytosine content from 0.45 to 0.42. In addition RSF1040 now has only one site on its DNA suscep-tible to cleavage by the EcoRI restriction endonuclease, whereas the parental R6K plasmid possesses two such sites. Thus RSF1040 DNA can be cleaved to a single linear molecule by EcoRI action which simplifies the examination of replicative forms by electron microscopy and, because of its lower guanine + cytosine content, can be distinguished from the bacterial chromosome in density gradients. By exploiting these technical advantages we have been able to examine the general mode of RSF1040 replication.

Figure 2 summarizes the replicative properties of RSF1040. RSF1040 can initiate replication at two distinct sites on the plasmid genome. The two distinct origins of replication can be identified at 23% (origin α) and 39% (origin β) relative to one end of an EcoRI cleaved molecule (Fig. 2).

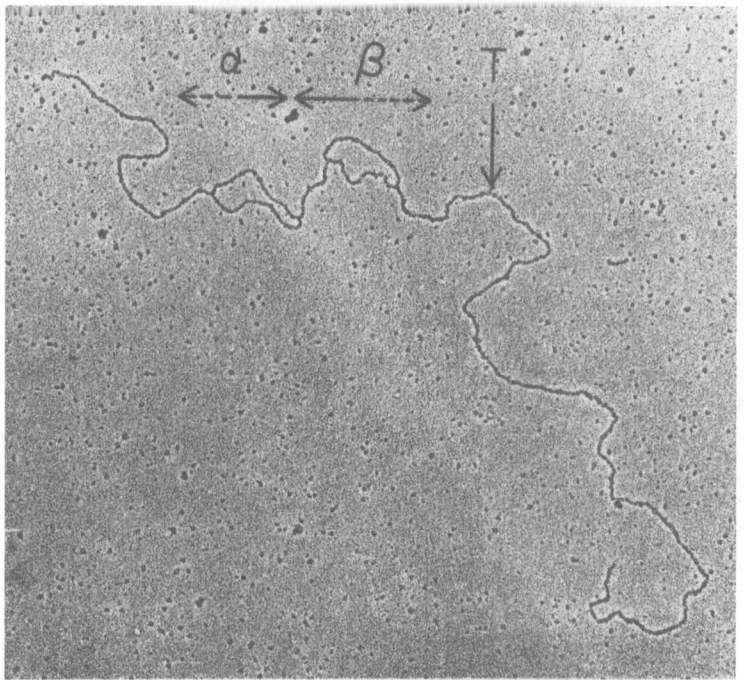

Fig. 2. Summary of the replication properties of RSF1040.

In most cases, replication is initiated exclusively from one or the other of the two origins although, as illustrated in Figure 2, a proportion of molecules are found in which both replication sites are employed simultaneously. On average however, initiation proceeds from α at a higher frequency. Perhaps the most unique feature of RSF1040 replication is that it is asymmetric and bidirectional. In other DNA species known to undergo bidirectional replication (for example, SV40 virus, polyoma and E. coli), the bidirectional replication is symmetrical and the two replication forks reach a termination point at roughly the same time. Moreover, the termination point in these cases appears to be nonspecific. In the case of RSF1040, however, replication is bidirectional but sequential /12/. In the case of the α origin, replication first proceeds unidirectionally in one direction to a specific terminus (T) and then proceeds from the origin in the opposite direction to T to complete the replicative process. Replication from the β origin is largely unidirectional but also appears to possess a component that replicates in the opposite direction to the main growth of the replication fork. However, replication initiated from either α or β proceeds to the same unique terminus.

Initially it was thought that R6K possessed only the α origin and that β might represent a "silent" origin that had become activated as a consequence of the 9×10^6 dalton deletion that accompanied the formation of RSF1040 /12/, /22/. More recent studies have established that R6K possesses both the α and β origins and that the mode of replication of R6K and RSF1040 are comparable (in preparation). The finding that R6K and RSF1040 possess two origins of replication is not unique. Studies from several laboratories have shown that some R plasmids, which exist in E. coli as a single unit of replication may dissociate in other bacterial hosts into component replicons /9/, /16/, /21/, /25/. Not unexpectedly such plasmid cointegrates may initiate replication at either of the two origins of the cointegrated replicons /26/. More recent work has shown that a constructed hybrid plasmid can possess two distinct sets of replication functions which are each operationally competent under appropriate conditions /7/. R6K is not known to dissociate into component replicons in any bacterial host although it may represent the in vivo fusion or recombinational product between two distinct replicons. At any rate it seemed of considerable interest to attempt to dissect the essential replicative features of R6K and RSF1040 and identify, if possible, the factors that regulate the utilization of discrete replicative origins as well as the nature of the segmented control of replication and its specific termination. As a preliminary step towards this goal we have concentrated upon the isolation of DNA recombinant molecules containing essential regions of the R6K genome.

4. Isolation of DNA Recombinant Molecules Containing Essential Replication
   Regions of R6K

Recent developments in DNA biochemistry have made possible the in vitro joining of DNA segments from diverse sources. The isolation of such DNA recombinant molecules has involved the ligation of an enzymatically cleaved DNA fragment to a similarly cleaved but still functional plasmid or phage genome. Such DNA recombinant molecules may then be introduced into a suitable host cell by transformation where they replicate autonomously, serving to "clone" the ligated DNA fragment(s). This methodology has already been employed to examine the functional properties of F /28/ and has also been employed to examine replication initiation site selection following the ligation of the plasmids pSC101 and ColE1 /7/. In the latter instance, under normal conditions of cellular growth the ColE1 replication apparatus and initiation site are used exclusively for replication of the composite plasmid. In cells lacking a functional DNA polymerase I (polA$^-$), however, ColE1 replication does not normally occur and the pSC101 replication machinery acts to duplicate the composite plasmid. The important point is that either replication system can accomplish replication of the entire plasmid composite molecule. In the following sections we describe the use of a similar strategy to isolate the essential replication components of R6K and RSF1040.

As noted earlier, R6K DNA is cleaved by the EcoRI endonuclease into two fragments. The two fragments are 10×10^6 and 16×10^6 daltons in mass respectively (Fig. 3C). Initially we wished to determine whether the replicative functions of R6K were localized exclusively on one of these fragments. To accomplish this end, EcoRI cleaved R6k fragments were mixed with EcoRI cleaved fragments of the plasmid pML21 /19/; Fig. 3E). pML21 is cleaved by

EcoRI into a functional ColEl derivative and a fragment carrying genes for kanamycin resistance. The pML21 fragments and R6K fragments were ligated and transformed into E. *coli* K-12 polA⁻ recipient cells with selection for Km^r transformants. Since the ColEl component of pML21 cannot replicate in the absence of DNA polymerase I while R6K can replicate in the absence of this enzyme, it is clear that Km^r transformants should contain a Km^r fragment derived from pML21 and the fragment of R6K which contained one or more of its replication functions. When the plasmid DNA from Km^r transformants was isolated and cleaved with EcoRI it was found (Fig. 3D) that they contained the Km fragment and the 10×10^6 dalton R6K fragment. In no case was the 16×10^6 dalton R6K fragment found suggesting that the replication functions of R6K were solely contained on the 10×10^6 dalton R6K fragment.

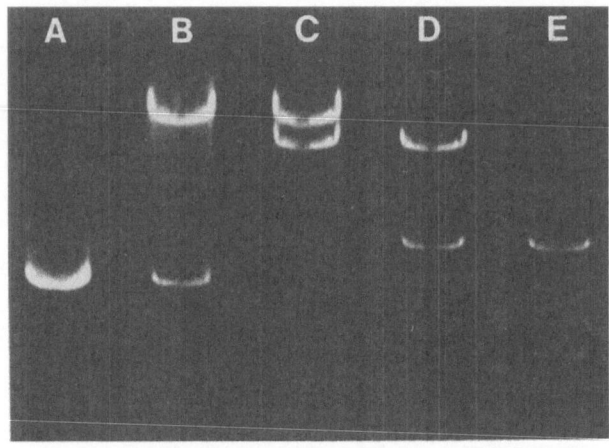

Fig. 3. Agarose gel electrophoresis of EcoRI treated cloned EcoRI fragments of R6K DNA.

R6K encodes for resistance to ampicillin and streptomycin. Yet the Km^r transformants containing the 10×10^6 dalton R6K fragment expressed neither of these resistance traits. In order to confirm that the 16×10^6 R6K fragment contained the antibiotic resistance determinants for ampicillin and streptomycin resistance, EcoRI cleaved R6K was mixed and ligated with EcoRI cleaved pMB9 DNA. pMB9 contains a single EcoRI site (Fig. 3A) and contains the replication machinery and colicin immunity genes of ColE1 and a determinant conferring resistance to tetracycline (Tc^r) /3/. The ligated mixture of R6K and pMB9 DNA was transformed into an E. coli K-12 pol A$^+$ recipient with selection for Tc^r Sm^{r}Ap^r transformants. When the plasmid DNA was extracted from these clones and cleaved with EcoRI it was found (Fig. 3B) that they contained pMB9 and the 16 x 10^6 dalton R6K fragment. Attempts to transform these hybrid plasmids into E. coli K-12 pol A$^-$ cells was not successful indicating that the 16 x 10^6 dalton fragment does not contain functional replication genes. It is of further interest to note that recombinant molecules containing the 10 x 10^6 or 16 x 10^6 dalton R6K fragments were non-conjugative indicating that essential transfer functions are present on both fragments.

In order to assess the degree of homology between RSF1040 and the cloned 10 Mdal EcoRI fragment of R6K, we prepared heteroduplex molecules and examined them in the electron microscope. Figure 4 shows one of such hetero-duplex molecules. There is a double stranded region comprising most of the 10 Mdal R6K EcoRI fragment which includes one of the EcoRI ends of RSF1040. The small single stranded tail is the portion of the 10 Mdal R6K EcoRI fragment that was deleted when RSF1040 was formed while the larger single stranded tail corresponds to the rest of the RSF1040 genome.

The data obtained in these preliminary experiments not only served to con-firm that the essential replication functions of R6K were clustered in a discrete region of R6K but further documented that these genes could function as a part of a hybrid molecule in a pol A$^-$ host. Consequently, we attempted to more precisely dissect the essential replicative functions of R6K by molecular cloning.

R6K has 23 sites susceptible to cleavage by the restriction endonuclease Hind III while RSF1040 is cleaved at 18 sites. We attempted to isolate each of the R6K fragments by ligation to the cloning vehicle pBR313 (Ap^{r}Tc^r; 5.8

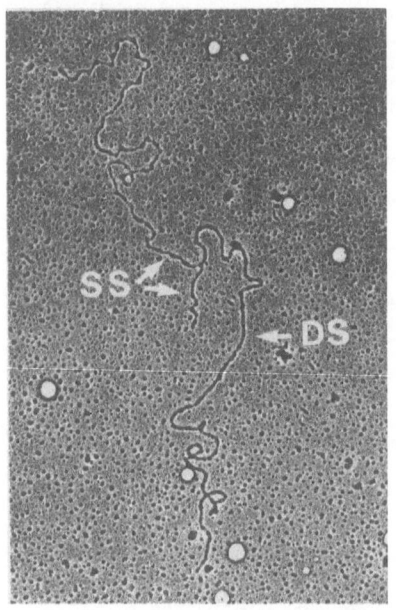

Figure 4.   Heteroduplex between EcoRI cleaved RSF1040 and the small R6K

               EcoRI fragment.   (SS: single-stranded DNA; DS: double-stranded DNA)

x 10^6 daltons) /4/, /5/ which possesses a single Hind III site.   Ligation

of a DNA fragment into the Hind III site of pBR313 generally results in the

inactivation of the Tc^r phenotype.   Hence the isolation of transformants

carrying pBR313 which contain an inserted DNA fragment is considerably sim-

plified by screening for $Ap^r Tc^s$ cells in contrast to cells containing the

parental PBR313 plasmid ($Ap^r Tc^r$).   R6K DNA digested with Hind III was ligated

with similarly digested pBR313 DNA.   When the ligation mixture was transformed

into E. coli polA⁻ recipient cells with selection for ampicillin resistance,

no transformants were obtained.   These findings suggested that no single

Hind III fragment contained sufficient information to permit replication.

Transformation of such ligated mixtures into E. coli polA⁺ cell did permit

us, however, to obtain a number of transformants which contained pBR313

into which the various R6K Hind III fragments had been ligated.   Inspection

of Table 1 indicates that Hind III fragment 1 carries the Ap^r genes while

253

Table 1. Properties of some of the R6K derivatives obtained by either molecular cloning or partial digestion and ligation of Hind III cleaved R6K DNA

| Derivative | Properties of cloned fragment or derivative | | | | Properties of Recombinant | |
	MW Mdal	Hind III fragments	EcoRI sites	Drug resistance determinants	Replication E. coli-K12 pol A⁻	Transfer
R6K	26	1-9;10**;11;12**;13-23	2	$Ap^r Sm^r$	+	+
RSF1040	17.3	1*;4-9;10**;15;16;18-20;22	1	Ap^r	+	+
Small R6K EcoRI fragment (cloned with Km² fragment)	10	2-5;7-9;10**;12**;14; 15;18-20	---	---	+	---
Large R6K EcoRI fragment (cloned with PMB9)	16	1;3;6;10**;11;12**;13; 16;17;21;23	---	$Ap^r Sm^r$	---	---
Hind III fragments 3;17;21 (cloned with PBR313)	1.9	3;17;21	---	Sm^r	---	---
Hind III fragment 1* (cloned with PSC101)	9.5	1*	---	Ap^r	+	---
RJHC73	5	3;4;9;15	---	Sm^r	+	---
RJHC26	7.2	2;3;9;12**;13-17;21	1	Sm^r	+	---
RJHC12	10	2;3;4;9;12**;13-18;21	1	Sm^r	-	---

* Because of the deletion that originated RSF1040, Hind III fragment 1 obtained from RSF1040 DNA is of a smaller size than R6K Hind III fragment 1. In addition it is fused to part of the R6K Hind III fragment 2 (part of this fragment was also deleted when RSF1040 was originated).
** Fragments 12 and 10 contain EcoRI sites 1 and 2 respectively. The 10 and 15 MdaI R6K EcoRI fragments have then a fraction of Hind III fragments 12 and 10.

Hind III fragment 3 carries the Sm^r determinants. EcoRI sites 1 and 2 are present on Hind III fragments 10 and 12 respectively.

Since complete Hind III digestion and insertion into pBR313 was not successful, an alternative experimental approach was employed. R6K DNA was treated with Hind III for short periods of time so that many of the R6K molecules were only partially cleaved. These partial digests were ligated and the ligated mixture used to transform E. coli pol A$^-$ cells with selection for either the Sm^r or Ap^r phenotype. This procedure permitted us to isolate a series of plasmids which had lost a considerable number of Hind III fragments but which retained sufficient genetic information for replication. These R6K derivatives capable of self-replication in the polA$^-$ background ranged from 5×10^6 daltons to 10×10^6 daltons in mass. The smallest of these self-replicating "mini" R6K derivatives, RJHC73 contained Hind III fragments 3, 4, 9 and 15 and possessed the Sm^r phenotype and no EcoRI site. Two other of these Sm^r mini R6K derivatives were RJHC26 (Hind III fragment 2, 3, 9, 12, 13, 14, 15, 17, 21 and one EcoRI site) and RJHC12 (Hind III fragments 2, 3, 4, 9, 12, 13, 14, 15, 17, 21 and one EcoRI site).

Measurements of EcoRI cleaved replicating structures indicate that the origin α should be located in Hind III fragment 4 while the β origin should be located on fragment 2 (which appears to contain the terminus T) or fragments 15-9 (a preliminary mapping of the Hind III fragments indicate that there are two possibilities for their sequence in the vicinity of the replication origin, that is: 2-15-9-4 or 2-9-15-4, most of the evidence indicates that the first possibility is more probable).

It is interesting to note that mini R6K RJHC26 does not have Hind III fragment 4, RJHC73 does not have fragment 2 and that RJHC12 has both fragments 2 and 4. The implications are then that RJHC26 should have lost the α origin (or replication functions associated with it) and conserved the terminus T and that RJHC73 has probably only the α origin and lost the terminus T. RJHC12 should have conserved both α and β as well as the terminus T.

We are now analyzing the topology and replication of the mini R6K derivatives and from these studies we hope that insight into the specificity and interactions of origins of replication in naturally occurring multiple replicons will be gained.

Acknowledgments

This research was supported by grant PCM-75-14174 A01 of the National Science Foundation.

Literature

1. Berk, A. J., and Clayton, D. A. Mechanisms of mitochondrial DNA replication in mouse L-cells: Asynchronous replication of strands, segregation of circular daughter molecules, aspects of topology and turnover of an initiation sequence. J. Mol. Biol., 86, 801-824 (1974).

2. Berk, A. J., and Clayton, D. A. Mechanisms of mitochondrial DNA replication in mouse L-cells: Topology of circular daughter molecules and dynamics of catenated oligomer formation. J. Mol. Biol., 100, 85-102 (1976).

3. Betlach, M. C., Hershfield, V., Chow, L., Brown, W., Goodman, H. M., and Boyer, H. W. A restriction endonuclease analysis of the bacterial plasmid controlling the EcoRI restriction and modification of DNA. Fed. Proc., 35, 2037-2043 (1976).

4. Bolivar, F., Rodriquez, R., Betlach, M., and Boyer, H. W. Construction and characterization of new cloning vehicles. Gene, in press (1977).

5. Bolivar, F., Rodriquez, R. L., Greene, P. J., Betlach, M. C., Heymeker, H. L., Boyer, H. W., Crosa, J. H., and Falkow, S. A multipurpose cloning system: Construction and characterization. Gene, in press (1977).

6. Bourgaux, P., and Bourgaux-Ramoisy, D. Is a specific protein responsible for the supercoiling of polyoma DNA? Nature, 235, 105-107 (1972).

7. Cabello, F., Timmis, K., and Cohen, S. N. Replication control in a composite plasmid constructed by in vitro linkage of two distinct replicons. Nature, 259, 285-290 (1976).

8. Champoux, J. Evidence for an intermediate with a single-strand break in the reaction catalyzed by the DNA untwisting enzyme. Proc. Nat. Acad. Sci. U.S.A., 73, 3488-3491 (1976).

9. Champoux, J., and Dulbecco, R. An activity from mammalian cells that untwists superhelical DNA. A possible swivel for DNA replication. Proc. Nat. Acad. Sci. U.S.A., 69, 143-146 (1972).

10. Cohen, S. N., and Miller, C. A. Non-chromosomal antibiotic resistance in bacteria. II. Molecular nature of R factors isolated from Proteus mirabilis and Escherichia coli. J. Mol. Biol., 50, 671-687 (1970).

11. Crosa, J. H., Luttropp, L. K., Heffron, F., and Falkow, S. Two replication initiation sites on R plasmid DNA. Mol. Gen. Genet. 140, 39-50 (1975).

12. Crosa, J. H., Luttropp, L. K., and Falkow, S. Mode of replication of the conjugative R-plasmid RSF1040 in Escherichia coli. J. Bacteriol., 126, 454-466 (1976).

13. Crosa, J. H., Luttropp, L, K., and Falkow, S. Covalently closed circular DNA molecules deficient in superhelical density as intermediates in the plasmid life cycle. Nature, 261, 561-519 (1976).

14. Eason, R., and Vinograd, J. Superhelix density of intracellular Simian Virus 40 deoxyribonucleic acid. J. Virol, 7, 1-7 (1971).

15. Espejo, R., Espejo-Canelo, F., and Sinsheimer, R. L. A difference between intracellular and viral supercoiled PM2 DNA. J. Mol. Biol. 56, 623-626 (1971).

16. Falkow, S., Tompkins, L. S., Silver, R. P., Guerry, P., and LeBlanc, D. S. The replication of R-factor DNA in Escherichia coli K-12 following conjugation. Ann. N. Y. Acad. Sci., 182, 153-171 (1971).

17. Gellert, M., Mizuuchi, K., O'Dea, M. H., and Nash, H. A. DNA gyrase: the enzyme that introduces superhelical turns into DNA. Proc. Nat. Acad. Sci. U.S. 73, 3872-3876 (1976).

18. Gellert, M., O'Dea, H. H., Itoh, T., and Tomizawa, J. Novobiocin and coumermycin inhibit DNA supercoiling catalyzed by DNA gyrase. Proc. Nat. Acad. Sci. U.S. 73, 4474-4478 (1976).

19. Herschfield, V., Boyer, H. W., Chow, L., and Helinski, D. R. Characterization of a mini-colEI plasmid. J. Bacteriol. 126, 447-453 (1976).

20. Kontomichalou, P., Mitani, M., and Clowes, R. C. Circular R-factor molecules controlling penicillinase synthesis, replicating under either relaxed or stringent control. J. Bacteriol. 104, 34-55 (1970).

21. Kopecko, D. J., and Punch, J. D. Regulation of R-factor replication in Proteus mirabilis. Ann. N. Y. Acad. Sci., 182, 207-216 (1971).

22. Lovett, M., Sparks, R. M., and Helinski, D. R. Bidirectional replication of plasmid R6K DNA in Escherichia coli; correspondence between origin of replication and position of single-strand break in relaxed complex. Proc. Natl. Acad. Sci. U.S.A., 73, 2905-2909 (1975).

23. Pritchard, R. H., Barber, P. T., and Collins, J. Control of DNA synthesis in bacteria. XIX Symp. Soc. Gen. Microbiol., 19, 263-297 (1969).

24. Pritchard, R. H., Chandler, M. G., and Collins, J. Independence of F replication and chromosome replication in Escherichia coli. Mol. Gen. Genet. 138, 143-155 (1975).

25. Rownd, R. H., and Nickel, S. Dissociation and reassociation of RFT and r-determinants of the R-factor NR1 in Proteus mirabilis. Nature New Biol., 234, 40-43 (1971).

26. Rownd, R. H., Perlman, D., and Goto, N. Structure and replication of R-factor DNA in Proteus mirabilis. Microbiology 1974 (D. Schlessinger ed.), p. 76-95, Washington, D.C. American Society for Microbiology (1975).

27. Sakakibara, Y., and Tomizawa, J. Termination point of replication of colicin El plasmid DNA in cell extracts. Proc. Nat. Acad. Sci. U.S.A., 71, 4935-4939 (1974).

28. Skurray, R. A., Nagaishi, H., and Clark, A. J. Molecular cloning of DNA from F sex factor of Escherichia coli K-12. Proc. Nat. Acad. Sci. U.S. 73, 64-68 (1976).

29. Staudenbauer, W. L. Replication of colicinogenic factor El DNA: evidence for a discontinuous replication mechanism. Nucleic Acids Res., 1, 1153-1164 (1974).

30. Timmis, K., Cabello, F., and Cohen, S. N. Covalently closed circular DNA molecules with low superhelical density as intermediates in plasmid DNA replication. Nature, 261, 512-516 (1976).

31. Wang, J. C. Interaction between DNA and an Escherichia coli protein W. J. Mol. Biol. 55, 523-533 (1971).

32. Yu, K., and Cheevers, W. P. DNA synthesis in polyoma virus infection. IV. Mechanisms of formation of closed-circular viral DNA deficient in superhelical turns. J. Virol. 17, 402-414 (1976).

Discussion

Richmond: What about the incompatibility properties of the fragments?

Falkow: We are just beginning to work on this question. It
appears that the fragments α and β, if put on different plasmids,
show some degree of incompatibility, but at this point it is
still unclear.

Richmond: And what about the fragments in relation to plasmids
of standard incompatibility groups?

Falkow: We have no information on that as yet.

Anderson: To what point is the transferability retained?

Falkow: Neither of the two fragments, if cloned individually,
retained transferability and we have not yet been able to find
a combination which will allow us to obtain transfer.

Anderson: But you can mobilise them?

Falkow: Yes, we can.

Anderson: Can you get recombination between the two fragments
to restore transferability?

Falkow: We tried this, but so far we have not been successful.

Davies: Are both fragments, that is, are both the α and β origins
sensitive to novobiocin?

Falkow: We have not done this yet, we are probably first going
to examine DNA gyrase activity in vitro.

Starlinger: Do you know how the asymmetry of replication is
achieved?

Falkow: No, we don't understand what signals may be involved.

Starlinger: I am referring to the situation where there is first
replication in the direction of the terminator and only then in
the other direction. Is the terminator involved and is there a
similar phenomenon seen in the recombinant that has no terminator region?

Falkow: No, it is not. If there is no terminator region the

plasmid appears to replicate in a unidirectional mode.

Starlinger: So there must be a signal coming from the terminator when it has been reached in one direction?

Falkow: Presumably so. There is, however, another possibility: when there are tandem repeats close by, these may act as terminators. That is to say, replication forks will accumulate there.

Davies: Does R6K replicate in most of the dna mutants of E. coli?

Falkow: It does not replicate in dna B. It was reported that it replicated in dna E, but we found this not to be correct. R6K replicates normally in dna A and polA⁻ cells.

Levy: I was going to make a comment: you were saying that you would try to introduce the different fragments, containing α and β into minicells. I would be very interested in knowing about the segregation patterns you observe. R6K itself does not segregate as efficiently as other plasmids, and the question is whether there will be a difference in segregation if a recombinant has either the α or the β fragment. It would be interesting to find out, since we know that incompatibility does not seem to correlate with the segregation of plasmids into minicells, but is apparently more related to the replication machinery.

Falkow: The problem with R6K is that it belongs to incompatibility group X, and it is the sole member of the group.

Richmond: I wonder whether there may not even be a dual incompatibility resulting from the dual origin of replication?

Falkow: This may well be the case.

Levy: Just forgetting incompatibility: one should be able to determine whether replication from one origin or the other does determine the site of replication in a cell. This question could be answered by using the minicell system.

Falkow: Yes.

Dissociation and Recombination of Fragments with Defined Functions of the Antibiotic Resistance Factor R1

W. Goebel[1], W. Lindenmaier[2], H. Schrempf[1], R. Kollek[1], and D. Blohm[2]

The antibiotic resistance factor R1drd-19 determines resistance to ampicillin (Ap), kanamycin (Km), sulfonamid (Sa), streptomycin (Sm) and chloramphenicol (Cm). It is derepressed in its transfer (drd) and occurs in the E. coli cell in few copies. As previously demonstrated by Sharp et al. /1/ R1 shares extensive sequence homologies with R6 and NR1 (R100-1). As shown in Table 1 most of the EcoRI fragments obtained with R1drd-19 are, however, different from those of NR1 /2/. Nordström et al. /3/ have isolated several copy mutants (cop) of R1drd-19, named R1drd-19B2 (new nomenclature pKN) which have 3-10 fold increased copy numbers. One of them R1drd-19B2 (pKN102) which does not seem to determine resistance to kanamycin has been studied in our laboratory and shown to give rise to the frequent generation of mini-plasmids, which we named Rsc plasmids /4/. Table 1 shows that R1drd-19B2 differs from R1drd-19 by the loss of three EcoRI fragments (F, J and O) and a slight alteration of EcoRI fragment D which carries the ampicillin resistance. The lost EcoRI fragments are present in a R1-derivative R1drd-16, previously isolated by E. Meynell. This plasmid carries resistance to kanamycin but has lost the other four antibiotic resistances, determined by R1drd-19 which apparently results in the loss of EcoRI-fragments D, G, H, I, L and N. R1drd-16/1 is a kanamycin-sensitive mutant of R1drd-16, which has been isolated in our laboratory. This deletion mutant which appears to be identical to the RTF unit of R1 again looses the three EcoRI-fragments F, J and O, which are also absent in R1drd-19B2. This indicates that kanamycin resistance is located on a fragment of $\sim$6x10^6 dalton (9kb), which seems to be lost as a unit in R1drd-19B2 and R1drd-16/1. In addition heteroduplex analysis between R1drd-16 and R6-5 (Fig. 1 a) shows a single stranded loop of 9 kb. Such a segment has

[1]Institut für Genetik und Mikrobiologie, Universität Würzburg, Germany.
[2]Gesellschaft für Biotechnologische Forschung, Stöckheim, Germany.

262

Table 1

EcoR1 Fragments of R1 and its derivatives compared to EcoR1 fragments of NR1 (R100)

NR1 Tc, Sm, Sa, Cm Mw(x10⁶ d)	Fragment	R1drd-19 Ap, Km, Sa, Sm, Cm Mw(x10⁶ d)	Fragment	Fragment	R1drd-19B2 Ap, Sa, Sm, Cm Mw(x10⁶ d)	R1drd-16 Km Mw(x10⁶ d)	R1drd-16/1 – Mw(x10⁶ d)	Plasmid Antibiotic resistances
13,5	A	11,6	A	A	11,6	11,6	11,6	
8,0	B	11,5	B	B	11,5	11,5	11,5	
7,55	C	8,5	C	C	8,5	8,5	8,5	Ampicillin
7,2	D	6,0	D	D	6,5	–	–	
5,0	E	5,1	E	E	5,1	5,1	5,1	Kanamycin?
4,0	F	4,2	F	F	–	4,2	–	
3,5	G	3,5	G	G	3,5	–	–	Streptomycin (2)
3,2	H	2,8	H	H	2,8	–	–	
2,7	I	1,85	I	I	1,85	–	–	Chloramphenicol (2)
1,79	J	1,70	J	J	–	1,70	–	Kanamycin?
		1,35	K	K	1,35	1,35	1,35	
1,10	K	1,3	L	L	1,3	–	–	Sulfonamid (2)
1,01	L	0,95	M	M	0,95	0,95	0,95	
		0,8		N	0,8	–	–	
0,75	M	0,6		O	–	0,6	–	Kanamycin?

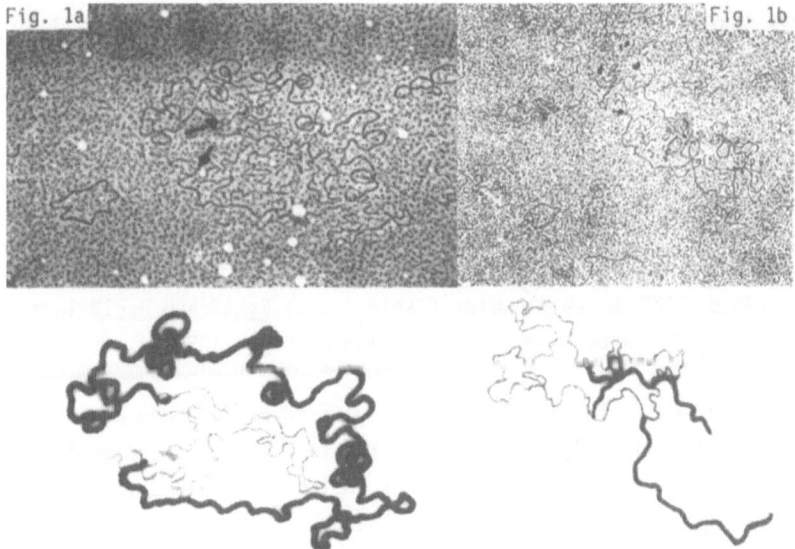

Fig. 1: Heteroduplexes of R1drd-16 with a) R100-1 and b) R1drd-19B2

not been seen in the previous heteroduplex map between R6-5 and R1 /1/ and
indicates that this segment is absent in the R1 factor used previously by
Sharp et al. /1/ for the heteroduplex analyses. The heteroduplex between
R1drd-19B2 and R1drd-16 (Fig. 1b) exhibits one ss-loop of 23 kb at the
R1drd-19B2 part which has the size found by Sharp et al. /1/ for the
R-determinant of R1 and a ss-loop of ~9 kb at the R1drd-16 part, which
appears to be the same as that observed in the R1drd-16/R6-5 heteroduplex
and may therefore be again attributed to the kanamycin resistance segment
of R1drd-16. We do not know at present whether these alterations of
R1drd-19B2 compared to R1drd-19 are responsible for the generation of the
mini-R1 plasmids (Rsc), which one frequently observes in strains carrying
R1drd-19B2, but not in strains carrying either R1drd-19 or R1drd-16. As a
consequence of the loss of the 9 kb segment carrying Km-resistance, the
ampicillin transposon Tn3 of R1 moves close to IS1, which separates the
r-determinant and the RTF unit of R1.

To date four different size classes of Rsc plasmids designated as Rsc10, 11,
12 and 13 have been isolated and transformed into E. coli C. There they
replicate as autonomous replicons rendering the transformants resistant to
high doses of ampicillin /4, 5/ indicating that they all contain the β-
lactamase gene. Their copy numbers in E. coli C are very high /4, 5/.
Heteroduplex analyses (performed in collaboration with E. Ohtsubo) of the
individual Rsc plasmids with the parental R1drd-19B2 plasmid and the
comparison of the restriction enzyme patterns pf Rsc plasmids and R1drd-19B2

indicate that they can be divided into two groups (Fig. 2). a) Rsc10 and Rsc11 représent circularized continuous sequences of the parental R1 factor extending from the end of the ampicillin transposon Tn3 to a site 20 kb apart in the case of Rsc10 and 12 kb in the case of Rsc11. These plasmids thus include the whole ampicillin transposon (Tn3) and 90 % and 30 %, respectively, of the EcoRI fragment which has been shown to carry the replication functions of R6-5 /6/. This fragment of R1 is identical to R6-5 according to the heteroduplex map of Sharp et al. /1/ and to the EcoRI fragments obtained with these plasmids (Table 1). b) Rsc13 and Rsc12 lack a segment between Tn3 and the replication region of R1drd-19B2.

The physical map of Rsc13 indicates that this plasmid arises spontaneously from Rsc11. The deletion may be triggered by the terminal sequence of Tn3. The deletion does not affect the structure of Tn3, since Tn3 can still be translocated from Rsc13 to other replicons. The generation of Rsc12, in contrast, is more complex. The comparison of the restriction maps of Rsc12 with Rsc11 or R1drd-19B2 (pKN102) readily shows that the orientation of Tn3 relative to the replication region is inverted. Therefore Rsc12 can not arise by a deletion from one of the continuous Rsc plasmids as Rsc13 does.

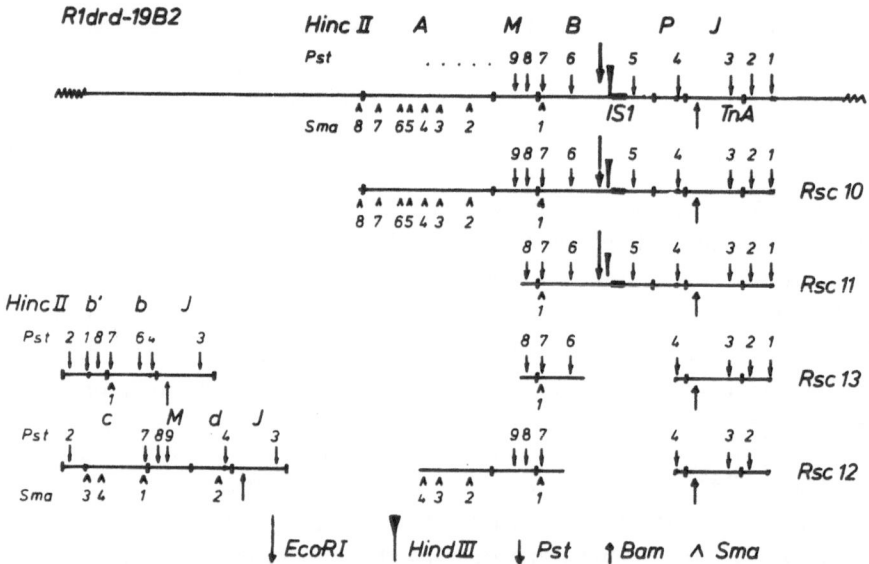

Fig.2:
Physical maps of Rsc10-13 plasmids and that part of the parental plasmid R1drd-19B2 from which the Rsc plasmids derive. The maps are drawn in a linear scale, indicating those parts of R1drd-19B2 with which the Rsc plasmids hybridise. On the left site of the figure the linear continuous maps of Rsc13 and Rsc12 are given.

Generation of Rsc12 and Rsc13

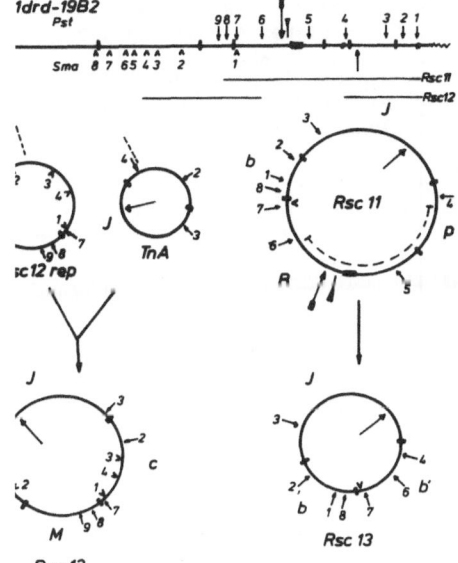

Fig.3:
Models for the generation of Rsc12 and Rsc13. Rsc13 derives from Rsc11 by a spontaneous deletion of a segment indicated by the dashed line in Rsc11. Rsc12 is assumed to be generated by transposition of Tn3 to a circularized autonomously replicating fragment of R1drd-19B2 including SmaI sites 1-4 (see uper line). The site of insertion of Tn3 into this fragment is given by the dashed line in Rsc12 rep.

physical map rather suggests that Rsc12 is generated by transposition of to a circularized autonomously replicating fragment of R1drd-19B2 (102) (Fig. 3). The site of insertion of Tn3 is between the two SmaI es of HincII-fragment M. It is interesting to notice that in Rsc12 the I-site 1 at the end of Tn3 is lost during this insertion, which indicates t this PstI site may be located very close to the terminal sequence of Tn3.

11 and Rsc10 are incompatible with R1drd-19. The segregation rate of rd-19 which always segregates from the corresponding pairs is rather fast, ecially for Rsc10/R1drd-19, as indicated in Fig. 4. Both plasmids are also ompatible with R1drd-19B2. However, in this case the segregation rate is h more slowly. Rsc13, in contrast, is by and large compatible with R1drd-19 R1drd-19B2. Even after more than 100 generations all clones analysed tain both plasmids, whereas no Rsc11/R1drd-19 or Rsc10/R1drd-19 clones, taining both plasmids, could be isolated after this period of growth. s indicates that the segment which is deleted in Rsc13 carries essential ction(s) for incompatibility.

previously shown Rsc11 can be used as a vector for insertion of EcoRI gments into the single EcoRI site of this plasmid /7/.The replication all composite elements tested, like Rsc11-pSC101, Rsc11-ColE1, Rsc11-

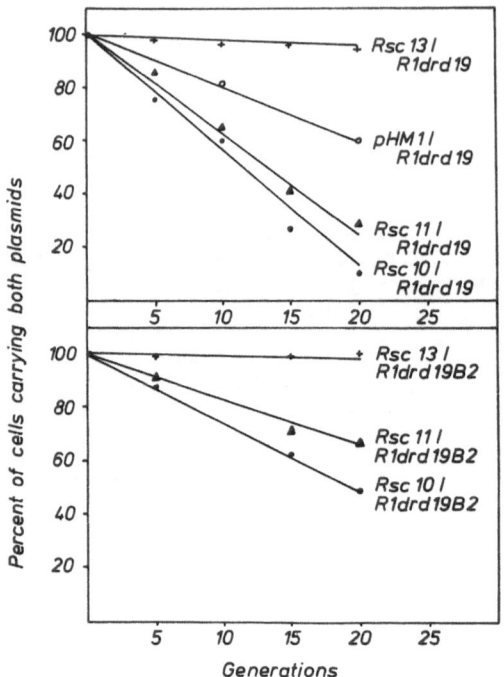

Fig.4:
Segregation rates of
R1drd-19 and R1drd-19B2
from clones containing the
indicated Rsc plasmids, or
Rsc-hybrid plasmids and
either R1drd-19 or R1drd-
19B2

Comparison of the physical maps of Rsc 11 and pWB5

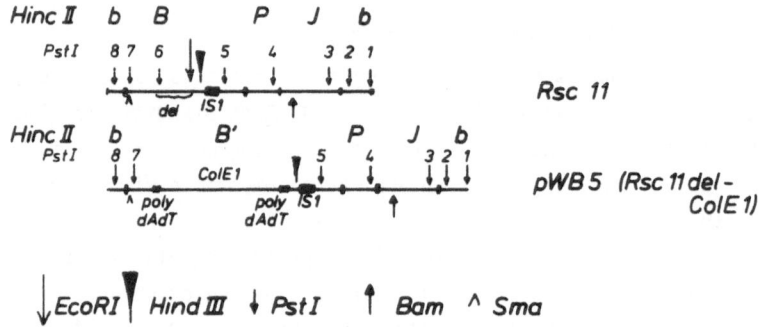

Fig.5:
Physical map of hybrid plasmid pWB5. The upper map represents Rsc11 and
shows the deletion introduced into this plasmid before joining it to ColE1
by the polydAdT linker method /5/, which results in the generation of pWB5

mini_Col_E1 comes under the control of the _Rsc_11-part, which is independent
of high levels of _pol_A1 and dependent on de novo protein synthesis. _Rsc_11
hybrid plasmids constructed by the _Eco_RI/ligase procedure are more compatible
with R1_drd_-19 and R1_drd_-19B2, suggesting that the insertion of the foreign
DNA regardless of whether it represents a replicating or a non-replicating
_Eco_RI-fragment, lowers the incompatibility with the parent plasmids R1_drd_-19
and R1_drd_-19B2. Since these plasmids are present in lower copy numbers than
the original _Rsc_11 plasmid /7/, it is difficult to decide whether the decreased incompatibility is due to the lower copy number of the _Rsc_-hybrids
or to a partial destruction of a function required for incompatibility by
the insertion into the _Eco_RI site of _Rsc_11. The latter possibility is more
likely since _Rsc_10 which is also present in _E. coli_ C in a lower copy number
than _Rsc_11, is still as incompatible with R1_drd_-19 as _Rsc_11.

Using the polydAdT linker method /8/ we could also construct _Col_E1 hybrids
which carry only parts of the _Rsc_11 plasmid. The varying _Rsc_11 parts were
generated by adding polydA on nicked _Rsc_11 with the aid of terminal transferase (TT). TT will add polyA on all single strand nicks, thus producing
tails which can then be linked to polydT-tailed _Col_E1. By selection for Ap^R,
Col^{imm} transformants we could isolate a variety of plasmids which have lost
more or less extended parts of the _Rsc_11 plasmid /9/. For the present
discussion concerned with replication and incompatibility, the hybrid plasmid
pWB5 is most interesting. This hybrid plasmid (Fig. 5) has lost a segment of
1.8 kb starting at the _Eco_RI site of _Rsc_11. The HindIII site is still retained.
It can no longer replicate under the control of _Rsc_11. This indicates that an
essential function of replication must be located 450 base pairs from the
_Pst_I site 6 which is dispensable for replication as indicated by the physical
map of _Rsc_12. This hybrid plasmid is also fully compatible with _Rsc_11.

To further characterise the minimal fragment required for autonomous replication of the Rsc plasmids and hence of the R1 factor the following procedure
was applied. A _Rsc_13-Km hybrid was constructed by in vitro joining of the
_Eco_RI Km-fragment of pML21 /10/ to $EcoRI^+$-cleaved _Rsc_13. The physical map of
_Rsc_13-Km (Fig. 6) shows that the Km fragments is inserted into the _Hinc_II-J-
fragment of the ampicillin transposon at a site 380 base pairs from the
BamI site which is located outside the β-lactamase-gene. The joining of these
two fragments creates a new _Eco_RI site (Fig. 6). This plasmid, which is a
suitable _Hind_III vector for cloning _Hind_III-fragments, was degraded by _Bam_I
and _Eco_RI to remove the 7 kb segment including the Km-fragment. The
remaining fragment carrying the replication region has non-complementary

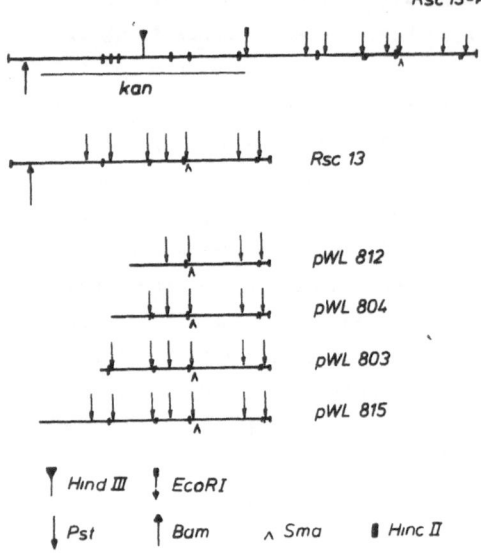

Fig.6:
Physical maps of
Rsc13-Km, Rsc13 and
of the miniRsc13
plasmids, pWL812,
pWL804, pWL803 and
pWL815. The con-
struction of Rsc13-Km
(pWL6) and the
generation of the
miniRsc13 plasmids
are described in the
text

termini. It was transformed in E. coli C and Ap^R-transformants were selected.
Plasmid DNA which was present in all of the obtained transformants were
mapped with HincII and PstI. The physical maps of these plasmids are shown
in Fig. 6. It is quite evident that even the smallest plasmid pWL812 contains
the segment of Rsc13 including the SmaI site a HincII site and the PstI sites
7 and 8. This structure is present in all Rsc plasmids. Since Pst-site 6 is
not present in Rsc12 it can not be located in a sequence required for autonomous replication. By subtracting the part which derives from Tn3 the segment of pWL812 which carries the rep function can have at the most a mass
of 1.2x10^6 dalton (about 1.8 kb). The incompatibility gene(s) is (are)
located outside of this segment, as indicated by the compatibility of pWL812
and Rsc13 with R1drd-19. As seen in Fig. 6 plasmid pWL812 which obviously
contains a replication unit of R1 is cleaved by PstI into four fragments of
1.6 kb, 1.2 kb, 0.6 kb and 0.55 kb. The origin of replication which has been
mapped by Ohtsubo (personal communication) is located on the largest PstI
fragment. The 1.6 kb fragment alone or the 1.6 kb together with the 0.55 kb
fragment may therefore be required for autonomous replication. These two
fragments were cloned with the recently developed plasmid vector pBR322
(Boyer et al., personal communication). Three different clones were obtained (Fig. 7). Clone I contains hybrid DNA (pRK101) with the large PstI
fragment inserted into pBR322 (Fig. 7d-f), whereas clone II carries a hybrid
plasmid (pRK102) with the small (0.55 kb) PstI fragment inserted into pBR322
(Fig. 7b). Clone III (Fig. 7c) contains a hybrid plasmid pRK103 with a PstI

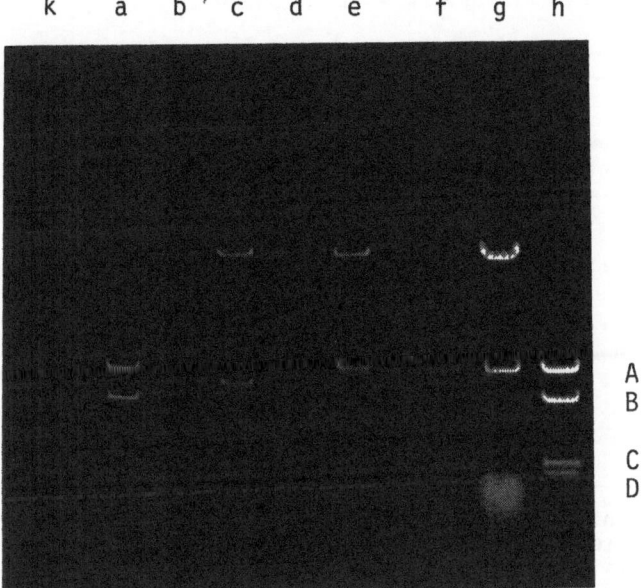

k   a   b   c   d   e   f   g   h

A
B
C
D

Fig.7:
Cloning of the two PstI fragments of the replication region of pWL812 by
pBR322. The miniRsc13 plasmid pWL812 was cut with PstI endonuclease and
ligated to pBR322 which was also linearised by PstI. After transformation
of the recombinant DNA in E. coli C, transformant colonies were selected
which were Tet^R, Ap^S. Plasmid DNA of such clones was isolated and cleaved
with PstI. a) and h) pWL812 cut with PstI. Note that the largest (A) and
the smallest PstI fragment (D) derive from the replication region of pWL812.
b) pRK102 (hybrid plasmid between pBR322 and the small PstI fragment) cut with
PstI, c) pRK103 (hybrid plasmid between pBR322 and the large PstI fragment
with a deletion in this fragment) cut with PstI, d-f) pRK101 (hybrid plasmid
between pBR322 and the large PstI fragment) cut with PstI, g) pRK101 after
extended growth in MM383 at 43 C, cut with PstI, k) pBR322 cut with PstI

fragment inserted into pBR322 which is smaller than PstI fragment A but
larger than PstI-B. Since this fragment has still the PstI termini it must
have a deletion in the PstI-A fragment. These hybrid plasmids were transferred into E. coli MM383 which carries the polA12 mutation causing a
temperature-sensitive DNA polymerase I. This strain is therefore not able
to replicate pBR322 (ColE1 replicon) at the restrictive temperature (43 C).
The capability of autonomous replication of a fragment inserted into pBR322
can therefore easily be detected by plating the transformants of MM383
carrying the hybrid pBR322 plasmids on tetracycline containing media at 43 C.
As shown in Table 2 pRK101 which contains the large PstI fragment forms
colonies at 43 C, but not pRK102 which contains only the small PstI fragment.
pRK103 can also not replicate at 43 C in MM383. This indicates that the
information carried by the large PstI fragment is sufficient for autonomous

TABLE 2   CAPABILITY OF REPLICATION OF HYBRID PLASMIDS PRK1 AND PRK2 IN A POLA12 MUTANT AT 43 C

PLASMID	GROWTH ON ENB PLATES CONTAINING 30 UG/ML TETRACYCLINE AT		GROWTH ON ENB PLATES CONTAINING MMS AT	
	30 C	43 C	30 C	43 C
pBR 322	+	-	+	-
pRK 101	+	+	+	-
pRK 102	+	-	+	-

Cultures with clones containing pRK101 or pRK102 were grown at 30 C and plated on media containing tetracyclin (30 µg/ml) which were incubated at 43 C. As control media containing methane methylsulfonate (MMS) at a concentration of 0.05 % were used. (+) indicates complete growth, (-)indicates normal growth

replication at least when covalently joined to the ColE1 replicon. Together with the results obtained with Rsc12 and pWB5 this suggests that the minimal fragment required for autonomous replication of R1 may not be larger than 1 kb. No colonies are formed by either of the two clones when plated at 43 C on nutrient agar containing methane methylsulfonate, which indicates that the DNA polymerase I is still temperature-sensitive in these strains.

Gene products of the Rsc plasmids can be expressed and analysed in minicells of E. coli P678-54 (Fig. 8 A). Rsc10 expresses 10 proteins, 3 of which (2, 6 and 9) are located outside of the sequence of Rsc11. Proteins 3, 4 and 5 must be located in or close by the segment which is deleted in Rsc13 since these proteins are missing in Rsc13. Insertion of a EcoRI fragment into Rsc11 abolishes protein 4 and alters slightly protein 5 (Fig. 8 B). This alteration could be responsible for the decreased incompatibility observed with this hybrid plasmid. The deletion of the 1.8 k base segment between the EcoRI site and PstI site 6 in pWB5 abolishes the capability of replication and in-compatibility and leads to the loss of proteins 4 and 5 (Fig. 8CC). These proteins must be therefore determined by this segment. Protein 5 may be involved in the incompatibility property. Protein 7 (β-lactamase) and possibly 3 minor proteins, 1', 4' and 6' (Fig. 9), having similar but not

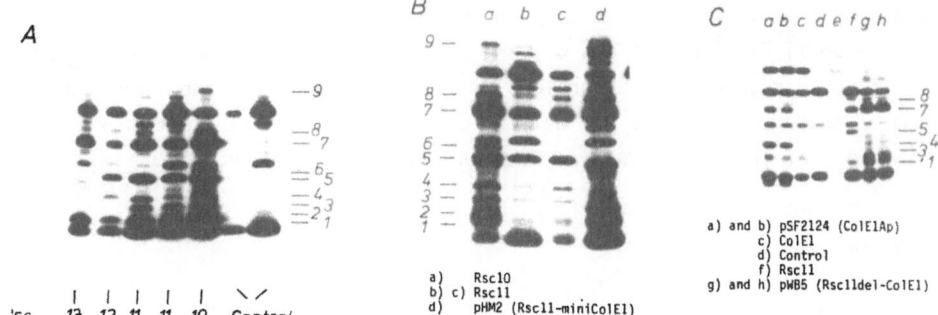

A

| | | | | | ʌ ⁄
'sc 13 12 11 11 10 Control

B a b c d

a) Rsc10
b) c) Rsc11
d) pHM2 (Rsc11-miniColE1)

C a b c d e f g h

a) and b) pSF2124 (ColE1Ap)
c) ColE1
d) Control
f) Rsc11
g) and h) pWB5 (Rsc11del-ColE1)

Fig. 8:
Radioautograms of SDS-polyacrylamid-gels of proteins expressed in mjni cells
of E. coli P678-54 containing the Rsc plasmids 10-13 (A), hybrid plasmid pHM2
(minicolE1-Rsc11)(B), and hybrid plasmid pWL5 (Rsc11del-ColE1) (C)

TABLE 3   PROTEINS OF RSC-PLASMIDS AND RSC11-HYBRID PLASMIDS EXPRESSED IN

MINICELLS OF E. COLI

PROTEINS	No	1	2	3	4	5	5'	6	7	8	9
	MW x 10⁻³	11.3	12.0	14.5	16.2	18.4		19.5	27.2	28.8	60
Rsc10		+	+	+	+	+	+	+	+	+	+
Rsc11		+	-	+	+	+	-	+	+	+	-
Rsc12		+	-	-	-	-	+	-	+	+	-
Rsc13		+	-	-	-	-	-	-	+	+	-
pHM2 (Rsc11-MINICOLE1)		+	-	+	(+)	V	-	-	+	+	-
pWB5 (Rsc11DEL-COLE1)		+	-	+	-	-	-	-	+	+	-

Table 3:
The molecular weights of the proteins expressed in mini cells containing the
various Rsc plasmids and the distribution of these proteins on the Rsc plasmids. (V) indicates, that this protein is altered in its migration rate in
the SDS-polyacrylamid-gel (see Fig. 6b). (+) indicates that only small
amounts of this protein are visible on the gel

identical molecular weights as proteins 1, 4 and 6, seem to be determined by
the ampicillin transposon (Tn3) as shown by comparing the gene products of
CoIE1, CoIE1Ap and Rsc11. The proteins 1 and 8, which are common to all Rsc

plasmids seem to be determined by the common 2,0 kb segment which is composed
of the small Pst fragment and of part of the large Pst-fragment the latter
of which is required for autonomous replication. Their functions are unknown.
One of these two proteins may well be determined by the replication region.
A summary of these results are given in Table 3 and Fig. 9.

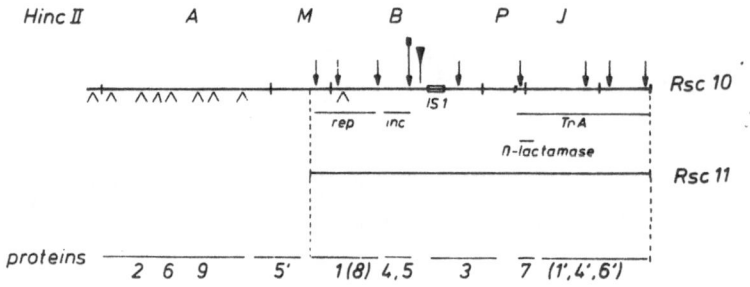

Fig.9:
Location of the genes determining the various proteins expressed by Rsc
plasmids in mini cells. The location of proteins in brackets is rather
preliminary

References

1. Sharp, O.A., Cohen, S.W., Davidson, N.: Electron Microscope Heteroduplex
   Studies of Sequence Relations among Plasmids of E. coli II. Structure
   of Drug Resistance (R)Factors and F.Factors. J. Mol. Biol. 75, 235-255
   (1973)

2. Tanaka, N., Cramer, H.J., Rownd, R.H.: EcoRI Restriction Endonuclease
   Map of the Composite R Plasmid NR1. J. Bacteriol. 127, 619-636 (1976)

3. Nordström, K., Ingram, L.C., Lundbäck, A.: Mutations in R-Factors of
   E. coli Causing an Increased Number of R-Factor Copies per Chromosome.
   J. Bacteriol. 110, 562-569 (1972)

4. Goebel, W. and Bonewald, R.: Class of Small Multicopy Plasmids Originating
   from the Mutant Antibiotic Resistance Factor R1drd-19B2. J. Bacteriol.
   123, 658-665 (1975)

5. Luibrand, G., Blohm, D., Mayer, H. and Goebel, W.: Characterization of
   Small Ampicillin Resistance Plasmids (Rsc) Originating from the Mutant
   Antibiotic Resistance Factor R1drd-19B2. Molec. gen. Genet. 152, 43-51
   (1977)

6. Timmis, K., Cabello, F., Cohen, S.N.: Cloning, Isolation and Characterization of Replication Regions of Complex Plasmid Genomes. Proc. Nat. Acad.
   Sci. USA, 72, 2242-2246 (1975)

7. Mayer, H., Luibrand, G., Goebel, W.: Replication of the Mini-R1 Plasmid Rsc11 and Rsc11 Hybrid Plasmids. Molec. gen. Genet. (in press)

8. Wensink, P.C., Finnegan, D.J., Donelson, J.E., Hogness, D.S.: A System for Mapping DNA Sequences in the Chromosomes of Drosophila melanogaster. Cell <u>3</u>, 315-325 (1975)

9. Boidol, W., Siewert, G., Lindenmaier, W., Luibrand, G., Goebel, W.: Properties of Hybrid Plasmids Consisting of Parts of the Mini-R1 Factor Rsc11 and ColE1. Molec. gen. Genet. (in press)

0. Hershfield, V., Boyer, H.W., Chow, L., Helinski, D.R.: Characterization of a Mini-ColE1 Plasmid. J. Bacteriol. <u>126</u>, 447-453 (1976)

Discussion

Davies: May I refer to your last slide (Fig. 9): where does protein 3 come from?

Goebel: This obviously comes from what is called TnS (or Tn3). The Kanamycin segment obviously starts at the end of TnS and goes to Is1.

Davies: But it does not overlap Is1?

Goebel: We don't know yet. We don't know whether the kanamycin segment has the properties of a transposon. Maybe it is just a deletion; but it would be a deletion which always starts at the end of TnS and reaches to Is1. Anyway, the protein 3 obviously comes from this area.

Starlinger: Could you comment on this extremely non-random distribution of restriction cleavage sites? You have a strong cluster of very closely spaced Pst sites on the right and you have a nearly equally strong cluster of Sma sites on the left. Has anybody else seen something like this?

Goebel: I have to confess that we have not mapped the Pst cleavage sites on the right side. I don't know why there are so many Sma cleavage sites on the other side, that certainly is a cluster.

Starlinger: The clustering is interesting; in the whole lambda phage there are only three or four Pst cuts. Another question: are you sure that there is no Pst cut in Is1? Because in the usual Is1 there is a Pst cut.

Goebel: It's quite possible that this is a typical Is1 and contains a Pst site.

Levy: Which of the proteins that are coded for by miniplasmid in minicells are also seen as products of large parental plasmids from which the miniplasmid has been derived?

Goebel: We have not checked this.

Levy: I am particularly interested in protein 1 and whether it is a membrane protein or not.

Goebel:It does not seem to be a membrane protein. We have checked this point and we see a good part of the protein 1 in the cytoplasm.

Levy: What was the molecular weight of protein 1?

Goebel: 12.000 daltons.

Richmond: Just an informational point: are those 4 Pst sites in TnA?

Goebel: There are only 3.

Richmond: But they are all within TnA, are they not?

Goebel: It may be interesting to notice one thing: when one examines plasmid Rsc 12 which obviously is derived from the second step of transposition to a replicating fragment, it uses the last Pst site. So it seems to be very close to one of the ends and during tranposition it may be lost.

Richmond: As you realise, not all TnAs are the same. The one we work with makes the TEM II enzyme and is supposedly derived from RP 1. I think all this is adding up to the fact that there is a much greater variety of TnA than people readily admitted.

Levy: I thought that the term TnA was reserved for a particular ampicillin determinant from a particular plasmid.

Richmond: That's the trouble. You are right, but people don't use it that way.

Bennett: It tends to be used very loosely.

Drews: Since you have such an extremely high copy number of TnA genes, does the ampicillin resistance rise accordingly?

Goebel: There is resistance to saturating levels of ampicillin.

Falkow: The minimum length of a self-replicating unit in your experiments was around 1 million?

Goebel: Around 700 000.

Falkow: I don't want to get into any contest, but is there any-one who has obtained something smaller? The smallest self-repli-cating piece isolated by Boyer from Co1E1 was about 600 000. That does not mean that this is essentially all what is re-quired for autonomous replication.

e Molecular Nature of R-Factors in Different Bacterial Hosts

G. O. Humphreys[1]

Introduction

etic and molecular studies of R-factors have led to the definition of
 classes of plasmid transfer systems (3,4,19,23,36,40). The resistance
d/or colicin) determinant(s) and transfer factor of Class 1 transfer
tems are covalently linked, and are transferred to new hosts as a single
kage group. The R-factor T-Δ^2 and the colicinogenic factor ColIb-P9 are
mples of Class 1 transfer systems (2,3,23). In Class 2 systems, the
nsfer factor and non-autotransferring resistance (or colicin) determin-
(s) are independent replicons, which can be transferred separately to
ipient cells, and which rarely recombine. The resistance determinant
 and transfer factor Δ form a Class 2 transfer system (2,3,·23).

 physical properties of the F-like R-factors NR1, R1 and R6 have been
ensively studied, mainly in _Proteus mirabilis_ and _Escherichia coli_ K12
12) hosts (12,13,15,27.29,31,32,35). The chromosomal DNA of _P.mirabilis_
 a guanine plus cytosine content of 40% which is sufficiently different
m the base composition of many R-factors to permit physical separation
host and plasmid DNA by centrifugation in a caesium chloride density
dient. When isolated· from _P.mirabilis_, the DNA of NR1, R1 or R6 consists
three molecular species. In the case of NR1 the molecular weights of
se species are approximately 14×10^6, 49×10^6 and 63×10^6·(32). It
 been concluded that in _P. mirabilis_, the largest species represents the
plete R-factor (63×10^6) and it can dissociate into two components

---

[1] The work described in this paper was carried out in the laboratory
of Prof. E.S. Anderson, at the Central Public Health Laboratory,
Colindale, London, in collaboration with Drs. G.A. Willshaw and
H.R. Smith.

[2] Symbols for drug resistances: A, ampicillin; C, chloramphenicol;
K, kanamycin; S, streptomycin; Su, sulphonamides; T, tetracycline.

corresponding to the transfer factor (49×10^6) and the region coding for the drug resistances CSSu, termed the r-determinant (14×10^6). Throughout the present paper this process will be referred to as dissociation. When P.mirabilis carrying NR1 is grown in the presence of any of the antibiotics to which the r-determinant gives resistance, there is an amplification of the r-determinant plasmid species, generating complex poly-r-determinants or poly-r-determinants linked to the transfer factor (see 32). This process, which is reversible on removal of the cells to drug-free medium has been termed "transition".

When R-factors such as NR1, R1 and R6 were first isolated from E.coli K12 they were generally found to exist as a single molecular species corresponding to the complete R-factors. However, detailed electron microscopy of the DNA of R1 isolated from K12 cells grown in the presence of chloramphenicol revealed that 3-6% of the molecules observed had a molecular weight of 10×10^6 and the others were 65×10^6 (12,13). More recently it has been observed that the F-like R-factor R100 (probably identical to NR1), dissociates in a minicell-producing strain of Salmonella typhimurium (34). These studies were complicated by the presence in the parent strain of two cryptic plasmids.

This paper describes the genetic and molecular properties of R factors in E.coli K12 and S.typhimurium phage-type 36; several of the R factors exist as single molecular species of DNA in K12 but dissociate into two or more molecules in S.typhimurium in a way that is superficially similar to the dissociation of R1, R6 and NR1 in P.mirabilis.

Methods

The bacterial strains and plasmids used in this study are listed in tables 1 and 2. The media used and the methods employed for conjugation, extraction of plasmid DNA, transformation and electron microscopy experiments have been described previously (1,2,17,18,24,25).

Chloramphenicol acetyl transferase was assayed as described by Foster and Shaw (16). Streptomycin adenylate synthetase by the procedure of Benveniste et al. (9) and beta-lactamase by the microacidimetric method of Saz et al. (33).

Table 1. List of strains

Enteric Reference Laboratory No.	Other designations	Description and relevant markers	Source (reference)
1R 713	K12-703	E.coli K12 prototrophic	W. Hayes (18)
14R 525	-	1R713 Nal^r	E.R.L. (18)
34R 99	-	S.typhimurium phage type 36: plasmid - free	E.R.L. (38)
42R 700	JC 7623	E.coli K12 recB$^-$ recC$^-$ sbcB	M.Oishi (14)
42R 000	C600 str^r	E.coli K12 Str^r	B. Bachman

Table 2. List of plasmids

Plasmid No.	Compatibility group	Resistances and other markers	Molecular Weight (x10^{-6})	Strain from which isolated	References
R1-19K$^-$	F$_{II}$	ACSSu	54.2	S.paratyphi	17,18
TP 129	F$_{IV}$	T	77.6	S.typhimurium	-
T-Δ	I$_1$	T	65.4	S.typhimurium	2,3,17,18
TP 110	I$_1$	KColIb	64.8	S.typhimurium	17,18
TP 114	I$_2$	K	40.8	E.coli	17,18
TP 113	B	K	56.7	S.typhimurium	17,18
TP 125	B	CSSuT	64.0	Shigella dysenteriae	17,18
TP 123	H	CSSuT	123.2	S.typhi	17,18

Results

Dissociation of Plasmids in S.typhimurium

The genetic and molecular properties of F-like R-factors have been extensively studied in E.coli K12 and P.mirabilis and to a lesser extent in S.
typhimurium hosts, but there is little information on the molecular properties of R-factors belonging to other compatibility groups in these strains.
R-factors specifying a range of antibiotic resistances and belonging to six

compatibility groups (table 2), were transferred to plasmid-free strains of E.coli K12 (1R713) and S.typhimurium phage type 36 (34R99). Plasmid DNA was extracted from these strains and examined by electron microscopy; plasmid molecules on electron microscope grids were counted to estimate the relative proportions of the DNA species of different sizes. Both open circular and supercoiled molecules were included.

The plasmids R1-19K[-], TP125 and TP123, belonging to compatibility groups F_{II}, B and H respectively, are present in E.coli K12 almost exclusively as single molecular species (see figure 1). We have not found any small circles present in several DNA preparations of the plasmids TP125 or TP123 when extracted from the strains 1R713 or 42R800. However, a large proportion of the DNA of each of these plasmids is recovered from S.typhimurium as a small circular species, 7-8μm in length. So far, we have only observed dissociation of this nature with plasmids coding for resistance to at least the three antibiotics chloramphenicol, streptomycin and sulphonamides. The plasmids TP129, T-Δ, TP110, TP114 and TP113 were not found to dissociate at all in S.typhimurium or E.coli hosts.

Watanabe and Ogata (41) observed that the drug resistance markers of fi[+] R-factors were stably maintained in E.coli K12, but some were easily lost in S.typhimurium LT2. Thus, chloramphenicol (C), streptomycin (S) and Sulphonamide (Su) resistances were lost together at a high frequency while the tetracycline (T) marker was retained. Our observed dissociation of plasmids coding for CSSuT resistances suggested a reason for such loss of markers. We examined the loss of drug resistance markers from E.coli and S.typhimurium carrying the plasmid TP125 (see figure 2). The T resistance marker of TP125 is lost at a similar frequency to the marker for C. The rate of joint loss of T and C is less than that for the loss of either alone. The segregants were tested for retention of transfer functions. All the (CSSu)[+]T[-] and (CSSu)[-]T[+] segregants were still auto-transferring. The transferring behaviour of (CSSu)[-]T[-] segregants was tested by the triparental-cross method(1); the non auto-transferring plasmid in the intermediate strain was NTP2 (SSu) and mobilisation of this determinant to a nalidixic acid resistant final recipient was measured. Approximately 50% of the (CSSu)[-]T[-] segregants mobilised the plasmid NTP2. Thus, it appears that all the markers can be lost without loss of the transmissibility of the plasmid remaining in the strain. We have not observed any independent loss of C, S or Su resistances: they were always lost as a group.

To determine if we could correlate spontaneous loss of resistances with loss of any species of DNA, spontaneous segregants of the plasmid TP125

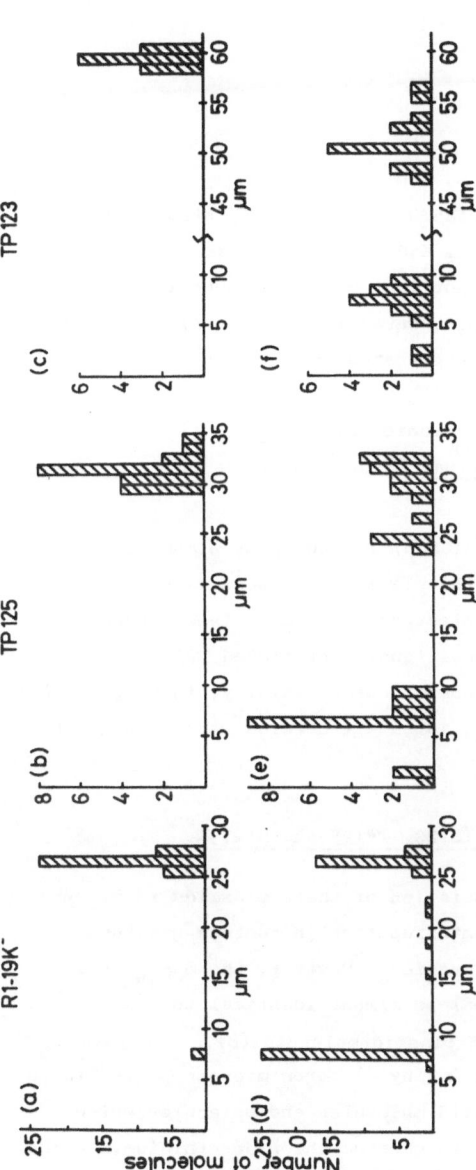

Fig. 1. Contour lengths of the circular DNA molecules observed in electron microscope preparations of the plasmids R1-19K⁻, TP125 and TP123. The DNA was prepared from both E. coli K12 and S. typhimurium strains carrying each plasmid:

a) R1-19K⁻ in K12 (152 large, 1 small); b) TP125 in K12 (150 large, 0 small); c) TP123 in K12 (132 large, 0 small);

d) R1-19K⁻ in S. typhimurium; e) TP125 in S. typhimurium; f) TP123 in S. typhimurium

(62 large, 140 small)   (30 large, 100 small)   (53 large, 105 small)

Numbers in parentheses represent total numbers of molecules of the different sizes counted, both OC and CCC forms included: large ≡ > 20 μm long; small ≡ < 10 μm long.

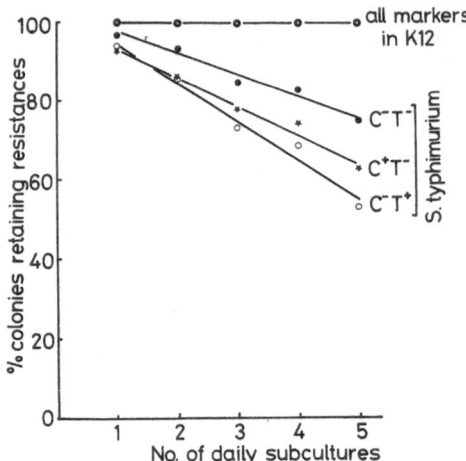

Fig. 2. Drug-sensitive segregants of TP125. Freshly cloned strains of
S. typhimurium type 36 or E. coli K12 (42R800) carrying TP125 were
grown in stationary culture in nutrient broth and subcultured daily.
At the time of subculture, samples were plated on nutrient medium
and the colonies obtained were replicated onto plates containing
chloramphenicol or tetracycline.

⊛ All markers in K12; ◯ C^-T^+ colonies of S. typhimurium;
✸ C^+T^- colonies of S. typhimurium; ⬤ C^-T^- colonies of S. typhimurium.

were isolated. $(CSSu)^+T^+$, $(CSSu)^-T^+$ and $(CSSu)^+T^-$ segregant plasmids were
transferred into S.typhimurium 36, and the plasmid DNA species isolated
from these strains was examined in the electron microscope (see figure 3).
The data show that loss of the (CSSu) resistances correlated with complete
loss of the 7μm DNA species. We have looked, unsuccessfully, in preparations
of $(CSSu)^-$ TP125 DNA from S.typhimurium, for small circles representing the
T resistance region.

The Extent of Dissociation of TP123, TP125 and R1-19K$^-$

We have attempted to quantify the dissociation of these plasmids in S.typh-
imurium in several ways. Initially, centrifugation in sucrose gradients
was employed to separate the different species. However, the $S_{20,w}$ values
of the CCC form of the 7μm molecule (38S) is almost identical to that of the
open circular form of the complete TP125 plasmid molecule (8). The method of
counting different molecular species of DNA by electron microscopy is biased
by the preferential loss of larger plasmid molecules and molecules which
are present in relaxation complex form, in caesium chloride-ethidium bromide

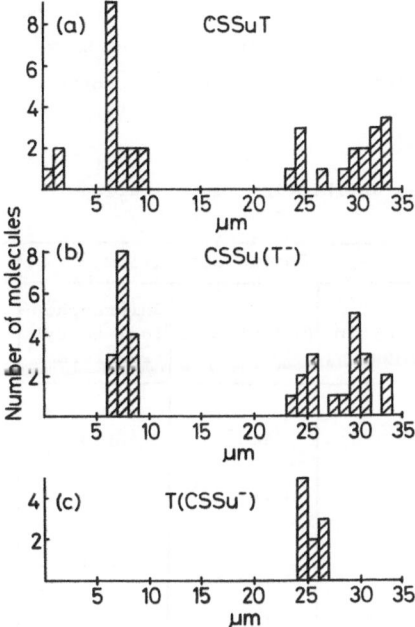

Fig. 3. Contour lengths of circular DNA molecules in electron micrographs of preparations of the parent plasmid TP125 and drug sensitive segregants. All were prepared from S. typhimurium type 36. a) Parent R-factor (30 large, 100 small); b) Tetracycline sensitive segregant (45 large, 100 small); c) Segregant sensitive to chloramphenicol, streptomycin and sulphonamide (151 large, 0 small).

density gradients. We have repeatedly found a greater loss of large plasmids when their DNA is prepared from S.typhimurium as opposed to E.coli hosts. This may be due to a greater proportion of plasmid molecules being in "relaxation complex" forms (10) in S.typhimurium (Humphreys G.O., Willshaw G.A. and Anderson E.S., unpublished observations).

Several workers have shown that there is a direct relationship between the expression of resistance genes of plasmids and their copy number in the bacterial cell (see 20,28,39). Furthermore, growth of Proteus mirabilis strains carrying NR2 in the presence of antibiotics leads to an amplification of the resistance genes (r-determinant) of the plasmid (see 32). We assayed the level of antibiotic-inactivating enzymes in exponentially-growing cultures of S.typhimurium and E.coli carrying R1-19K⁻, grown with or without antibiotics. The results are shown in table 3. There was very little change in the enzyme activities under these conditions. When extracts were prepared

from cultures in stationary phase and after prolonged growth in the presence
of the antibiotics there were slight increases in activity but never more
than 2-fold compared with control cultures grown in the absence of antibiotics.

Table 3. Activities of R1-19K⁻ plasmid-coded antibiotic - inactivating
enzymes[1]

Host strain	Additions to M9 minimal medium + glucose	Enzyme activities		
		Streptomycin adenylase	β- lactamase	Chloramphen-icol acetyl transferase
E.coli K12-C600	None	100^2	100	100
	100µg/ml penicillin G	163	151	143
	100µg/ml chloramphenicol	76	121	108
	100µg/ml streptomycin	151	193	162
S.typhimurium type 36	None	100	100	100
	100µg/ml penicillin G	127	64	154
	100µg/ml chloramphenicol	109	101	133
	100µg/ml streptomycin	136	77	166

[1] The enzyme activities were measured on sonicated extracts of cells
grown to late exponential growth phase.

[2] The activities are expressed as percentages of the activity of
extracts prepared from cells grown in the absence of antibiotics
(=100%).

Properties of TP125 in recombination-deficient strains of E.coli K12

While investigating transformation of E.coli K12 with plasmid DNA, we introduced DNA of R1-19K⁻ into strain JC7623 which has mutations in the recombination genes recB⁻ recC⁻ sbcB⁻. Plasmid DNA isolated from the transformed
bacteria included a significant number of molecules of length 7-8µm.

Extraction and examination of DNA of the plasmids TP125 and TP123 from
JC7623 also showed 7-8µm molecules. These molecules were present whether

Table 4. Dissociation of TP125 in host strains bearing mutations affecting recombination-proficiency

Strain No.[1]	recA	recB	recC	sbcA	sbcB	end	large	small
HF 4733	+[3]	+	+	+	+	-	95	0
JC 4588	-	+	+	+	+	-	101	0
JC 4586	+	-	+	+	+	-	104	0
JC 4585	+	+	-	+	+	-	104	0
SDB 1311	+	+	+	-	+	-	100	0
JC 5174	+	-	+	-	+	-	101	4
JC 5176	+	-	-	-	+	-	112	2
AB 1157	+	+	+	+	+	+	90	6
MO 609	+	+	+	+	+	-	110	0
MO 627	+	+	+	+	-	+	109	9
JC 7623	+	-	-	+	-	+	99	45
MO 675	+	-	-	+	-	-	91	14

The "Relevant genetic markers" columns span recA–end; "Molecular species present (Nos)[2]" spans large and small.

[1] All host strains are E. coli K12 F⁻. HF 4733 was the parent of the first 7 isogenic strains listed and they were kindly provided by Dr. S.D. Barbour. The remaining strains were derived from AB 1157 and were the gift of Dr. M. Oishi. Their derivation and additional properties are described in refs. 6,7,14 and 21.

[2] The molecules were counted in random fields viewed in the electron microscope. Molecules in the 'large' category include the complete R-factor and molecules containing the RTF. 'Small' molecules included mainly molecules of the r-determinant region (7μm). Both OC and CCC molecules were included in the counts.

[3] + indicates wild-type allele and - mutant allele.

the plasmids were introduced into the strain by conjugation or transformation. In this strain (JC 7623), recombination is thought to occur by the recF pathway (21), and it seemed possible that the pathway of recombination operative in a strain of E.coli might affect the physical state of the plasmids carried by it. The molecular nature of the plasmid TP125, which we have never observed to dissociate in standard, recombination-proficient strains of E.coli K12 was examined in a range of strains carrying mutations in their rec genes. The results of an electron microscope study of the DNA isolated from the various rec strains are shown in table 4, and are considered further in the discussion. All circular (OC and CCC) molecules seen on the grids were counted.

Attempts to Isolate the CSSu DNA Species of TP125

The observation that more than 50% of the CCC DNA in a cleared lysate of S.typhimurium carrying TP125 consists of CSSu (7μm) DNA led us to attempt to isolate this DNA species to determine whether it could survive on re-introduction into an E.coli strain by transformation.

We isolated a large quantity of DNA from a cleared lysate of S.typhimurium by the PEG precipitation method (24). 60% of the DNA molecules were 7μm long. We used this DNA to transform strains of JC7623 carrying the plasmids (CSSu)⁻TP125, (CSSu)⁻TP123, (CSSu)⁻R1-19K⁻, TP113 or no plasmid at all. 10μg DNA was used in transformation mixtures containing 10^{10} bacteria in a volume of 0.5 ml. In no case did we find any transformants which had received the CSSu genes. The concentration of intact TP125 molecules was probably too low to give transformants of the complete plasmid. However, transformation by smaller molecules such as the 7μm CSSu species is 10-100 fold more efficient and should have been detectable. The recipient bacteria were shown to be competent by transforming them with NTP3 (M.Wt.8.1x10^6) and TP125 (M.Wt.64x10^6) plasmid DNA at appropriate concentrations.

Discussion

The results presented show that the DNA of the plasmids R1-19K⁻, TP125 and TP123 dissociates in S.typhimurium phage-type 36, whereas the plasmids TP129, T-Δ, TP110, TP113 and TP114 are found as one DNA species in this strain of S.typhimurium. The plasmids which dissociate all produce a DNA species approximately 7μm in length and another species corresponding to the difference in length between the whole plasmid and this 7μm molecule. In the case of TP123, we did not find molecules corresponding to the complete R factor in plasmid DNA preparations from S.typhimurium. All three lengths of molecule were always found in the preparations of plasmid DNA (except in the case of TP123) but we cannot tell if all forms co-exist within each cell or whether some cells contain only dissociated molecules. Previous molecular studies on plasmids which dissociate in different hosts have been confined to F-like plasmids, and in this study we have shown that other plasmids (TP125, compatibility group B and TP123, compatibility group H) can also dissociate in S.typhimurium and some E.coli strains. The genes of TP125 which code for resistance to chloramphenicol, streptomycin and sulphonamides (CSSu) are located on the 7μm circle of DNA which is therefore analogous to the r-determinant region of the F-like plasmids previously studied (13,15,27, 32). This was proved by studying the DNA species present in S.typhimurium carrying spontaneously mutant plasmids lacking some of the resistance markers, and there was correlation of lack of the 7μm DNA species with loss of CSSu resistances.

We have attempted to quantify the dissociation of the plasmid TP125 by various methods. Every method employed had its problems and we failed to arrive at a reliable estimate of the extent of dissociation. The recently described method of Falkow and co-workers (26) for analysing plasmid DNA species by agarose gel electrophoresis should give unambiguous results as it should separate the species of DNA of different molecular weights. However, the results of enzyme assays of extracts of S.typhimurium carrying R1-19K⁻ suggest that there is little detectable amplification of the CSSu genes in this host, whether grown in the presence or absence of antibiotics. This result is in contrast to those of Rownd and co-workers, studying the plasmid NR1 in Proteus mirabilis (see 32), where they have shown that in the presence of antibiotics the plasmid DNA population shifts from the basic plasmid to consist of molecules which have multiple copies of the r-determinant either independent of the transfer factor or linked to a single copy of it. A model to explain this amplification in molecular terms has been proposed (30).

Another manifestation of the plasmid dissociation is the occurrence of spontaneous drug-sensitive segregants of plasmids which arise, and the increased frequency of such segregants in S.typhimurium (fig.2). Assuming that the distribution of the transfer factor region of the plasmid is closely regulated at cell division, the production of segregant clones reflects the fact that the transfer factor replicon was dissociated from its r-determinant region at cell division. In this context, it has not been directly shown in S.typhimurium or E.coli that the r-determinant can replicate autonomously. Figure 2 shows that the rate of loss of (CSSu) resistances from TP125 in S.typhimurium is constant per subculture, and 40-50% of the culture had lost these resistances after 5 subcultures in antibiotic-free nutrient broth. The tetracycline resistance is lost at about the same frequency as (CSSu). As expected, the rate of joint loss of T and (CSSu) markers was less than either alone, but was still significant. Approximately 50% of these segregants with no resistances still carried their transfer genes.

The foregoing results demonstrate that even between closely related bacteria
such as E.coli and S.typhimurium there are host factors which can affect
the structures of plasmids. The finding that R1-19K also dissociates to
a significant extent in E.coli JC7623, a strain with mutations in genes
affecting recombination, led us to explore the behaviour of TP125 in a range
of different strains defective in their recombination genes, (table 4).
TP125 was chosen for this experiment as we have never observed small circles
of DNA (7μm) when this plasmid is extracted from wild-type K12 strains. It
was unfortunate that the lines carrying the rec mutations belonged to two
series of mutants which are derived from different parent K12 strains (6,7,
14,21). The dissociation was most marked in strains which carried the gene
for endonuclease I. However, there was a further influence on dissociation,
and strain JC7623, in which the rec F, pathway is believed to be responsible
for recombination, shows the most dissociation. When the endonuclease I
gene is absent, this dissociation is however reduced. Further studies with
a series of recombination-defective strains derived from the same parent
strain would be interesting and would clarify whether host recombination
functions are involved in dissociation.

All our attempts to introduce the (CSSu) fragment alone into E.coli (by
transfer or transformation) and S.typhimurium (by transfer) were unsuccessful. Similar findings have been obtained by other workers (Chandler M.,
Silver, L., Frey J. and Caro L., personal communication). These workers
showed that on integrative suppression of an E.coli dnaA strain by the plasmid R100-1, a small plasmid species corresponding to the r-determinant
region of the plasmid was located in the cytoplasm. This enabled the purification of this species free from other DNA. However, it was not possible
to introduce this molecule stably into K12 by transformation, whether or
not there was a resident transfer factor in the strain.

Further General Comments on Plasmid Dissociation in Different Hosts

Dissociation and/or amplification of resistance genes of plasmids has now
been observed in several species of bacteria including Proteus mirabilis,
Salmonella typhimurium, Escherichia coli and Streptococcus faecalis (31,32,
13,12,34,42). The phenomenon is influenced in both Proteus and Streptococcus
species by the presence of appropriate antibiotics, but this has not been
shown in E.coli or S.typhimurium.   The plasmid dissociation takes place in
a reproducible, site-specific way, and the dissociating r-determinants are
flanked by insertion sequences (22,30). We have not shown the presence of
insertion sequences in TP123 or TP125 but it seems likely that these plasmids do have insertion sequences flanking the resistance genes. Transpos-

ition of resistance genes from one replicon to another has recently been
shown to be an important factor in the evolution of resistance plasmids
(see 11), and transposable genes (transposons) are bounded by repeated homologous sequences. However, there has not yet been a demonstration of the
free existence of transposons in the cytoplasm. The dissociation of the
CSSu segment of plasmids differs therefore in this respect from resistance
gene transposition in that the r-determinant has an apparently stable cytoplasmic existence. Moreover, we have been unable to transpose the CSSu
resistances to any compatible plasmid present in the same cell (results not
shown) or to pick up the genes on any transfer factor present in cells transformed with DNA of the r-determinant.

The enzymatic mechanism of dissociation or transposition of genes is so far
unknown. We have shown that plasmids belonging to different compatibility
groups, and coding for resistance to CSSu can dissociate. Plasmids from
groups B and H share very little sequence homology (18) and it is likely
that any homology between TP123 and TP125 is in the r-determinant region
(Humphreys G.O., G.A. Willshaw and E.S. Anderson, unpublished observations).
It is probable that there are gene products coded by the r-determinant region
which are involved in dissociation. The fact that the same plasmid can
dissociate to different extents in different hosts also implies that the
activity of any such plasmid-coded gene products are influenced by cellular
factors. Thus characterisation of a plasmid in one standard host does not
necessarily allow one to predict how this plasmid will behave in other, even
closely-related bacterial species.

Summary

R-factors belonging to several different plasmid compatibility groups were
transferred to plasmid-free E. coli K12 and S. typhimurium hosts. The DNA
of each plasmid was prepared from the strains and the molecular species
that were present were examined by electron microscopy. The plasmids TP129
(compatibility group F_{IV}), T-Δ and TP110 (group I_1), TP114 (group I_2) and
TP113 (group B) were each isolated from both hosts as single DNA species.
In contrast R1 (group F_{II}), TP123 (group H) and TP125 (group B) which were
present in 'wild-type' E. coli K12 as single DNA species, were found in
S. typhimurium to form two DNA molecules in addition to the parent plasmid
molecule. These dissociated species correspond to the transfer factor plus
tetracycline resistance marker and an r-determinant species (7-8 μm in length).
The r-determinant of TP125 was shown to code for resistance to chloramphenicol,
streptomycin and sulphonamides.

We examined the behaviour of TP125 in S. typhimurium and in various strains of E. coli K12 deficient in DNA recombination. Dissociation was most marked in S. typhimurium but was also appreciable in a strain of E. coli in which recombination is believed to take place by the rec F pathway. However, other nucleases in the cell also appear to affect the process.

From our results and those of other workers it is apparent that the same plasmid can behave differently when present in even closely-related bacterial species. Plasmid dissociation must in part be determined by plasmid genes, in this case, genes on the r-determinant DNA species. However, the activity of such genes must be subject to some control by host-determined conditions and the study of plasmids in different bacterial species may be important to our understanding of the distribution of plasmids and resistance genes in natural systems.

References

1. Anderson, E.S: A rapid screening test for transfer factors in drug-sensitive Salmonella typhimurium. Nature (London) 208, 1016-1017 (1965).

2. Anderson, E.S. and M.J. Lewis: Drug resistance and its transfer in Salmonella typhimurium. Nature (London) 206, 579-583 (1965).

3. Anderson, E.S. and N. Natkin: Transduction of resistance determinants and R factors of the Δ transfer systems by phage P1kc. Molec. gen. Genet. 114, 261-265 (1972).

4. Anderson, E.S. and E.J. Threlfall: Change of host range in a resistance factor. Genet. Res. (Camb.) 16, 207-214 (1970).

5. Anderson, E.S. and H.R. Smith: Fertility inhibition in strains of Salmonella typhimurium. Molec. Gen. Genet. 118, 79-84 (1972).

6. Barbour, S.D. and A.J. Clark: Biochemical and genetic studies of recombination proficiency in E. coli. I. Enzymatic activity associated with rec B[+] and rec C[+] genes. Proc. Natl. Acad. Sci. U.S.A. 65, 955-961 (1970).

7. Barbour, S.D., H. Nagaishi, A. Templin and A.J. Clark: Biochemical and genetic studies of recombination proficiency in E. coli. II. Rec[+] revertants caused by indirect suppression of Rec[-] mutations. Proc. Natl. Acad. Sci. U.S.A. 67, 128-135 (1970).

8. Bazaral, M. and D.R. Helinski: Characterisation of multiple circular DNA forms of colicinogenic factor E1 from Proteus mirabilis. Biochemistry 7, 3513-3520 (1968).

9. Benveniste, R., T. Yamada and J. Davies: Enzymatic adenylylation of streptomycin and spectinomycin resistance. Infection and Immunity 1, 109-119 (1970).

10. Clewell, D.B. and D.R. Helinski: Supercoiled circular DNA-protein complex in Escherichia coli: purification and induced conversion to an open-circular DNA form. Proc. Natl. Acad. Sci. U.S.A. 62, 1159-1166 (1969).

11. Cohen, S.N.: Transposable genetic elements and plasmid evolution. Nature (London) 263, 731-738 (1976).

12. Cohen, S.N. and C.A. Miller: Multiple molecular species of circular R-factor DNA isolated from Escherichia coli. Nature (London) 224, 1273-1277 (1969).

13. Cohen, S.N. and C.A. Miller: Non-chromosomal antibiotic resistance in bacteria. II. Molecular nature of R-factors isolated from P. mirabilis and E. coli. J. Mol. Biol. 50, 671-687 (1970).

14. Cosloy, S.D. and M. Oishi: Genetic transformation in Escherichia coli K12. Proc. Natl. Acad. Sci. U.S.A. 70, 84-87 (1973).

15. Falkow, S., R.V. Citarella, J.A. Wohlheiter and T. Watanabe: The molecular nature of R-factors. J. Mol. Biol. 17, 102-116 (1966).

16. Foster, T.J. and W.V. Shaw: Chloramphenicol acetyltransferases specified by fi⁻ R-factors. Antimicrob. Ag. Chemother. 3, 99-104 (1973).

17. Grindley, N.D.F., J.N. Grindley and E.S. Anderson: R-factor compatibility groups. Molec. Gen. Genet. 119, 287-297 (1972).

18. Grindley, N.D.F., G.O. Humphreys and E.S. Anderson: Molecular studies of R-factor compatibility groups. J. Bacteriol. 115, 387-398 (1973).

19. Guerry, P.,J. Van Embden and S. Falkow: Molecular nature of two non-conjugative plasmids carrying drug resistance genes. J. Bacteriol. 117, 619-630 (1974).

20. Hashimoto, H. and R.H. Rownd: Transition of the R factor NR1 in Proteus mirabilis: Level of drug resistance of non-transitioned and transitioned cells. J. Bacteriol. 123, 56-68 (1975).

21. Horii, Z. and A.J. Clark: Genetic analysis of the Rec F pathway to genetic recombination in Escherichia coli K12: isolation and characterization of mutants. J. Mol. Biol. 80, 327-344 (1973).

22. Hu, S., E. Ohtsubo, N. Davidson and H. Saedler: Electron microscope heteroduplex studies of sequence relations among bacterial plasmids: identification and mapping of the insertion sequences IS1 and IS2 in F and R plasmids. J. Bacteriol. 122, 764-775 (1975).

23. Humphreys, G.O., N.D.F. Grindley and E.S. Anderson: DNA-protein complexes of Δ-mediated transfer systems. Biochim. Biophys. Acta. 287, 355-360 (1972).

24. Humphreys, G.O., G.A. Willshaw,and E.S. Anderson: A simple method for the preparation of large quantities of pure plasmid DNA. Biochim. Biophys. Acta. 383, 457-463 (1975).

25. Humphreys, G.O., G.A. Willshaw, H.R. Smith and E.S. Anderson: Mutagenesis of plasmid DNA with hydroxylamine: isolation of mutants of multi-copy plasmids. Molec. Gen. Genet. 145, 101-108 (1976).

26. Meyers, J.A., D. Sanchez, L.P. Elwell and S. Falkow: Simple agarose gel electrophoretic method for the identification and characterization of plasmid deoxyribonucleic acid. J. Bacteriol. 127, 1529-1537 (1976).

27. Nisioka, T., M. Mitani and R. Clowes: Composite circular forms of R factor deoxyribonucleic acid molecules. J. Bacteriol. 97, 376-385 (1969).

28. Nordstrom, K., L.C. Ingram and A. Lundback: Mutations in R-factors of Escherichia coli causing an increased number of R-factor copies per chromo-some. J. Bacteriol. 110, 562-569 (1972).

29. Perlman, D. and R.H. Rownd: Transition of R factor NR1 in Proteus mira-bilis: Molecular structure and replication of NR1 deoxyribonucleic acid. J. Bacteriol. 123, 1013-1034 (1975).

30. Ptashne, K. and S.N. Cohen: Occurrence of insertion sequence (IS) regions on plasmid deoxyribonucleic acid as direct and inverted nucleotide sequ-ence duplications. J. Bacteriol. 122, 776-781 (1975).

31. Rownd, R., R. Nakaya and A. Nakamura: Molecular nature of the drug-resis-tance factors of the enterobacteriaceae. J. Mol. Biol. 17, 376-393 (1966).

32. Rownd, R., D. Perlman and N. Goto: Structure and replication of R-factor deoxyribonucleic acid in Proteus mirabilis. In D. Schlessinger (Ed.) Microbiology 1974, American Society for Microbiology, Washington. 76-94 (1975).

33. Saz, A.K., D.L. Lowery and L.J. Jackson: Staphylococcal penicillinase. I. Inhibition and stimulation of activity. J. Bacteriol. 82, 298-304 (1961).

34. Sheehy, R.J., A. Perry, D.P. Allison and R. Curtiss III: Molecular nature of R factor deoxyribonucleic acid isolated from Salmonella typhi-murium minicells. J. Bacteriol. 114, 1328-1335 (1973).

35. Silver, R.P. and S. Falkow: Studies on resistance transfer factor deoxy-ribonucleic acid in Escherichia coli. J. Bacteriol. 104, 340-344 (1970).

36. Smith, C.E., E.S. Anderson and R.C. Clowes: Stable composite molecules of an R-factor. Bact. Proc. p60, (1970).

37. Smith, H.R., G.O. Humphreys and E.S. Anderson: Genetic and molecular characterization of some non-transferring plasmids. Molec. Gen. Genet. 129, 229-242 (1974).

38. Smith, H.R., G.O. Humphreys, N.D.F. Grindley, J.N. Grindley and E.S. Anderson: Molecular studies of an fi[+] plasmid from strains of Salmonella typhimurium. Molec. Gen. Genet. 126, 143-151 (1973).

39. Smith, H.R., G.O. Humphreys, G.A. Willshaw and E.S. Anderson: Characteri-
    zation of plasmids coding for the restriction endonuclease Eco R1. Molec.
    Gen. Genet. 143, 319-325 (1976).

40. Van Embden, J. and S.N. Cohen: Molecular and genetic studies of an R
    factor system consisting of independent transfer and drug resistance
    plasmids. J. Bacteriol. 116, 699-709 (1973).

41. Watanabe, T. and Y. Ogata: Genetic stability of various resistance factors
    in Escherichia coli and Salmonella typhimurium. J. Bacteriol. 102, 363-368
    (1970).

42. Yagi, Y. and D.B. Clewell: Identification and characterization of a small
    sequence located at two sites on the amplifiable tetracycline resistance
    plasmid pAMα1 in Streptococcus faecalis. J. Bacteriol. 129, 400-406 (1977).

Discussion

Anderson: I just wanted to add the comment that, as you must be well aware, TP 123, the typhoid R-plasmid, shows a very interesting segregation pattern in its own host strain. In fact, what happens is that there is segregation of the transfer factor with a T-marker, the tetracycline marker, or the transfer factor with the CSSu marker. There is another interesting point there and that is the following: all wild examples of the group H1 plasmids of whatever origin, whether from typhoid or from typhimurium, are incompatible with the F-factor, but it's a unilateral incompatibility. The H1-factors will kick out the F-factors, but F cannot kick out the H1-factors. When segregation occurs, the incompatibility with F almost invariably disappears. If the transferable CSSu factor remains, it is not incompatible with the F-factor. But a segregant containing the T-determinant with the R-factor, is still incompatible.

Saedler: You have studied the influence of various recombination alleles on the segregation patterns: was there any influence?

Humphreys: No, there did not seem to be any specific influence. The best correlation, in fact, was with the endonuclease I gene. In the end$^+$ strains we tended to get dissociation, although not very much. In the end$^-$ strains we did not seem to observe much segregation at all.

Saedler: And the recB and recC contributed to that?

Humphreys: Yes, it seemed to be superimposed, but there seemed to be no direct correlation.

Falkow: JC 7623 has what phenotype? Was it a recA$^+$ cell?

Humphreys: Yes, but it did not have a recB/C pathway.

Davies: Have you tested a variety of drugs for amplification in those cases where you observed dissociation?

Humphreys: We have tried all antibiotics.

Davies: Separately?

Humphreys: Yes.

Davies: And they all worked?

Humphreys: No, they didn't work, there was no amplification.

Davies: Not in any of these cases?

Humphreys: No.

Davies: So that's quite different from Proteus.

Humphreys: Yes.

Falkow: There is no amplification of drug resistance enzymes?

Humphreys: No.

Davies: What I was going to ask specifically is: do you see an increase in the R determinants?

Humphreys: We did not look specifically.

Starlinger: Quite apart from dissociation, if you have several copies of the same plasmid in the cell and the cell is recombination-proficient, there should be dimers and multimers simply by recombination. Sometimes these are found but most people don't find them and you don't seem to have seen them. Why do you think there are no oligomers? Do you think there is some disentanglement upon termination of replication which is independent of recombination?

Anderson: I am sorry, would you mind repeating that?

Starlinger: I am asking: if you have a cell with several copies of the same plasmid and if this cell is recombination-proficient, then by just simple recombination one should observe the formation of dimers and other multimers. These are usually not found. The question is: Do you think that there is a specific dissociation step at the end of replication? Otherwise there must be multimers because recombination of such long stretches of DNA is certainly very effective.

Humphreys: I have no real idea, but I agree there must be some dissociation step which is as yet unrecognised.

Anderson: Quite early in these studies, we got a strain of S. typhimurium which was part of our normal screening programme. This strain had the most remarkable property of "falling into pieces" every time we looked at it. It was resistant to chloramphenicol, streptomycin, sulphonamides and kanamycin and - I cannot remember what else - but certainly those. The strain kept segregating in the most remarkable way. One could get kanamycin resistant segregants or CSSu resistant segregants. If one applied selection pressure with all the antibiotics, all the R-determinants remained together. However, as soon as selection pressure was let up, it would "fall to pieces" again. This thing remained a mystery for a very long time until we discovered what was actually happening: Dr. Humphreys referred to a so-called "cryptic plasmid". It is the plasmid which we called MT10. It is fi$^+$; it is, in fact, a defective transfer factor. It is present in the majority of S. typhimurium strains from all over the world. Why this is so, we don't know, but we concluded that it has some evolutionary connexion with S. typhimurium. MT10 is a plasmid which will interact with other plasmids and what was happening in our strain was this: CSSu was recombining with MT10, but kanamycin was also recombining with MT10, though not with the same copy. The result was that there were two plasmids within the same cell which were incompatible with each other. The result is, of course, that the plasmids segregated. There was obviously a high recombinant facility in the CSSu determinants and there was obviously a high recombinant facility in the K (kanamycin) determinant and, if you combine that with the recombinant facility of the MT10, what results is a cell which contains several incompatible plasmids. They keep "falling to pieces" unless there is selection for all the resistance determinants present in both plasmids. This was the explanation. At that time, however, we were not educated to study this problem in greater detail and to look, for example, for multimers of the CSSu or the K plasmid.

We had no evidence, as a matter of fact, that this phenomenon was occurring. This was very early in the development of the resistance plasmid field and, in retrospect, this was a beautiful example of the CSSu operon (now replicon) floating around and looking for something to recombine with - and finding it - and the K (kanamycin) doing exactly the same.

Humphreys: One thing we did try to do with no success, was the following: we attempted to transfer the CSSu fragment from TP125 onto the RTF fragment of TP 123. We failed to get any recombinants.

Falkow: I am happy that someone followed up this S. typhimurium dissociation phenomenon, I enjoyed your talk very much. In Proteus, Robert Rownd proposed that one should not find many single R-determinants and, in fact, he found what Peter Starlinger has suggested one should see, namely multimers. If Bob Rownd was here, he would probably say that you did not see these multimers because they were so enormous and I was just wondering whether his could be the case.

umphreys: We did not look for structures that big.

tarlinger: What Bob Rownd finds, is one RTF and several R-eterminants.

alkow: That's right, but he finds very large structures indeed nd, remember, the H1-plasmids are already in the 100 million alton range. Does the S. typhimurium type 36 have a cryptic lasmid? Let us not call it a cryptic plasmid. What I mean is he 30 megadalton plasmid? Apparently not?

umphreys: No.

nderson: It had lost the plasmid?

umphreys: Yes.

nderson: But it started off with it?

umphreys: Yes.

alkow: Can I change topics and ask you about the transduction f small plasmids? Do you think that the transduction of small -determinants might be a way of rescuing them? I don't know hether you could try it with this particular system. One might xpect that with a P1-like phage or P22 one might be able to ransduce the resistance replicon into a cell with a transfer actor and rescue it that way.

umphreys: I don't know if that would work.

alkow: Can one actually transduce the small ampicillin and mall Su-Sm plasmids?

umphreys: Yes.

aedler: Did you ever try to isolate the RTF and the CSSu unit nd to check whether or not they contain an Is1?

umphreys: No. That's something we have not gotten to.

eadler: This has a significant implication for the model we ave been devising, and for which there is essentially no proof. e assumed that dissociation occurs by recombination of the wo copies of Is1 on the composite plasmid, but actually it ould be a mechanism like a transposition event. Actually, Is1 ecombination occurs but whether it is the natural event, no-ody can tell. It can occur as soon as there are two Is1 se-uences in tandem but whether this is the natural mechanism of ow an R-determinant gets integrated or trapped by an RTF unit, r the means by which dissociation occurs, must remain uncertain.

nderson: I would like to come back to this business with the SSu and the K. These were, I suppose, transposons floating round, looking for something to recombine with. What I cannot

remember is the rate of spontaneous loss of one and the other.
For that I will have to go back to the records.

Starlinger: Has anybody done an experiment where he selected
for tetracycline resistance in E. coli which carried R1 or R100
to see whether there was an accumulation of cells which carried
RTF and had lost R-determinants? If they would segregate, if
they would recombine in E. coli and just the R-determinant was
not stable, then at least selection for the RTF and its tetracycline resistance marker should accumulate in cell which had
lost the other resistance determinants.

Davies: You do get miniplasmids with tetracycline resistance.
That experiment was first done by Lebek.

Starlinger: But shouldn't you get the RTF?

Davies: I don't think that situation has ever been looked at.

Anderson: But take the well-known case of T-Δ? This plasmid
does not normally segregate in S. typhimurium. That is to say
in terms of what observes in extracted DNA. On the other hand,
if one simply performs a transfer of T-Δ without antibiotic
selection, one finds that about 1% of the recipient cells will
get the Δ factor alone, without the tetracycline resistance
determinant.

Levy: The mechanism by which the Salmonella seems to increase
the dissociation of what seems to be F II R-plasmids is
related to the fact that the MT10 plasmid is F II and that
pieces of it may be left in the chromosome of Salmonella even
though you have isolated a Salmonella which now no longer has
that plasmid?

Humphreys: The MT10 is not incompatible with F II plasmids.

Levy: Which were the S. typhimurium cryptic plasmids that were
FII? Was it not demonstrated - that was the reason for the segregation of F-plasmids in Salmonella!?

Falkow: Those plasmids were merely shown to share some homologous sequences with F II R-plasmids on the basis of DNA-DNA
hybridisation, but that observation does not imply that they
had the F II incompatibility gene.

Anderson: Just to complete the story: if you put TnA into the
cell carrying MT10, you have a complete R-factor which will
transfer.

Copy Mutants of the Plasmid R 1 as a Tool in Studies of Control of Plasmid Replication

Kurt Nordström, Birgitta Engberg[1], Petter Gustafsson, Søren Molin, and **Bernt Eric Uhlin**

Introduction

Replication of bacterial chromosomes and plasmids is carefully regulated; their cellular concentration is kept constant in an exponentially growing population of bacteria /4/, /13/. Replication is controlled at the level of initiation /38/. The initiation mass (cell mass per origin) of the Escherichia coli chromosome is constant at least at growth rates above one generation per hour suggesting that initiation mass is the parameter used to control replication /10/, /36/, /38/. This is a reasonable idea since it requires measurement of a concentration, a principle often used in biochemical processes. Two main models have been proposed to explain the coupling between replication and growth, the one suggesting positive /19/, the other negative control /37/, /39/. Many experiments have been performed in order to distinguish between these two models, but almost no definitive answers have so far been obtained. Control of DNA replication differs from the control of synthesis of other cellular macromolecules in that the number of molecules that are synthesized per cell (and per cell generation) is limited; in some cases this number is only one. This particularly applies to the chromosome but also to many plasmids. On the other hand, it is absolutely necessary that the process is carefully controlled, otherwise cells lacking the DNA molecule could become abundant. In contrast to other macromolecules, loss of DNA is irreversible since the cells no longer contain the genetic information of

---

[1] Department of Microbiology, University of Umeå, Sweden.

synthesis of the lacking molecule. Therefore, DNA replication
cannot possibly be regulated by chance processes, such as those
of the promoter type.

We have for several years worked with the system that controls
the replication of the plasmid R1. Our aim is to describe the
control system in as much detail as possible. To our mind, a
number of questions have to be answered before any really useful model can be constructed. Some of these important questions
will be discussed in this paper. Proper answers do not exist
for all of them and we are not at this stage going to present
any model.

1. On the average, during one cell generation, every plasmid
    in a population replicates exactly once. During most of the
    time it does not replicate. What is the mechanism that for-
    bids/allows replication ?

2. In a fused replicon with two functional origins only one
    origin is normally used /3/, /40/. What is the mechanism
    that forbids the use of the other origin ?

3. If the plasmid content in a cell deviates from the steady
    state level, what is the mechanism that brings the plasmid
    content back to the normal value ?

4. What is the parameter used to control replication such that
    it keeps pace with growth ?

5. Several replications occur on the average per cell during
    one cell generation. How are plasmid copies selected for
    replication ?

6. What is the timing of plasmid replication, is it related to
    the chromosome replication cycle and to the cell division
    cycle ? Do all plasmid replications in a cell coincide in
    time or is there a time spread ?

7. How many control genes are involved in the control process ?

8. What is the function of the control genes and their gene
    products ?

The System Used

Escherichia coli K-12 was used throughout this work; the relevant strains have been listed in Table 1. The plasmid investigated is the R plasmid R1drd-19 /28/, /29/ (in the following
denoted R1); its properties are listed in Table 2, which also
contains information about the mutants of plasmid R1 studied.
Plasmid copy number is defined as plasmid copies per chromosome
equivalent (2.5 x 10^9 dalton (7)). Plasmid-borne mutations
affecting the copy number of the plasmid are referred to as
copy mutations (phenotype Cop, genotype cop). The ratio between
the copy number of a copy mutant and that of the wild type has
been denoted copy effect.

Table 1. Strains in E. coli K-12 used.

Strain	Markers	Source
EC1005	met, nal, relA	Grinsted et al. (15)
D1 [a]	his, pro, trp	Meynell and Datta (28)

[a] Strain RC711 of Meynell and Datta (28)

Plasmid Replication Is Controlled Independently of Chromosome Replication

Several types of experiments have been used to correlate plasmid
replication with chromosome replication and with the bacterial
cell cycle. It is now well documented that plasmid replication
is independent of these two processes; it neither coincides with
termination or initiation of chromosome replication nor does it
take place (at all growth rates) at the same cell age. This is
apparent from analysis of the plasmid (F'lac and R1) content in
balanced cultures growing at different growth rates, the growth
rate being varied by using different carbon sources (Fig. 1)
/5/, /12/, /38/. The growth rate seems to be the parameter that
defines the copy number since we obtained exactly the same results as in Fig. 1 when the growth rate was varied by adding

Table 2. Plasmids used.

Plasmid[a]	Derivation	Genotype	Copy effect[b]	Reference
R1drd-19	Mutant of naturally occurring plasmid R1, derepressed for transfer	bla$^+$ cat$^+$ aphA$^+$ aadA$^+$, sul$^+$ tra$^+$ fin	1.0	Meynell and Datta (29)
pKN102 (B2)			3.7	Nordström et al. (33)
pKN103 (B3)	Copy mutants of	cop	2.0	
pKN104 (B4)	R1drd-19		8.2	Uhlin and Nordström (48)
pKN142 (B42)			5.0	
pKN301		cop(td)	1 (4 - 6)	Our laboratory, unpublished
pKN303		cop(am)	1 (4 - 6)	
pKN401		cop(td)	2 (very high)	
R100	Naturally occurring	cat$^+$ aadA$^+$ sul$^+$ tet$^+$, tra$^+$ fin$^+$	1.0	Egawa and Hirota (11)

a) Mutant denotation previously used: R1drd-19B2 for pKN102, etc.

b) cop(td) and cop(am) denote temperature-dependent copy mutants and amber copy mutants, respectively.

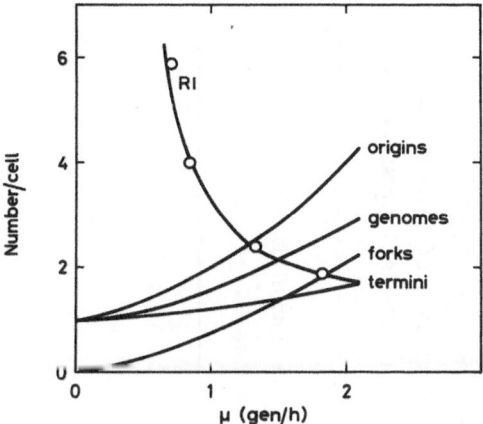

Fig. 1. Plasmid R1drd-19 content in E. coli EC1005-R1drd-19 growing exponentially at various growth rates. The plasmid data were taken from Engberg and Nordström (12) and the theoretical values for the chromosome from Cooper and Helmstetter (7), assuming a C period of 40 min and a D period of 20 min.

different concentrations of α-methylglucoside to glucose-minimal media. The independence of plasmid replication is also evident from the existence of copy mutants of plasmids /33/. It is possible by mutation in the genome of several plasmids to increase the plasmid copy number. Hence many plasmids control their own replication (Table 3). There are also chromosomal mutations that affect plasmid copy number (Table 3). This matter will be further discussed under the heading genetic control.

Selection and Timing of Plasmid Replication

An understanding of the mechanism that controls plasmid replication requires information about the relation between successive plasmid replications in a cell or a series of cells formed from a parent cell. Different approaches have been tried; several research groups have used synchronous cultures and pulse induction by IPTG (isopropyl-ß-thiogalactoside) of the lac operon of plasmid F'lac to place plasmid replication in the bacterial cell cycle /6/, /9/, /49/. Although these groups have used the same system (host strain and plasmid) they have arrived at different conclusions. However, they all claim that

Table 3. Mutations affecting plasmid copy number.

Location of mutation	Plasmid	Wild type copy number	Mutation[a]	Copy effect[b]	Reference
Plasmid	R1drd-19	Low	cop	1 - 10	Nordström et al. (33) Uhlin and Nordström (48)
	MarA	Low	?	2 - 4	Timmis and Winkler (47)
	R100	Low	ror	2 - 4	Rownd et al. (30)
	CloDF13	High	?	7	Nijkamp et al.(21)
	λdv	High	cro	varying	Matsubara and Takeda (26)
	P1	Low	seg	?	Jaffe-Brachet, unpublished
Chromosome	A few F,P1	Low	pkn	2 - 4	Cress and Kline (8)
	R6K	High	?	22 - 3	CurtissIII et al. (24)

a) ? indicates that no symbol has been proposed.

b) ? indicates that the copy effect has not been determined.

plasmid F'<u>lac</u> replicates at a defined cell age in all cells
growing exponentially in a given medium. It is also evident
from their results that the timing of plasmid replication is
less precise than that of chromosome replication. It should
also be stressed that, in those studies, plasmid DNA was never
measured directly.

Another approach has been to use density-shift experiments /27/.
These have shown that plasmids ColE1 /1/, NR1 /43/, R1 /17/,
and F'<u>lac</u> (Gustafsson and Nordström, Lunteren Lectures 1975)
are selected randomly for replication. This means that one plasmid copy is selected and then replicated. The daughter plasmids
formed have the same probability as the unreplicated ones of
being selected for the next replication.

We have also performed density shift experiments with plasmid-
carrying cultures /17/. We want to discuss critically the assumptions made and also forward the idea that such experiments
can be used to measure the average time interval between successive replications (Gustafsson and Nordström, Lunteren Lectures 1975). In these experiments, plasmid content has been determined as covalently closed circular (CCC) DNA; this is justified because the turnover of replicating plasmid DNA into
CCC-DNA only takes a few minutes (Gustafsson and Nordström, unpublished). Density shift experiments give information about
large populations of plasmid molecules in exponentially growing populations of bacteria. Therefore, the values obtained
are average values. It should be much more informative if it
were possible to analyze plasmid replication in individual cells.
Unfortunately, there is no method available that allows this.

The calculations are based upon the assumption that there is
very little variation with respect to plasmid content in different cells. Two types of evidence support this idea. If the
segregation of plasmid copies at cell division were random and
determined by a Poissonian distribution, a copy number determined fraction of the cells should be plasmidless, but the actual figure is 100-fold less than the calculated value /17/.
The other piece of evidence refers to antibiotic resistance.
Resistance to ampicillin is proportional to the gene dosage
/33/, /48/ (<u>cf</u>. Fig. 9). Resistance is measured by spreading
cells on plates containing different concentrations of ampi-

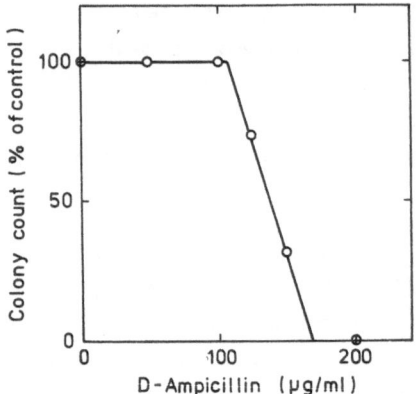

Fig. 2. Single-cell resistance to ampicillin of strain EC1005-
R1drd-19. The bacteria were grown exponentially in LB medium.
At a cell density of about 2×10^8 cells/ml, about 200 cells were
spread per plate containing LA medium and different concentrations
of D-ampicillin. Survival was measured after incubation over
night (32).

cillin /32/. Up to a certain concentration of the drug (the
resistance level) all cells form colonies (Fig. 2). At still
higher concentrations the number of colony formers decrease
by 20% at an increase of 10% in ampicillin concentration, i.e.
no colonies are formed at a drug level 1.5 times the resistance
level. This strongly indicates that there is very little variation in the plasmid content of individual cells.

We have performed density shift experiments using glycerol-
minimal medium. The average plasmid R1 content in this medium
is three copies per newborn cell. It can be concluded from the
discussion above that a vast majority of the newborn cells
carry three plasmid R1 copies and that three replications occur
per cell and cell cycle /17/. Here we will present results only
for plasmid R1 but we have arrived at similar results and conclusions also for plasmid F'lac. In a density shift from dense
(H) to light (L) medium, nonreplicated (HH), once-replicated
(HL), and at least twice-replicated (LL) DNA are determined by
density gradient centrifugation (Fig. 3). The result of such an
experiment performed with plasmid R1 is presented in Fig. 4,
that shows that HH-DNA decays rapidly, HL-DNA increases rapidly

DENSITY SHIFT EXPERIMENT
(Experimental procedure)

Density shift :

      Steady state culture in D_2O ^{15}N ^{14}C-thy
                Shift
      Steady state culture in H_2O ^{14}N ^{3}H-thy

          Samples

Purification of R1 DNA :

      PrI / CsCl density centrifugation

      Neutral sucrose velocity centrifug.

Isolation of heavy, hybrid and light DNA :

      CsCl density centrifugation

Fig. 3. Procedure used in density shift experiments with strain EC1005-R1drd-19.

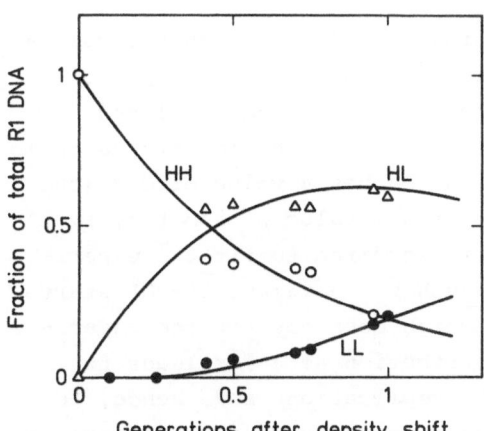

Fig. 4. Replication of plasmid R1drd-19 during density shift experiment with strain EC1005-R1drd-19 growing exponentially in glycerol-minimal medium. At zero time, the culture was shifted from dense (H) to light (L) medium. The frequency of HH (o), HL (Δ), and LL (●) plasmid DNA was measured at intervals. The curves correspond to the theoretical equations 9 - 11, assuming a delay time (t_d) of 0.22 generations.

and reaches a maximum about one generation after the density shift, while LL-DNA appears at about 0.3 generations after the shift and then increases with time (the curves in the Figure refer to equations 9-11 below). The appearance of LL-DNA shows that a considerable fraction of the plasmid R1 copies replicates at least twice during one cell generation. One possibility of getting LL-DNA appearing considerably earlier than one generation after a density shift would be that all replications in a cell coincided (the democratic model) /4/, but there was a great spread in the time interval between two successive triple replications. If we assume that the time interval (y) between successive replications follows a standardized normal distribution:

$$f(\underline{c}) = \frac{1}{\sqrt{2\pi}} \; e^{-\underline{c}^2/2}$$

where $c = (y - \tau)/\sigma$

τ = generation time of the population

σ = standard deviation of the mean

Two or more consecutive replications overlap at higher σ values giving rise to two or more replications during a test period considerably less than τ. Numeric analysis using tabulated values for $\int_{-\infty}^{c} f(\underline{c})d\underline{c}$ have been summarized in Fig. 5. The ratio LL-DNA/HL-DNA after one generation reaches a value of 0.3 (the experimentally found value) only at a σ value of about τ, i.e. an extremely broad distribution is required to fit the experimental results. Furthermore, at such big σ values LL-DNA starts to appear already at zero time, which does not fit the experimental results. Such a broad distribution as $\sigma = \tau$ leads to great overlaps between successive replications and, hence, to a high probability of a later event occurring before an earlier one. This is in contradiction to the delay found for the appearance of LL-DNA (cf. below). The extreme possibility of combining this delay (0.3 generations) with the democratic model would be the distribution shown in Fig. 6. However, numeric integration of this Figure shows that this distribution does not give enough LL-DNA to fit the experimental data. We therefore have to look for a more probable model than the democratic one.

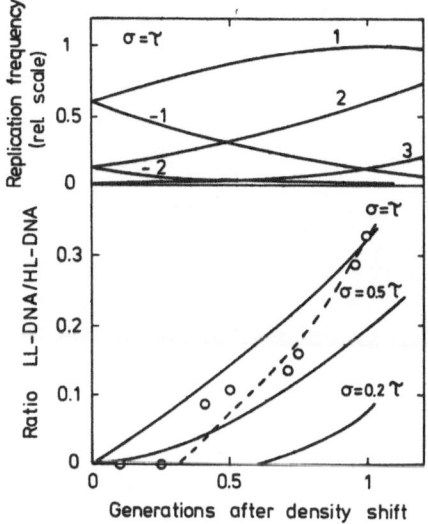

Fig. 5. Comparison of the result of the density shift experiment with plasmid R1drd-19 described in Fig. 4 (dotted line) with a model of plasmid replication in which all plasmid replications in a cell coincide in time, but in which there is a time spread (σ) in the length of the interreplication times (cf. equation 1). Curves are given for three different values of σ (as indicated in the Fig.). The upper part of the Figure demonstrates the distribution of replication probabilities if $\sigma = \tau$. The numbers given in that part of the Figure refer to the sequence of replications such that -2 and -1 are the replications that on the average occur 2τ and τ before the one appearing between time 0 and time τ, and those denoted 1 and 2 are the ones that on the average follow the generations thereafter.

The following scheme describes the replications:

$$HH + \text{deoxyribonucleotide triphosphates} \xrightarrow{k} 2HL$$

$$HL + \text{deoxyribonucleotide triphosphates} \xrightarrow{k} HL + LL$$

$$LL + \text{deoxyribonucleotide triphosphates} \xrightarrow{k} 2LL$$

We regard it as being justified to assume that the rate constant (k) is the same for all three reactions. The simplest assumption is that the rate of each reaction is determined only by the

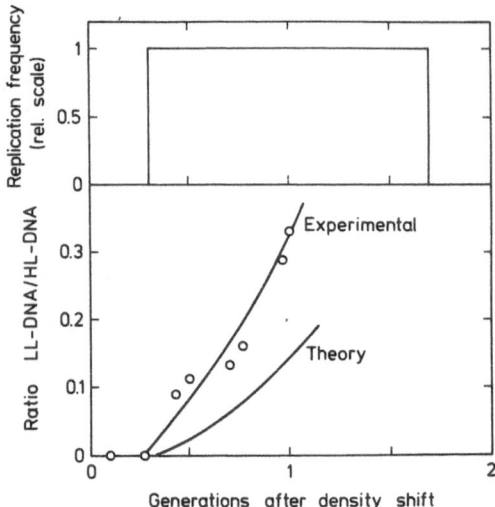

Fig. 6. Comparison of the result of the density shift experiment
with plasmid R1drd-19 described in Fig. 4 (circles) with a model
of plasmid replication in which all plasmid replications in a
cell coincide but where there is a period of 0.3 generations
after one set of replications during which further plasmid
replications in a cell are forbidden. The probability of the next
set of replications is assumed to be constant during the period
0.3 - 1.7 generations after the first replication (cf. top part
of the Figure).

rate constant and the concentration of the reactants. This gives
the following equations:

$$\text{Relative amount of HH-DNA} = \underline{x}_1 = 3^{-2kt} \tag{2}$$

$$\text{Relative amount of HL-DNA} = \underline{x}_2 = 2(e^{-kt} - e^{-2kt}) \tag{3}$$

$$\text{Relative amount of LL-DNA} = \underline{x}_3 = 1 - 2e^{-kt} + e^{-2kt} \tag{4}$$

The ratio between LL-DNA and HL-DNA, plotted in Fig. 7, increases directly from zero time. The theoretical results do not fit
the experimental results (circles in the Figure), but the data
indicate that a newly formed molecule cannot participate in a
second replication until a certain time later. The most general
formalism for making the kinetics dependent on the previous

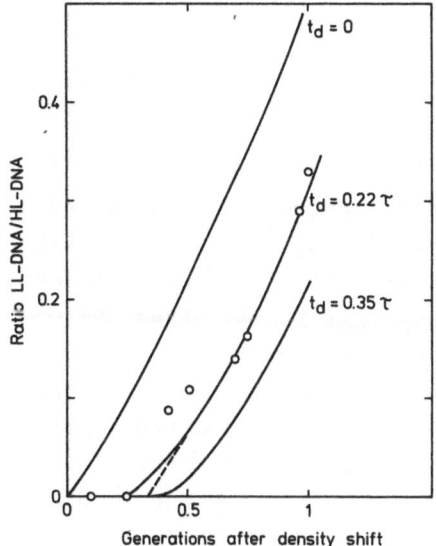

Fig. 7. Comparison of the result of the density shift experiment with plasmid R1drd-19 described in Fig. 4 (circles) with a model of plasmid replication in which the rate of formation of HH-, HL-, and LL-plasmid DNA is solely a function of the concentration of the corresponding substrates (cf. equations 2 - 4)(curve labelled $t_d = 0$), and with the same model in which there is a time delay (t_d) after the replication of a plasmid molecule during which further replications in the cell are forbidden (cf. equations 9 - 11).

history of the system consists of making the rate constant $k(s)$ a function of the previous time s, so that for instance

$$\frac{dx_1}{dt} = \int_0^\infty k(s) x_1 (t - s) ds \qquad (7)$$

Such equations are difficult to solve, and we have thus assumed that $k(s)$ is very sharply peaked about a specific value t_d, making

$$d(s) = k \, \sigma \, (s - t_d) \qquad (8)$$

where $\sigma(s)$ is the Dirac delta function. Then the rate equations become:

$$dx_1/dt = kx_1(t - t_d) \tag{9}$$

$$dx_2/dt = 2kx_1(t - t_d) \tag{10}$$

$$dx_3/dt = kx_2(t - t_d) + kx_3(t - t_d) \tag{11}$$

A program for integrating the equations above was constructed and computer calculations gave curves for x_1, x_2, and $x_3 = f(t)$ for various values of t_d. As is observed in Fig. 7, experimental results agreed with the calculated data if t_d was given the value of 0.22 τ. This means that there is a period of 0.22 τ after a replication during which further replications are forbidden. After this time the probability of a second replication rapidly increases. The extrapolated value from the curve (dotted line) shows that the second replication on the average occurs about 0.3 generations after the first one. Hence, a random selection model with a time interval of τ/n between successive replications fits with the experimental results. We therefore conclude that plasmid replication occurs in a sequence of single replications on the average separated by τ/n min. A spread of plasmid replication over the whole cell cycle is also supported by the analysis of plasmid replication in cells of different sizes (ages); plasmid replication was equally frequent in cells of all sizes (Fig. 8).

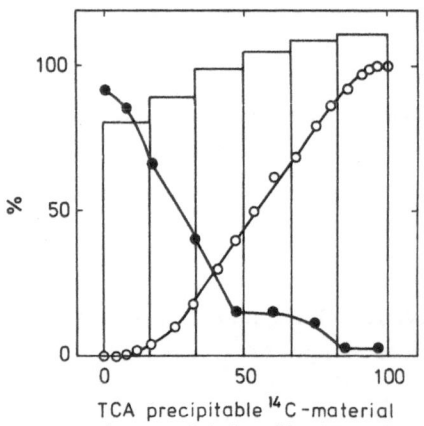

Fig. 8. Replication of plasmid R1 in cells of various sizes. Strain EC1005-R1drd-19 was grown exponentially in glycerol-minimal medium in the presence of ^{14}C-thymidine. The culture

was pulse-labelled for 1/10 of a generation time with ^{3}H-thymidine. The cells were then harvested by chilling and centrifugation and separated by low speed centrifugation in a sucrose gradient. The cells were analysed for trichloroacetate precipitable radio-activity (o), and for the frequency of septation of the cells (●). The material was then divided into six lots, which were analysed for plasmid DNA by alkaline sucrose gradient centrifu-gation. The relative rate of plasmid replication in these six lots is given as a histogram in the Figure.

The time at which LL-DNA starts to appear in a density shift seems to be $\tau/\underline{n}$ after the shift, i.e. the intercept in LL-DNA/HL-DNA = f($\underline{t}$) is a good measure of the average copy number in a new cell. Furthermore, the curves for LL-DNA/HL-DNA = f($\underline{t}$) at different $\underline{n}$ values are virtually parallel. This result in $\underline{n}$-determined distributions between LL-, HL-, and HH-DNA through-out a density shift experiment. The distribution after one gen-eration has been used by several groups to prove that selection for replication of a plasmid is random /1/, /42/ but we want to stress that this distribution can also be used to measure plas-mid copy number. A comparison of various methods of estimating plasmid copy number is presented in Table 4.

Genetic Control of Replication

Several years ago we described mutants of plasmid R1 which show-ed an increased copy number compared to the wild type plasmid, so-called copy mutants (Cop, cop) /31/, /33/. The existence of these mutants prove that plasmid R1 is in command of its own rep-lication. Since then, several research groups have isolated analogous mutants of other plasmids /21/, /26/, /30/, /47/. There-fore, plasmid-controlled plasmid replication seems to be a gen-eral phenomenon. There are also chromosomal mutations that affect the copy number of some plasmids /8/, /24/ (Table 3).

In most of the examples mentioned in Table 4, virtually nothing is known about the gene product of the mutated control gene. Plasmid λ$\underline{dv}$ is an exception. Its replication is under negative control by the $\underline{cro}$ gene product (see below) /2/, /25/. We have found similar results with some plasmid R1 copy mutants, a mat-

Table 4. Estimation of plasmid copy number.

Plasmid	Host	Plasmid copy number[a]			Reference
		Centrifugation	Intercept[b]	One generation value[c]	
R1drd-19	E. coli K-12	2.8[d]	3.0	2.9	This paper
F'lac	E. coli B/rA		5.0	4.2	e)
F'lac	E. coli K-12		4		Kline (20)
NR1	Proteus mirabilis	10[f]	10	10	Rownd (43)

a) Number of plasmid copies per newborn cell.

b) Intercept at LL-DNA/HL-DNA = 0 in Fig. 7 and analogous experiments.

c) From Fig. 7 and analogous experiments.

d) Ethidium Bromide CsCl gradient centrifugation.

e) P. Gustafsson and K. Nordström, unpublished data.

f) CsCl gradient centrifugation. The result is given as copies per chromosome equivalent.

ter that will also be discussed below. The copy mutations have
not been properly mapped. Rownd /30/ has reported that the copy
mutation of the mutant R12 of plasmid R100 is located on the
RTF (resistance transfer factor) part. We have indications for
the location to the r-determinant of the copy mutation of the
plasmid pKN102 /33/. It should be stressed that plasmids R1 and
R100 are complex plasmids presumably consisting of two replicons,
the RTF and the r-determinant (resistance determinant); the former is a replicating molecule while it remains to be proven that
the r-determinant can replicate in the absence of other plasmids
/4/. Nevertheless, the RTF as well as the r-determinant contain
at least one origin of vegetative replication /35/. It remains
to be demonstrated which origin is used by the various copy mutants of plasmid R1. We have isolated a considerable number of
copy mutants of plasmid R1 /48/. They have been selected by plating a plasmid R1 containing population on plates containing different concentrations of penicillin - penicillin resistance is
directly proportional to the gene dosage /33/, /48/.
The copy mutants form a more or less continuous series of copy
effects ranging from that of the wild type to a tenfold higher
value (Table 2, Fig. 9). We have never in a one-step selection

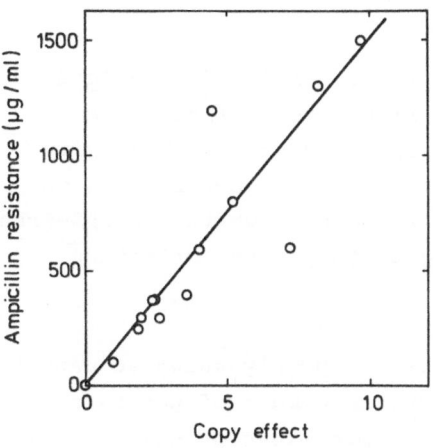

Fig. 9. Ampicillin resistance on solid medium as a function of
the gene dosage. Strain EC1005 carrying plasmid R1drd-19 or
copy mutants of this plasmid were tested as described in Fig. 2.
Resistance is defined as the highest drug concentration at which
100% of the cells plated were able to form colonies (32).

process starting with a wild type plasmid been able to isolate
copy mutants with a copy effect higher than ten. The frequency
of clones found on ampicillin plates decreases rapidly with increasing concentrations of the drug /31/. As an example, Fig. 10
shows the results obtained with an EMS (ethyl methanesulphonate)
treated culture; the resistance level of the wild type population is 100 µg/ml. About 10^{-3} of the population resisted 300-
500 µg/ml, while only 10^{-6} grew in the presence of 1000 µg/ml.
This could suggest that the latter are double-mutants. Similar
indications will be discussed below in connection with conditional copy mutants. We have never found any chromosomal mutations affecting the copy number of plasmid R1.

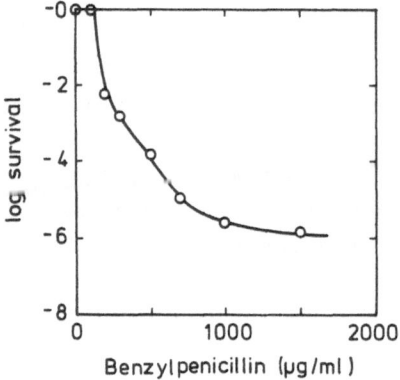

Fig. 10. Survival of EMS-treated cells of strain EC1005-R1drd-19
on LA plates containing benzylpenicillin. The bacteria were
grown in LB medium. EMS (10 µg/ml) was added at a cell density
of about $2x10^8$ ml^{-1}. The mutagen was removed by centrifugation
after about 2 hours. The cells were further incubated in EMS-free
LB medium for 3 hours before plating on LA plates containing
benzylpenicillin.

Since the genetics of the copy effects is poorly known we cannot
make any definitive conclusions about the number of genes involved in the system that controls the plasmid copy number. However, an analysis of plasmid incompatibility indicates that at
least two plasmid genes are involved (Table 5) /48/.

Two types of conditional copy mutants have been isolated(Table 6)
(Gustafsson and Nordström, Lunteren Lectures 1975). One type is

Table 5. Incompatibility properties of copy mutants of plasmid R1drd-19.

Incoming plasmid	Resident plasmid	Copy effect of resident plasmid	Frequency of loss (% per cell doubling)[a]	
			R1	R100
R100	R1drd-19	1.0	8	8
R100	pKN103	2.0	<1	19
R100	pKN102	3.7	<1	26
R100	pKN104	8.2	5	<1
R100	pKN142	5	<1	<1

[a] A clone carrying both plasmids was selected by double antibiotic selection. This clone was then grown in LB medium without any antibiotic. Samples were plated at intervals and the colonies obtained were tested for the presence of the plasmids R1 and R100 (48).

Table 6. Conditional copy mutants of plasmid R1drd-19.

Plasmid[a]	Parent	Growth conditions	Copy effect
R1drd-19	-	30°C	1
		40°C	1
pKN301 (td)	R1drd-19	30°C	1
		40°C	4 - 6
pKN401 (td)	pKN301	30°C	2 - 3
		40°C	very high, lethal
pKN303 (am)	R1drd-19	SuIII	1.5 - 2
		Su⁻	4 - 6

[a] td = temperature-dependent, am = amber.

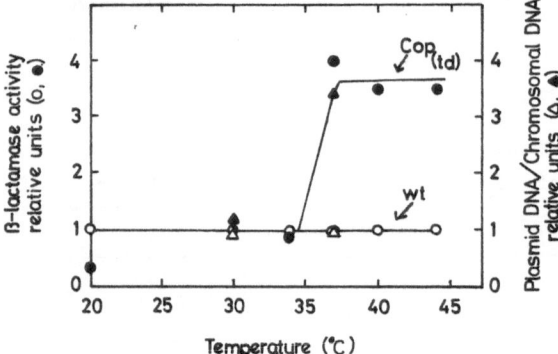

Fig. 11. Temperature-dependence of copy effect of the plasmid copy mutant pKN301.

temperature-dependent; at 30C the copy effect is wild type but it is 4-6-fold higher than that of the wild type at 40°C(Fig. 11). The transition between the two levels of copy effects is very sharp, which to our mind, is fairly uncommon among temperature-sensitive gene products. Perhaps it could indicate that a poly-mer protein is involved. The other conditional copy mutants are amber mutants. In the presence of a strong amber suppressor the copy effect is 1-2 times that of the wild type plasmid while in the absence of any amber suppressor it is 4-6-fold higher. These results prove that a protein with a negative control function is involved in the control of plasmid R1 replication. The two types of conditional copy mutants (temperature-dependent and amber) show the same result, namely that the copy effect is 4-6-fold higher in the absence than in the presence of the control protein. This suggests that one protein exerts its control at this level. The fact that the nonconditional copy mutants may show considerably higher copy effects indicates that other con-trol functions also exist. To test this possibility we isolated from a temperature-dependent copy mutant (pKN301) a double mu-tant (pKN401) which at 30°C showed a copy effect of 2-3 but at higher temperatures had a drastically increased copy effect (Fig. 12). At 36°C about 70% of the total DNA was plasmid DNA and at still higher temperatures the cells did not form colonies. About 10^{-5} - 10^{-6} of the cells carrying plasmid pKN401 formed colonies at 42°C (Table 7). These thermo-resistant clones formed two classes, the one showing a copy effect similar to that of

plasmid pKN301 (the parent of pKN401), while the other was almost wild type with respect to copy number at all temperatures.

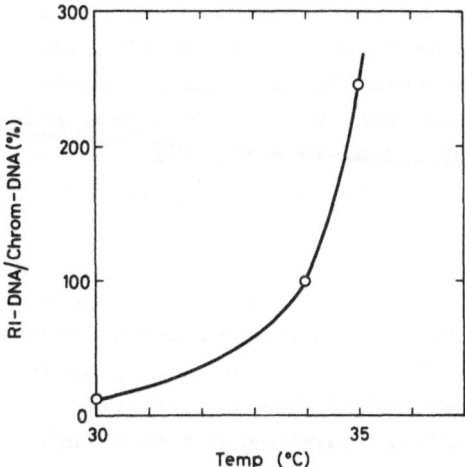

Fig. 12. Temperature-dependence of the copy effect of the plasmid copy mutant pKN401.

Table 7. Temperature-resistant derivatives obtained from strain
D1-pKN401[a].

Class	Frequency	Copy effect	
	(%)	$30^{\circ}C$	$40^{\circ}C$
A	70	1	4
B	30	1	1
C	10	0	0

[a] Strain D1-pKN401 was grown exponentially in LB medium at $30^{\circ}C$.
At a cell density of about 10^8 ml^{-1}, samples were spread on LA
plates and incubated over night at $42^{\circ}C$. About 10^{-5} - 10^{-6} of the
cells plated gave rise to colonies. These were tested for copy
effect by determination of their ampicillin resistance.

Control Functions

Replication of plasmid λdv is under its own negative control /2/, /25/. The control does not operate directly at the origin of DNA replication but is exerted by the cro gene product which acts as an (auto)repressor of its own synthesis /2/, /25/. The cro gene is an early gene located on an operon, which also contains the genes O and P. The products of these genes are positive factors involved in DNA replication. Berg /2/ has described the functioning of the λdv control system in terms that are very similar to those of the Pritchard negative control model /37/, /39/.

Control of plasmid R1 replication also contains a negative control protein (Fig. 11, Table 6) (Gustafsson and Nordström, Lunteren Lectures 1975). We do not know at what level this protein operates. Some information has been gained from experiments in which a logarithmically growing culture carrying a temperature-dependent copy mutant of plasmid R1 (pKN301) is shifted from one temperature to another; this means that the culture shifts from one level to another with respect to copy number (Fig. 13).

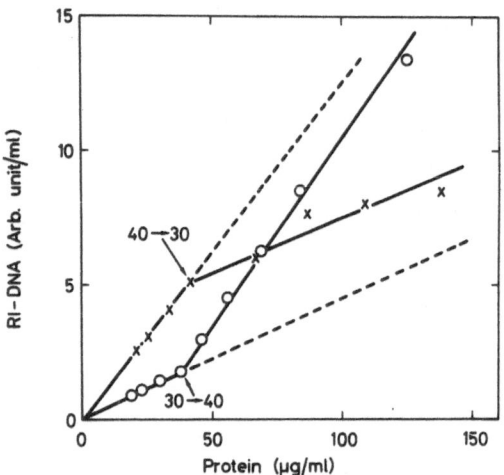

Fig. 13. Specific rate of replication of the temperature-dependent plasmid copy mutant pKN301 in temperature shifts. The dotted lines refer to steady state growth at 30°C and 40°C, respectively.

In up-shifts as well as in down-shifts the result was virtually identical: The frequency of plasmid R1 replication rapidly adjusted to that characteristic of the post-shift temperature.

In shifts from 30°C to 40°C there was no period during which the frequency of plasmid R1 replication was higher than at steady state at 40°C (Fig. 13). This indicates that the mutant protein is not simply a temperature-sensitive repressor acting on initiation of DNA replication. Several possibilities are open: i) the synthesis of the repressor is temperature sensitive, ii) the repressor is temperature sensitive during its formation (e.g. during the building up of a complex structure) but not after this structure has been formed, and iii) the repressor acts somewhere else than at the replicative origin, maybe by forming a negative loop in analogy to the cro gene product in the λ dv system /2/, /25/. In shifts from 40°C to 30°C plasmid R1 replication was never less frequent than in balanced growth at 30°C (Fig. 13). This indicates that the denatured protein does not renature rapidly. The results rather fit any of the other possibilities discussed in the previous paragraph.

At present we cannot exclude any of the alternatives regarding the level where the repressor acts. We are currently trying to identify and purify the repressor protein in order to be able to investigate by in vitro techniques if and where the protein binds to plasmid DNA.

Control Parameters

One idea about the replication control process that is favoured by many authors is that the control parameter is the concentration of replicative origins (or initiation mass, i.e. cell mass per origin) /10/, /36/, /38/. We want to present data that seem to rule out this possibility at least for plasmid R1. Several years ago we reported that the copy number of plasmid R1 decreased with increasing growth rate (Fig. 14) /12/. By supplementing a culture growing in minimal-glycerol medium with casamino acids-glucose, the growth rate doubled and the population was transferred from one copy number to a threefold lower copy number. During the transition period, plasmid R1 replication was never less frequent than in the steady state in the post

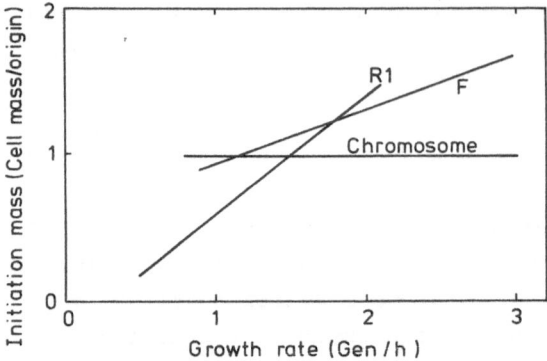

<u>Fig. 14</u>. Initiation mass of the <u>E. coli</u> chromosome and of plasmids F'<u>lac</u> and R1<u>drd</u>-19. The values for the chromosome were taken from Cooper and Helmstetter (7), those for plasmids F'<u>lac</u> and R1<u>drd</u>-19 from Collins and Pritchard (5), and Engberg and Nordström (12), respectively.

shift medium, <u>i.e.</u> for a very long time the plasmid content of the shifted culture was higher than in the steady state. Hence, the origin concentration cannot be the control parameter used. We have repeated these experiments by using a less drastic shift, based upon the fact that α-methylglucoside is a glucose antagonist. This enables up-shifts as well as down-shifts under conditions where the basic features of the metabolism are unchanged. The results obtained in such shifts verify the conclusions mentioned above and can be phrased in the following way: in a shifted culture there is a rapid adjustment of the frequency of replication to that characteristic of the post-shift conditions. Hence, in a shift from a low to a high plasmid copy number the concentration of the plasmid for a very long period is lower than that of a steady state culture and in a shift from a high to a low plasmid copy number the opposite is true. Hence, the control system knows how frequently to replicate but does not know or measure the concentration of the plasmid. In other words the control system has got a device to count replications (or time). The resolution of our experiments does not allow us to conclude or disprove that the first plasmid replication after a shift takes place at the preshift frequency or, in other words, that the frequency of a replication is determined by the condi-

tion at which the previous replication occurred. One consequence
of the sequential replication of plasmids has to be stressed.
Once one copy of a plasmid has started to replicate, neither
this nor any of its sister molecules in the cell can replicate
until a certain time later. Hence, the control system reacts
very rapidly. This can be phrased as if the replication control
was a function separate from initiation of replication. For example, in a simple positive control system, it is assumed that
an initiation complex is built from many molecules. Replication
is initiated as soon as the complex is completed. Our results
show that, if this were the control system used by plasmids R1
and F'lac, the complex cannot be built around the origin of replication since replication is initiated at only one origin at
a time. In a simple negative control system, the repressor concentration has to increase rapidly; this requirement is perhaps
fulfilled by the plasmid λdv system in which a pulse of repressor
synthesis precedes initiation of replication /2/, /25/. Since
it takes some time to synthesize protein at derepression of an
operon, the Pritchard /37/, /39/ model in which initiation of
replication is followed by derepression of the repressor gene
does not safeguard against multiple initiations neither at the
replicating molecule nor at the other ones. Particularly the
origin of the replicating copy should be open and hence prone
to serial initiations. These do not occur. Therefore, in the
Pritchard model there must be a mechanism that blocks these origins. The uncoupling between replication control and the initiation process discussed has to be considered in analyzing the
control system and in constructing control models. In many cases,
replicons consist of two functional and independent replicons.
Examples of such fused plasmids are the Hfr chromosome, the
plasmid pSC134 /3/, etc. It appears as if in these cases only
one of the origins were used, namely the one which has the
smallest initiation mass (or highest copy number) /3/. Since the
initiation mass of plasmid F and of the chromosome show different growth response (Fig. 14) the plasmid F origin in an Hfr
strain seems to be used at low growth rates and the chromosomal
origin at higher (cf. Discussion by Pritchard et al. /40/). At
some intermediate growth rate the initiation mass of both origins may be expected to be equal. This could lead to problems,
particularly if the plasmid is integrated far away from the

chromosomal origin, particularly if termination of chromosome
replication triggers cell division. The system could become unstable, but to our knowledge no such instability has been reported.

Negative or Positive Control of Replication ?

Two main theories of control of replication have been proposed,
the one suggesting positive /19/, the other negative control
/37/, /39/. Lots of effort has been used to advocate for or
against the one or the other of these theories and to try to
fit experimental data with either of them. To our mind, this
has not led to any conclusive results. It is evident that replication of plasmids λ<u>dv</u> /2/, /25/ and R1 (Gustafsson and
Nordström, Lunteren Lectures 1975)(Table 6) is under negative
control in the sense that the control systems contain repressor
proteins. However, this fact does not at all rule out the possibility that positive factors exist. For plasmid λ<u>dv</u> there are
definitively such factors, the gene products of the genes O and
P /2/, /25/. It is likely that a system that operates with positive as well as negative elements is best suited for an effective replicational control. Hence, there may not even be any
controversy between positive and negative control models. It
seems to be more constructive not to talk about negative or
positive control but rather about the function of individual
elements of the control system.

The control genes (at least some of them) are present on the
plasmid itself and replication of plasmids R1 and F'<u>lac</u> seems
to be controlled such that each time the cell volume has increased by one initiation mass, one plasmid copy replicates
irrespective of the actual plasmid copy number. This means that
there is no gene dosage effect in the control system. In a
simple positive control system, activator cannot be formed constitutively from each activator gene, but at a constant, gene-
dosage-independent rate. The autorepressor model of Sompayrac
and Maaløe /45/ may supply a possible explanation. In a simple
negative control system the repressor cannot be formed constitutively from each repressor gene, but the data fit the idea
proposed by Pritchard /37/, /39/, namely that repressor formation is coupled to the initiation or replication event. In the

Pritchard /37/, /39/ system, replication is supposed to induce the synthesis of the repressor. The opposite is true of the λdv system in which derepression of repressor formation leads to triggering of replication /2/, /25/.

Stability of the System

Plasmid-carrying cells form a very stable system. Even if the plasmid copy number is low (2-5 copies/cell) plasmid-free cells are formed with a very low frequency. This indicates that the segregation of plasmids into daughter cells at cell division is strictly controlled but also that the copy number control is effective (see above). An important feature of the control system, therefore, is its stability.

The general assumption seems to be that in a balanced growing culture the plasmid copy number is kept at a constant value by a mechanism that delays replication if the concentration of the plasmid in a cell happens to be higher than the average value, the opposite being true if a cell happens to carry too few plasmid copies. Some quantitative properties of such a system were discussed by Sompayrac and Maaløe /45/. As far as we know these authors assumed that replication of all copies of a particular plasmid in a cell coincided in time. However, such a system, probing the plasmid concentration, does not seem to be used at least by plasmids R1 and F'lac (see above). These plasmids rather replicate in a stepwise manner in which the plasmid copy number is increased by one in each step. We have no indication that there is any negative or positive correlation between the length of successive replication intervals; there is a negative correlation between the individual generation times of mother and daughter cells /22/, /44/. A system like the one used by plasmids R1 and F'lac will of course be very stable since it can never lead to large, rapid changes in the plasmid content but rather give a small steady increase thereof.

One experimental control of the system that regulates replication would be to analyze plasmid replication under extreme conditions, e.g. at the introduction of one plasmid copy into a plasmid-free cell.

Plasmids as Models for Chromosomes

Plasmids are important biological entities and a study of their
replication is well justified in its own right /13/, /42/. However, a basic problem in cell biology is how chromosome replication is regulated. Although important and much studied, this
problem is almost unsolved. One reason for this is that the experimental freedom is limited when such an essential component
as the chromosome is being studied. Plasmids are dispensible
genetic elements. They are being replicated by the same proteins
as is the bacterial chromosome /14/, /15/, /34/, /47/. Many
plasmids are also present in a very small number of copies per
cell and their replication is strictly matched to the growth of
the cells. Hence, plasmids could possibly be used as model systems for chromosome replication. One basic feature of replication
of plasmids R1 and F'lac is that it is spread over the whole
cell cycle. At growth rates above one generation/h, two chromosome initiations occur per cell cycle and this number increases
to four at growth rates above two generations/h /7/, /18/. It
is generally assumed that these initiations coincide in time.
However, there are experimental data that seem to be in conflict
with this conclusion. The data of Lark et al. /23/ and Kline
/20/ show that in a density shift from heavy to light medium
double-replicated DNA starts to appear about 0.5 generations
after the shift. Pritchard and Lark /41/ have reported that re-
initiation at the addition of thymine to thymine-starved cells
only occurs at half of the chromosomal origins.

It should be stressed that if the generally accepted idea is
correct, namely that the chromosomal initiations coincide in
time, there is a qualitative difference between plasmid and
chromosome replication. This difference can be justified if
chromosome replication triggers cell division, but such a coupling has not been unambiguously proven. Rather, quite a few
data suggest that chromosome replication and the cell division
cycle form two parallel but uncoupled cycles that occur at the
same frequency.

Conclusions

The following picture emerges from our results. Replications
of plasmids F'lac and R1 occur one at a time. There is a period

after each replication during which further replications are
forbidden resulting, on the average, in a time interval of $\tau/\underline{n}$
between successive single replications. As soon as the cell volume has increased by one initiation mass one replication is
triggered. The control system measures the frequency of replication rather than the concentration of replicative origins.
The frequency of replication is determined by the conditions at
which the bacterial population actually is growing. At least
plasmid R1 replication is under negative control by a plasmid-
mediated control protein. It is not known at what level (DNA,
RNA, protein) this protein interacts. At least two plasmid genes
are involved in the control.

Acknowledgements

Our work was supported by the Swedish Medical Research Council
(project no. 4236), the Danish Medical Research Council (project no. 6866) and the Danish Natural Science Research Council
(project no. 6532 and 7077). John W. Perram, Department of Mathe-
matics, University of Odense, kindly helped us with the mathe-
matics.

References

1. Bazaral, M., Helinski, D.R.: Replication of a bacterial
   plasmid and an episome in Escherichia coli. Biochemistry 9,
   399-406 (1970).
2. Berg, D.E.: Genes of phage λ essential for λ<u>dv</u> plasmids.
   Virology 62, 224-233 (1974).
3. Cabello, P., Timmis, K., Cohen, S.N.: Replication control
   in a composite plasmid constructed by in vitro linkage of
   two distinct replicons. Nature (London) 259, 285-290 (1976)
4. Clowes, R.C.: Molecular structure of bacterial plasmids.
   Bacteriol. Rev. 36, 361-405 (1972).
5. Collins, J., Pritchard, R.H.: Relationship between chromosome replication and F'<u>lac</u> episome replication in Escherichia
   coli. J. Mol. Biol. 78, 143-155 (1973).
6. Cooper, S.: Relationship of F'<u>lac</u> replication and chromosome
   replication. Proc. Natl. Acad. Sci. U.S.A. 69, 2706-2710
   (1972).
7. Cooper, S., Helmstetter, C.E.: Chromosome replication and
   the division cycle of Escherichia coli B/r. J. Mol. Biol.
   31, 519-540 (1968).

8. Cress, D.E., Kline, B.C.: Isolation and characterization of Escherichia coli chromosomal mutants affecting plasmid copy number. J. Bacteriol. 125, 635-642 (1976).

9. Davis, D.B., Helmstetter, C.E.: Control of F'lac replication in Escherichia coli B/r. J. Bacteriol. 114, 294-299 (1973)

10. Donachie, W.D.: Relationship between cell size and time of initiation of DNA replication. Nature (London) 219, 1077-1079 (1968).

11. Egawa, R., Hirota, Y.: Inhibition of fertility by multiple drug-resistance factor (R) in Escherichia coli K-12. Jpn. J. Genet. 37, 66-69 (1962).

12. Engberg, B., Nordström, K.: Replication of the R-factor R1 in Escherichia coli K-12 at different growth rates. J. Bacteriol. 123, 179-186 (1975).

13. Falkow, S.: Infectious multiple drug resistance. Pion Ltd., London 1975.

14. Goebel, W.: The influence of dnaA and dnaC mutations on the initiation of plasmid DNA replication. Biochem. Biophys. Res. Commun. 51, 1000-1007 (1973).

15. Goebel, W.: Replication of plasmid DNA in Escherichia coli. Proc. Soc. Gen. Microbiol. 1, 1-2 (1973).

16. Grinsted, J., Saunders, J.R., Ingram, L.C., Sykes, R.B., Richmond, M.H.: Properties of an R-factor wich originated in Pseudomonas aeruginosa 1822. J. Bacteriol. 110, 529-537 (1972).

17. Gustafsson, P., Nordström, K.: Random replication of the stringent plasmid R1 in Escherichia coli K-12. J. Bacteriol. 123, 443-448 (1975).

18. Helmstetter, C.E., Cooper, S.: DNA synthesis during the division cycle of rapidly growing Escherichia coli B/r. J. Mol. Biol. 31, 507-518 (1968).

19. Jacob, F., Brenner, S., Cuzin, F.: On the regulation of DNA replication in bacteria. Cold Spring Harbor Symp. Quant. Biol. 28, 329-348 (1963).

20. Kline, B.C.: Mechanism and biosynthesis requirements for F plasmid replication in Escherichia coli. Biochemistry 13, 139-146 (1974).

21. Kool, A.J., van Zeben, M.S., Nijkamp, H.J.J.: Identification of messenger ribonucleic acids and proteins synthesized by the bacteriocinogenic factor CloDF13 in purified minicells of Escherichia coli. J. Bacteriol. 118, 213-224 (1974).

22. Kubitschek, H.: Generation times: ancestral dependence and dependence upon cell size. Exp. Cell. Res. 43, 30-38 (1966).

23. Lark, K.G., Repko, R., Hoffman, E.J.: The effect of amino acid deprivation on subsequent deoxyribonucleic acid replication. Biochim. Biophys. Acta 76, 9-24 (1963).

24. Macrina, F.L., Weatherly, G.G., Curtiss, R. III: R6K plasmid replication: influence of chromosomal genotype in minicell-producing strains of Escherichia coli K-12. J. Bacteriol. 120, 1387-1400 (1974).

25. Matsubara, K.: Genetic structure and regulation of a replication of plasmid λdv. J. Mol. Biol. 102, 427-439 (1976).

26. Matsubara, K., Takeda, Y.: Role of the tof gene in the production and perpetuation of the λdv plasmid. Mol. Gen. Genet. 142, 225-230 (1975).

27. Meselson, M., Stahl, F.W.: The replication of DNA in Escherichia coli. Proc. Soc. Natl. Acad. Sci. U.S. 44, 671-682 (1958).

28. Meynell, E., Datta, N.: The relation of resistance transfer factors to the F-factor (sex-factor) of Escherichia coli K-12. Genet. Res. 7, 134-140 (1966).

29. Meynell, E., Datta, N.: Mutant drug-resistant factors of high transmissibility. Nature (London) 214, 885-887 (1967).

30. Morris, C.F., Hashimoto, H., Mickel, S., Rownd, R.: Round of replication mutant of a drug resistance factor. J. Bacteriol. 118, 855-866 (1974).

31. Nordström, K.: Increased resistance to several antibiotics by one mutation in an R-factor, R1a. J. Gen. Microbiol. 66, 205-214 (1971).

32. Nordström, K., Eriksson-Grennberg, K.G., Boman, H.G.: Resistance of Escherichia coli to penicillins. III. AmpB, a locus affecting episomally and chromosomally mediated resistance to ampicillin and chloramphenicol. Genet. Res. 12, 157-168 (1968).

33. Nordström, K., Ingram, L.C., Lundbäck, A.: Mutations in R-factors of Escherichia coli causing an increased number of R-factor copies per chromosome. J. Bacteriol. 110, 562-569 (1972).

34. Nordström, U.M., Engberg, B., Nordström, K.: Competition for DNA polymerase III between the chromosome and the R-factor R1. Mol. Gen. Genet. 135, 185-190 (1974).

35. Perlman, D., Twose, T.M., Holland, M.J., Rownd, R.H.: Denaturation mapping of R-factor deoxyribonucleic acid. J. Bacteriol. 123, 1035-1042 (1975).

36. Pritchard, R.H.: Control of DNA synthesis in bacteria. Heredity 23, 472 (1968).

37. Pritchard, R.H.: Control of replication of genetic material in bacteria, 1969, 65-74. In G.E.W. Wolstenholme and M. O'Connor (ed.), Bacterial episomes and plasmids. A Ciba Foundation Symposium. J. & A. Churchill Ltd., London.

38. Pritchard, R.H.: On the growth and form of a bacterial cell. Philos. Trans. R. Soc. London 264, 303-336 (1974).

39. Pritchard, R.H., Barth, P.T., Collins, J.: Control of DNA synthesis in bacteria. Symp. Soc. Gen. Microbiol. 19, 263-297 (1969).

40. Pritchard, R.H., Chandler, M.G., Collins, J.: Independence of F replication and chromosome replication in Escherichia coli. Mol. Gen. Genet. 138, 143-155 (1975).

41. Pritchard, R.H., Lark, K.L.: Induction of replication by thimine starvation at the chromosome origin in Escherichia coli. J. Mol. Biol. 9, 288-307 (1964).

42. Reanney, D.: Extrachromosomal elements as possible agents of adaptation and development. Bacteriol. Revs. 40, 552-590 (1976).

43. Rownd, R.: Replication of a bacterial episome under relaxed control. J. Mol. Biol. 44, 387-402 (1969).

44. Schaechter, M., Williamson, J.P., Hood, J.R.,Jr., Koch, A.C.: Growth, cell and nuclear divisions in some bacteria. J. Gen. Microbiol. 29, 421-434 (1962).

45. Sompayrac, L., and O. Maaløe: Autorepressor model for control of DNA replication. Nature (London) New. Biol. 241, 133-135 (1973).

46. Thompson, R., Broda, P.: DNA polymerase III and the replication of F and ColVBtrp in Escherichia coli. Mol. Gen. Genet. 127, 255-258 (1973).

47. Timmis, K., Winkler, U.: Gene dosage studies with pleiotropic mutants of Serratia marcescens superactive in the synthesis of marcescin A and certain other exocellular proteins. Mol. Gen. Genet. 124, 207-217 (1973).

48. Uhlin, B.E., Nordström, K.: Plasmid incompatibility and control of replication: Copy mutants of the R-factor R1 in Escherichia coli K-12. J. Bacteriol. 124, 641-649 (1975).

49. Zeuthen, J., Pato, M.L.: Replication of the F'lac sex factor in the cell cycle of Escherichia coli. Mol. Gen. Genet. 111, 242-255 (1971).

Discussion

Goebel: You are mentioning that you had some evidence that a locus which is part of the R-determinant may also be involved in the regulation of the copy numbers. Could you comment on that?

Nordström: What we did was the following: we took the R-determinant of the same mutant you have, B2, and transformed it to a Salmonella typhimurium carrying the wild type RTF. The result of this experiment was a phenotype with respect to antibiotic resistance which was identical to the B2 mutant.

Goebel: Well, that's surprising because in our mutants we don't have anything of the R-determinant left, yet we retained the copy character of the mini plasmids.

Nordström: It appears that in your system you have lost something, because your copy number is far above what one normally finds in B2. What you transform with this R-determinant is the ability to fix the copy number at a higher level than the wild type but certainly not at the level which you find with your miniplasmids.

Goebel: But isn't a higher copy number something which one always observes if one goes from large plasmids to smaller plasmids?

Falkow: No, that's not necessarily true, you reach a point of diminishing returns. One can keep nibbling away at ColEI and suddenly the copy number, which had been going up, drops precipitously.

Drews: Does anything happen to the rate of DNA synthesis in these temperature shift situations? Is it just the number of replicatory events, i.e. initiation which changes or is the rate of DNA synthesis also affected?

Nordström: I have no real answer to this.

Drews: You had one curve where you showed the temperature shift and the sudden increase in the copy number and in the second curve the increase seemed to be much more gradual. Is there any reason for that?

Nordström: As a matter of fact, yes. If there are not two control levels involved, there is a very sudden transition; but in the double mutant two control mechanisms may be involved which provides for a more continuous increase of copy number with temperature.

Drews: In that double mutant, would you expect the presence of a clearly defined number of copies at each temperature?

Nordström: I suppose so, at least up to 34°C. Beyond that there is a tendency of the population to leave the steady state.

Saedler: In the very highly derepressed situation, do you see a corresponding increase in gene products coded for by the plasmid?

Nordström: Yes, as far as we can see the amount of gene products is absolutely proportional to the copy number.

Goebel: Did you check the incompatibility properties of these high copy mutants?

Nordström: No, we have not attempted this yet, it is going to be very difficult.

Drews: Coming back to your talk this morning, where you showed these impressive morphological changes in the multicopy mutants, did you do similar studies with this double mutant which is in a highly derepressed state? Would you expect an increase in these changes at the permissive temperature?

Nordström: We have not done that, but it is obvious that it should be done.

III. Round Table Discussion

a) Measures Against the Spread of R-Factors
(Chairman: M. H. Richmond)

The session concerned itself with three main topics:
1. What is the size of the reservoir of resistant bacteria and is it universally distributed across the world?
2. What are the factors which go to make that reservoir?
3. Are there any steps that we could take to reduce the size of the reservoir?

As far as the first point is concerned, there was general agreement that the incidence of resistant bacteria was high throughout the world. But the distribution was not uniform. In certain parts of the human environment, resistant organisms seem to be very common. In others they were less common. For example, there was no doubt that in the hospital community, resistant organisms were more prevalent than in the community. Similarly, in the group of animals that provide food for man and particularly those animals which are raised under intensive rearing conditions, the incidence of resistant bacteria and of R-factors in particular was high.

Even though the incidence of resistant bacteria across the world is uniformly high in hospitals, this does not necessarily mean that the same types of resistant organisms are prevalent in all hospitals or all geographical regions. This point had been stressed in the formal sessions of the symposium. For example, Prof. Mitsuhashi described the properties of resistant bacteria and of plasmids that he had studied in Japan. The pattern of resistance found there was similar but by no means identical

to that found in the United States or in Britain. Similarly,
Dr. Acar described how gentamicin-resistant strains of bacteria
were relatively common in French hospitals but Falkow and Richmond both pointed out that similar organisms were not encountered on a large scale in the United States or the British
Isles. The general conclusion, therefore, is that while resistant organisms certainly are widespread, there is a clonal distribution of such organisms in certain geographical locations.
Moreover, the distribution of the clones need not be even. For
example, Anderson in his formal presentation showed that strains
of Salmonella typhimurium carrying a particular class of plasmids had been encountered across the most of the Middle East.
On the other hand, other examples were provided where a single
clone of plasmids was restricted to a single hospital. Thus one
has a highly complicated situation in which some clones are
distributed widely,and some narrowly, and the total result is a
uniformly high level of resistance in certain locations but this
does not imply that the high level of resistance is caused by
the same organism.

The discussion now turned to the question of what causes the
emergence of resistant populations. The first question was
whether this could be attributed solely to the use of antibiotics. In practice, the discussion led one to believe that antibiotic use was not the sole force acting to produce resistant
populations. For example, the incidence of kanamycin-resistant
strains of Haemophilus was reported to be high in Paris and
yet the drug in question was used relatively little. Conversely,
a very large amount of kanamycin is used in the United States
but the kanamycin-resistant Haemophilus has not yet been found.
Other examples were given by other people. Levy, for example,
had sought carefully for the presence of gentamicin-resistant
organisms in Boston and has found them relatively uncommon
despite considerable use of that particular antibiotic. It
seems clear, therefore, that the use of antibiotics is not
necessarily the prime cause for the emergence of given resistant
populations. However, the evidence that the use of a particular
antibiotic does select resistant populations in individual
people, is unquestioned and one, therefore, once again has a
complicated relationship between the composition of the reservoir and the use of antibiotics.

At this point the discussion diverged to think about a question
posed by Dr. Drews as to whether the situation in the hospital
and in the community had changed significantly over recent
years. Acar felt that it was hard to generalise. In certain
cases, the incidence of resistance to a particular antibiotic
had not increased substantially. On the other hand, there were
clear examples where the introduction of an antibiotic had been
followed rather rapidly by the appearance of resistant strains.
There was even some evidence that the incidence of resistance
to certain antibiotics had decreased. For example, chloramphenicol-resistant Staphylococcus aureus strains were now much less
common than they had been in the 1950s and it was possible to
associate that change with a reduced use of the antibiotic in
question. Falkow quoted one or two examples from the US: for
example, the incidence of antibiotic-resistant group D streptococci, in the community, in the US, had increased substantially
in recent years and there was general reference to the appearance
of the ampicillin-resistant clones of Gonococcus which had
appeared in the Philippines and in the British Isles.

So in summary up to this point: there was a general feeling that
antibiotic use was one factor in the emergence of resistant
populations but was by no means the only factor. If the use of
antibiotics was not the only factor operating to select resistant populations, could one identify some of the other factors
that were at work?

The work of Anderson with Salmonella clearly shows that the
colonisation and invasive properties of the organism must be
looked at in this context. As far as his analysis of the situation goes, the evidence is strong that the spread of antibiotic
resistant Salmonella species is very substantially due to the
innate epidemic producing properties of these organisms. Thus,
the antibiotic in this case only plays a part at the beginning
of an epidemic. It seems to be responsible for the emergence
of the initial clone of resistant organisms, but their subsequent spread even sometimes on a world-wide scale, can be due
all but entirely to the properties of the organism itself. This
observation related back to some studies described by Richmond
in the first formal session where the survival of E. coli in
the human gut was found to be independent of antibiotic use

even though the organisms in question carried an antibiotic
resistance marker. In contrast to the observations of Anderson,
Acar stressed that in certain situations in French hospitals
it was clear to see that the use of antibiotics was the main
factor which seemed to maintain a resistant clone; and this
observation certainly accords well with work, published by
others previously, which shows that a cessation in the use of
antibiotics can lead to the disappearance of resistant organisms.
Another factor in the emergence of resistant populations is
certainly the colonising ability of the bacteria in question.
In some cases this is good, and in those circumstances, the
incidence of resistant bacteria will tend to increase independently of antibiotic use.

If one now has identified two factors which are responsible or
which play a part in the emergence of resistance populations,
can we discover any more? Certainly the colonising ability of
bacterial populations will be greatly influenced by the host
strain in which the colonisation has to take place. Thus, a
number of people suggested that the conditions under which the
population on which the antibiotic was being used were living,
was a relevant consideration.

Thus, there is little doubt that the accumulation of people in
hospitals, where the background of their life tends to be more
uniform, is a factor which tends to help the colonisation by
certain bacteria. Moreover this principle also applies even
more strongly to animals being raised under intensive rearing
conditions. Under these circumstances not only is the environmental background of the animals extremely uniform, the beasts
themselves commonly are of a similar genetic origin. Thus, in
these circumstances, the resistant bacteria have a more uniform
host population in which to operate and this seems in some cases
to enhance the chance of large populations of resistant organisms.

The meeting now turned to think for a short time about a specific question posed by the Chairman: if it is known that organisms resistant to a novel antibiotic already exist in the hospital population, should one go ahead and introduce that antibiotic into clinical use? The general feeling was that one

should go ahead, and introduce the compound. An example was the
us of amikacin where it was known that resistant organisms were
already detectable in the hospital population at the time that
the drug was first introduced. Nevertheless, the point was made
by several speakers that amikacin undoubtedly had helped in the
treatment of many patients. Thus, the knowledge that resistant
organisms do occur in the environment should not necessarily
inhibit the introduction of a new agent. On the other hand, it
must be accepted that the presence of such resistant organisms
is likely to shorten the commercial life of a new product.

The discussion now turned to the question of what might be done
to reduce the size of the resistant reservoirs. Acar made an
important statement about some steps that could be taken in
terms of therapy. He stressed that the use of antibiotics for
topical purposes should be reduced as far as possible. Thus in
France many antibiotics are used in dressings in the hope that
in this way they would reduce the chance of wound infection.
Acar feels, however, that the disadvantages of this method of
approach are very considerable since, amongst other things,
it tends to contaminate the environment. Similarly, in the past
the use of creams such as neomycin cream has been shown to be
a potent force in the selection of resistant staphylococci.
There was general agreement, therefore, that the topical use
of antibiotics should be restricted as much as possible.

The question was now considered as to whether the alternation
of antibiotic use was a useful step to try to minimise the
emergence of resistant populations. Starlinger felt that some
national or even international encouragement to use antibiotics
in defined ways could be helpful, though others doubted whether
it would be possible to get the degree of international accord
that would be necessary for such an approach to be successful.
Falkow pointed out that alternation of antibiotic use was already practiced in the treatment of tuberculosis and was certainly an effective method of reducing the emergence of resistant bacteria. In general, the consensus of view seemed to be
that this approach was one worth considering but that there
would be practical difficulties in implementing it. Undoubtedly,
the most important step that people felt could be taken to reduce

the emergence of resistant populations was to attempt to regulate the use of antibiotics in the human environment and particularly to limit the use of these compounds for purposes other
than human therapy. It was pointed out that large amounts of
antibiotics were still being used for plant protection and for
growth promotion in animals and that it would be desirable if
this use of human therapeutic antibiotics was reduced. It was
pointed out by a number of people that policy with respect to
the use of antibiotics for growth promotion was changing. At the
present time the emphasis increasingly was on compounds active
against gram-positive bacteria and these might be expected to
have less of an effect on gram-negative colonisers of the animal
gut. Although this was thought to be beneficial from the point
of view of the incidence of resistant coliforms in man, worries
were expressed, notably by Falkow, about the possibility of the
emergence of resistant gram-positive organisms. There was some
discussion as to whether the major source of resistant organisms
from man came from the animal reservoir or from the hospital as
a result of the use of antibiotics for therapeutic purposes in
man. Anderson insisted that the flow from the resistance reservoir in farm animals to man on meat was a significant source
of resistant organisms in the human population. On the other hand,
there did not seem to be in the human population a very high incidence of resistance to agents which were known to be prevalent
in the animal community. In particular, resistance to furazoli-
done and to chloramphenicol were relatively common in Britain
in the animal population but relatively uncommon in man. This
suggested that the flow from the animal reservoir to man might
not be so substantial; but it was agreed that it was still
difficult to reach a balanced judgement on this point.

If the use of antibiotics for human therapy is indeed the major
factor influencing the spread of resistant organisms and the
emergence of new ones, the question arises as to whether the
use of human therapeutic antibiotics could not be reduced. All
speakers with clinical insight stressed the fact that they felt
that antibiotics were often used inappropriately by the medical
profession. This led to a uniform view that there was an important
role for the educators to play in this problem. All attempts
must be made to educate the physicians in the appropriate and
careful use of antibiotics. Various speakers stressed the situ-

ation, as they saw it at the moment, in their own countries.
Falkow, for example, suggested that the importance of being
prudent with antibiotic use was reaching home to the physicians
in the United States and less antibiotics were being used. On
the other hand, there was still evidence that in certain countries of the world, antibiotics could be purchased freely across
the counters without a medical prescription and the general
feeling was that this was an unsatisfactory situation. Even in
the United States, as Falkow pointed out, some antibiotics
could be bought in large quantities for keeping ornamental
fish and he felt that this sort of outlet should also be restricted.

There were those amongst the discussants who felt that the
education should not be confined solely to the doctors using
antibiotics. It was pointed out that in some countries the
medical profession was under extremely strong pressure from
members of the general public to prescribe antibiotics when
they were not perhaps strictly necessary. Thus, the education must
be on a broad scale, on the one hand to educate physicians in
the most prudent possible use of antibiotics, but on the other
hand it was important to make the general public aware of the
potential dangers, not necessarily to themselves but to the population at large, of the indiscriminate use of antibiotics.
Anderson stressed the role of the pharmaceutical companies in
this particular matter and moreover he suggested that a heavy
responsibility lay with commercial representatives of firms
who very frequently were the interphase between the company
and the doctor or veterinary surgeon who used the antibiotics.
He felt strongly that these people should be included within the
education programme so that they could be made aware of some of
the undesirable consequences that could flow from too wide a use
of antibiotics in an inconsidered manner.

It was pointed out in connexion with the education of doctors
that it would be unreasonable to expect them to use antibiotics
in the highly precise way that was envisaged by the discussants
of this meeting, without also providing them with the necessary
laboratory back-up to make the analysis to support their work.
Moreover there was the feeling that the pharmaceutical industry
should do what it could to provide rapid identification and test

methods to facilitate this sort of work. It was at this point
in the discussion that one returned to a theme which cannot be
escaped in the whole of one's consideration of antibiotic resistance and its emergence as a threat to human health. It was
clear in the context of laboratory facilities that situations
vary widely from country to country and perhaps the theme that
the meeting felt in general was least well understood at the
moment was the local variations that were encountered from place
to place.Not only did this influence the type and incidence of
individual resistant organisms that were found in the environment, it also influenced the regulations which controlled the
use of antibiotics, the level of education of the people who
use the antibiotics and the sophistication of the laboratory
back-up available to people working in this field. There was
certainly a feeling that it would be very helpful if all these
aspects that were relevant to antibiotic use could be made more
uniform, but equally a number of people, at various stages in
the discussion, were none too sanguine about how easy this
would be to achieve.

In summary, one has the feeling that progress is being made in
understanding the underlying mechanisms which determine the
spread of antibiotic-resistant organisms and progress is also
slowly being made in reducing the pressures that are put on
organisms to become resistant and to occupy ever wider ecological
niches. However, progress is not rapid and the difficulties
against making rapid progress are very considerable. The most we
can hope for perhaps is that the situation will not get any
worse.

b) Possible Pharmaceutical Approaches to the Control of R-Factors
(Chairman: Julian Davies)

Strains carrying resistance plasmids (R^+) have become an integral
part of the bacterial population; although the proportions of
these strains, relative to those without resistance plasmids
(R^-), varies from place to place, it can be assumed that R^+
strains will continue to interfere with antibiotic therapy. The
object of this exercise was to consider what steps may be taken
to reduce or eliminate R^+ strains; the earlier discussion had
focussed on epidemiological aspects and the strategy of drug use.
This discussion asked questions about special properties of R^+
strains that might be exploited as targets of pharmaceutical
agents to eliminate R^+ strains and restore normal flora, or in-
capacitate their antibiotic resistance functions.

Those properties of R^+ strains that suggest themselves as sites
of attack include
   1) transmissibility and other properties of
      autonomous replicons, such as their indepen-
      dent replication machinery;
   2) specific surface structures such as pili
      or other antigens;
   3) antibiotic inactivating enzymes.

In considering gene transfer (transmissibility), the question
was first asked as to whether or not this is a significant aspect
of the development and spread of resistance plasmids in humans
and animals. The notion of contagious spread of R-plasmids by
conjugative transfer has probably been overemphasized; the high
incidence of R^+ strains in hospitals is not due to the passage
of plasmids throughout all hospital-associated bacteria by in-

fectious transfer. Rather, clonal selection under the pressure
of antibiotic use is a more likely explanation. Nonetheless,
there is little doubt that the property of transmissibility is
important, both in the evolution of resistance plasmids and in
their dissemination, but the gene transfer events are probably
rare and difficult to identify. For this reason alone, the development of anti-gene transfer agents was considered to be
unprofitable. However, it was pointed out that such agents might
be usefully applied to single patients or small groups; for
example in a burn ward where the same R-plasmid appears in a
succession of opportunistic pathogens during the development of
an epidemic of resistant infections, as was shown by the Birming-
ham group. An effective anti-transfer agent might be used to
prevent the appearance of resistant <u>Pseudomonas aeruginosa</u>
following the original <u>Klebsiella</u> infections. The problem is to
identify when and where the transfer event occurs; since the
patients are already infected with R$^+$ <u>Klebsiella</u> the therapeutic problem remains. It was pointed out that an anti-transfer
agent would have to be 100% effective and that many antibiotic
resistant organisms have been found to harbour non-transmissible
plasmids, which also argues against the requirement for conjugative transfer during the development of resistant infections.
Antibiotic resistant <u>Staphylococcus aureus</u> are widely disseminated
throughout hospital populations and have been the cause of a
number of serious clinical problems and have developed without
the benefit of transmissible plasmids, at least in terms of conjugative transfer. The role of pathogenicity in the development
of resistant populations should also be emphasized.

The conclusion was that gene transfer (of one kind or another)
is a critical but rare event in the development of resistant
bacterial populations; the availability of anti-gene transfer
agents might be of some utility in isolated cases but would not
be of general application.

It has long been known that certain chemicals, notably DNA inter-
calating agents such as acridines, can "cure" bacterial populations of their plasmids. The mechanism of action of these
agents is only partly understood but is believed to involve
specific inhibition of plasmid replication; during cell duplication therefore, the plasmid is prevented from segregating into

the daughter cells and an R$^-$ population results. Could agents of this type be used to remove R$^+$ strains from the bacterial population? Although at first sight this is an attractive proposition, there are many objections. The agent would have to be 100% effective otherwise the few remaining "uncured" R$^+$ cells in the population would be selected when antibiotic pressure was applied. In addition, R-plasmids are extraordinarily resistant to the action of "curing" chemicals, and it was considered unlikely that any such agent could be developed that would be effective against all R-plasmids of all compatibility types. The "curing" agent would of necessity be a prophylactic agent and would have to be provided to all potential recipients of antibiotic therapy; any pockets of untreated strains would propagate upon subsequent antibiotic use. If the curing agents were administered in combination with the antibiotic the presence of the selective force of the antibiotic would probably render "curing" ineffective. Finally, it was pointed out that the presence of transposable resistance elements would tend to negate the plasmid "curing" approach. Since the resistance determinants are not obliged to remain associated with plasmids they could retreat to the safety of the chromosome and in fact, the combined action of a curing agent and an antibiotic may create a new generation of resistant strains with resistance determinants as chromosomal functions.

In contrast to the pessimistic feelings about the "curing" approach it was suggested that an agent that would eliminate resistance plasmids, perhaps by taking advantage of a step in replication specific to R-plasmids, might be of some use in sensitising the bacterial population in single patients. The replication functions and apparatus of different types of plasmids differ and are unlikely to be susceptible to a single agent, but short nucleic acid sequences, possibly at replication origins, might be common to many plasmids and be possible targets for the development of agents that interfere with plasmid replication.

A more practical approach to sensitising the bacterial flora of hospital patients to antibiotics was that of population replacement, as described by Dr. Richmond. It may be possible, particularly in intensive care units, to colonise patients with sensitive bacteria (possibly their own flora sampled before entry to the hospital). This was discussed at some length in an earlier session.

A related approach was suggested by Dr. Levy, who indicated the
possibility of eliminating all the plasmid containing strains
in a given bacterial microenvironment. This would require
eradication of entire bacterial species in the gut, urine, or on
the skin by treatment with antibiotics, inducing pH changes, or
by changing the availability of essential nutrients. While there
was some concern about the effect of such drastic changes in the
human flora it was thought that alteration of the bacterial
microenvironment might be useful for short term use in limited
situations.

With respect to pharmaceutical agents specifically effective
against R^+ strains, Dr. Mitsuhashi mentioned macarbomycin, a
phospholipid antibiotic discovered in Umezawa's laboratory that
inhibits the growth of R^+ strains but has no effect on R^- strains.
The availability of such a compound is of considerable interest
but macarbomycin is effective against only a limited range of
R^+ strains (probably due to an effect on the sex pili) and resistance to the drug develops very rapidly. When one considers
the wide variety of plasmids and their properties in different
host strains it seems unlikely that broad spectrum agents of this
type would exist.

In spite of the fact that the mechanisms of plasmid-determined
antibiotic resistance remain, in many cases, poorly understood,
it is known that plasmid-coded enzymatic modification of antibiotics is required for the expression of resistance to ß-lactams,
aminoglycosides and chloramphenicol. These are important
classes of antibiotics and inhibitors of ß-lactamases,
aminoglycoside N-acetylating, O-phosphorylating or O-adenylylating
enzymes, or chloramphenicol transacetylase, administered in combination with the antibiotic, would restore these antibiotics to
their original effectiveness. In fact, this strategy has already
proved to be successful; clavulanic acid is a potent inhibitor
of ß-lactamases and has been demonstrated to improve the activity
of penicillin and other ß-lactam antibiotics against resistance
strains. The potential for the discovery and utility of compounds
of this type is very high. Inhibitors of chloramphenicol transacetylase exist and continued investigation of compounds of this
type is to be encouraged, particularly when one considers the
effectiveness of chloramphenicol in treating anaerobic infections

and meningitis. The situation in the case of the aminoglycoside antibiotics is complicated by the fact that the modifying enzymes are intracellular (as is also the case with chloramphenicol) and there may be difficulties in transporting the inhibitor to the enzymes. Inhibitors of some of the aminoglycoside-modifying enzymes are known, but they are effective at high concentrations only and are probably competitive inhibitors. What is needed is a systematic search for non-antibiotic, non-competitive inhibitors with appropriately low K_i constants that can be mixed with antibiotics in low concentrations (1:100 or less) and administered as a combination. In the case of the aminoglycoside antibiotics, the prospect of making kanamycin or gentamycin 100% effective against R^+ strains is attractive and important. Undoubtedly, resistant strains would still arise by mutation, as has been demonstrated for P.aeruginosa by Bryan and his colleagues, however, experience suggests that such resistant mutants may be a less serious infectious disease problem.

As an adjunct to the use of inhibitors of resistance enzymes, the search for suicide compounds was also discussed. As we learn more about the biochemistry of antibiotic modifying enzymes, it should be possible to devise substrates, that when cleaved or modified would produce compounds that were toxic to the cell.

In conclusion, there was general agreement that the control of R-factors would be best approached by screening for agents that directly inhibit the expression of the resistance mechanisms. However, the continuing need for new antibiotics with desirable properties and obvious advantages over existing drugs was also emphasized; such compounds may be new natural isolates, semi-synthetic compounds designed to be refractory to plasmid-determined resistance mechanisms, or totally synthetic anti-microbial agents. More research into structure-toxicity relationships (requiring rapid and accurate models for human toxicity), might lead to ways of making new antibiotics from old. However, the introduction of new antibiotics should always be accompanied by measures designed to reduce, as much as possible, the development of resistant strains. These measures have been discussed in much detail elsewhere. The responsibility of the pharmaceutical industry to the health and welfare of the public should be the primary concern with economic (profit) considerations subordinated as much as possible. When resistant strains are known to exist in hospital populations before the introduction of new antimicrobial agents, these agents should be used with discretion so as to avoid, at all costs, the creation of strong selective pressures in favour of the pre-existing resistant strains. Antibiotics are important and vital natural resources that must be conserved by prudent use.

List of Participants

Editors:

Prof.Dr.med. Jürgen Drews
Head, Section of Chemotherapy
SANDOZ Forschungsinstitut
Gesellschaft m.b.H.
Brunnerstrasse 59
A-1235 Vienna
Austria

Univ.-Doz.Dr. Gregor Högenauer
Department of Experimental
Chemotherapy
SANDOZ Forschungsinstitut Ges.m.b.H.
Brunnerstrasse 59
A-1235 Vienna
Austria

Active Participants:

Dr. Jacques F. Acar
Maitre de confêrence agrêgê
Biologiste des hôpitaux
Hopital Saint-Joseph
7, rue Pierre-Larousse
F-75674 Paris Cedex 14
France

Prof.Dr. Ephraim S. Anderson
Director, Enteric Reference
Laboratory
Central Public Health Laboratory
Colindale Avenue
London, NW9 5HT
England

Dr. Peter M. Bennett
University of Bristol
Department of Bacteriology
The Medical School
University Walk
Bristol BS8 1TD
England

Julian Davies, Ph.D.
Professor, Department of
Biochemistry
University of Wisconsin-Madison
College of Agricultural
and Life Sciences
420 Henry Mall
Madison, Wisconsin 53706
USA

Stanley Falkow, Ph.D.
Professor of Microbiology
and Genetics
University of Washington
School of Medicine
Department of Microbiology, SC-42
Seattle, Washington 98195
USA

Prof.Dr. W. Goebel
Institut für Genetik und Mikrobiologie
der Universität Würzburg
Lehrstuhl für Mikrobiologie
Röntgenring 11
D-87 Würzburg
Germany

Univ.-Doz.Dr. Gregor Högenauer
Department of Experimental
Chemotherapy
SANDOZ Forschungsinstitut
Gesellschaft m.b.H.
Brunnerstrasse 59
A-1235 Vienna
Austria

Dr. Gwynfor O. Humphreys
The University of Liverpool
Department of Microbiology
Life Sciences Building
P.O.Box 147
Liverpool L69 3BX
England

Stuart B. Levy, M.D.
Tufts University
School of Medicine
New England Medical
Center Hospital
Department of Medicine
Hematology Service
171 Harrison Avenue
Boston, Massachusetts 02111
USA

Prof.Dr. Susumu Mitsuhashi
Department of Microbiology
School of Medicine
Gunma University
Showa-machi
Maebashi City
Japan

Prof.Dr. Kurt Nordström
Odense University
Unit of Experimental Microbiology
Niels Bohrs Alle
DK-5000 Odense
Denmark

Mark H. Richmond, M.A., Ph.D.
Professor of Bacteriology
University of Bristol
Department of Bacteriology
The Medical School
University Walk
Bristol BS8 1TD
England

Dr. Heinz Saedler
Wissenschaftlicher Rat und Professor
Institut für Biologie III
Universität Freiburg
Schänzlestrasse 9-11
D-78 Freiburg i.Br.
Germany

Prof.Dr.P. Starlinger
Institut für Genetik
der Universität zu Köln
Weyertal 121
D-5 Köln 41
Germany

List of Authors

Subject Index